Cochlear Implants

Josef M. Miller Francis A. Spelman
Editors

Cochlear Implants

Models of the Electrically Stimulated Ear

With 142 Illustrations

Springer-Verlag
New York Berlin Heidelberg
London Paris Tokyo Hong Kong

Josef M. Miller
Kresge Hearing Research Institute
The University of Michigan
Ann Arbor, MI 48109-0506
USA

Francis A. Spelman
Center for Bioengineering
Regional Primate Research Center
University of Washington
Seattle, WA 98195
USA

Library of Congress Cataloging-in-Publication Data
Cochlear implants: models of the electrically stimulated ear/edited by Josef M. Miller and Francis A. Spelman.
p. cm.
1. Cochlear implants. I. Miller, Josef M. II. Spelman, Francis A.
RF305.C6294 1989
617.8′9—dc20 89-11256

Printed on acid-free paper.

Typeset by TCSystems, Inc., Shippensburg, Pennsylvania.

9 8 7 6 5 4 3 2 1

ISBN-13:978-1-4612-7936-5 e-ISBN-13:978-1-4612-3256-8
DOI: 10.1007/978-1-4612-3256-8

To Cheryl and Kay, who have endured dismal days and near endless nights of editorial grumbling with grace, support, and humor.

Acknowledgment

Support for aspects of the work incorporated in this volume, preparation of manuscripts, and the symposium, which permitted all important discussions by the contributing authors of this volume, was provided by NIH Grants NS-21440 and RR00166, and funds from The University of Michigan offices of the Vice-President for Research and Medical School Associate Dean for Research. The authors would like to thank Robert and Clara VanderKloot for their support. We also gratefully acknowledge the organizational care as well as manuscript preparation provided by Yvonne Beerens.

Contents

Contributors

PATRICIA M. BACKOFF
Kresge Hearing Research Institute, The University of Michigan, Ann Arbor, MI 48109-0506, USA

C.C. BLACKBURN
Department of Biomedical Engineering, Johns Hopkins School of Medicine, Baltimore, MD 21205, USA

G.M. CLARK
Department of Otolaryngology, Royal Victorian Eye and Ear Hospital, East Melbourne, Australia 3002

BEN M. CLOPTON, PH.D.
Kresge Hearing Research Institute, The University of Michigan, Ann Arbor, MI 48109-0506, USA

CHARLES C. FINLEY, PH.D.
Neuroscience Program Office, Research Triangle Institute, Research Triangle Park, NC 27709, USA

C. DANIEL GEISLER, SC.D.
Department of Neurophysiology, University of Washington-Madison, Madison, WI 53705, USA

RAINER HARTMANN, M.D.
Zentrum der Physiologie, Klin. J.W. Goethe-Universität, Frankfurt, Germany

CHRIS VAN DEN HONERT, PH.D.
3M Corporation, 3M Center, Saint Paul, MN 55144, USA

Eric Javel, Ph.D.
Boys Town National Institute, Omaha, NE 68131, USA

Brian M. Johnstone, Ph.D.
Department of Physiology, University of Western Australia, Crawley West, Australia

Rainer Klinke, Ph.D.
Zentrum der Physiologie, Klin. J.W. Goethe-Universität, Frankfurt, Germany

Dewey T. Lawson, Ph.D.
Division of Otolaryngology, Department of Surgery, Duke University Medical Center, Durham, NC 27710, USA

H.H. Lim
Department of Otolaryngology, Royal Victorian Eye and Ear Hospital, East Melbourne, Australia 3002

James D. Miller, Ph.D.
Central Institute for the Deaf, St. Louis, MO 63130, USA

Josef M. Miller, Ph.D.
Kresge Hearing Research Institute, The University of Michigan, Ann Arbor, MI 48109-0506, USA

Bryan E. Pfingst, Ph.D.
Kresge Hearing Research Institute, The University of Michigan, Ann Arbor, MI 48109-0506, USA

William M. Rabinowitz, Ph.D.
Massachusetts Institute of Technology, Cambridge, MA 02139, USA

Murray B. Sachs, M.D.
Department of Biomedical Engineering, Johns Hopkins School of Medicine, Baltimore, MD 21205, USA

Robert V. Shannon, Ph.D.
Boys Town National Institute, Omaha, NE 68131, USA

Guido F. Smoorenburg, Ph.D.
ENT Department, University Hospital Utrecht, Utrecht, The Netherlands

Sigfrid D. Soli, Ph.D.
House Ear Institute, Los Angeles, CA 90057, USA

MOSHE SOLOMONOW, PH.D.
Department of Orthopaedic Surgery, Louisiana State University, New Orleans, LA 70112, USA

FRANCIS A. SPELMAN, PH.D.
Center for Bioengineering, Regional Primate Research Center, University of Washington, Seattle, WA 98195, USA

Y.C. TONG, PH.D.
Department of Otolaryngology, Royal Victorian Eye and Ear Hospital, East Melbourne, Australia 3002

GREGORY H. WAKEFIELD, PH.D.
Kresge Hearing Research Institute, The University of Michigan, Ann Arbor, MI 48109-0506, USA

MARK W. WHITE, PH.D.
Department of Electrical Engineering, North Carolina State University, Raleigh, NC 27695, USA

JAMES A. WILER
Kresge Hearing Research Institute, The University of Michigan, Ann Arbor, MI 48109-0506, USA

BLAKE S. WILSON, PH.D.
Neuroscience Program, Research Triangle Institute, Research Triangle Park, NC 27709, USA

1
Introduction to Models of the Electrically Stimulated Ear

JOSEF M. MILLER AND FRANCIS A. SPELMAN

During the past two decades a therapeutic strategy for treatment of the profoundly sensorineural deaf, based on the cochlear prosthesis, has developed where none had previously existed. Environmental acoustic contact, an aid to lip-reading and a significant potential for some degree of open-set speech discrimination with the prosthesis alone, is now available for the deaf: one-half to one million in the United States and millions more worldwide. The obvious and growing benefits compared with the less obvious and/or readily controlled morbidity and risks make this strategy the therapy of choice for profound hearing loss (Hopkinson et al., 1986; NIH Consensus Meeting, 1988).

As an area of research, this field was initiated and largely driven by clearly stated clinical goals. Much of the initial strategy of study was defined specifically in terms of clinical concerns. Thus, initial study was designed to demonstrate the feasibility of the approach and to document its beneficial effects. This done, the investigators in this field now ask how to optimize the device and its attendant therapy, how to develop ideal devices, and how to meet the needs of the individual patient. Investigators ask how to evaluate patients and tailor prostheses to overcome a variety of pathologies and match their interpretive skills as well. In asking these questions, there has been a growing appreciation by investigators for scope and breadth of basic science areas upon which we must draw, if a systematic, comprehensive, and effective program of cochlear prosthesis development is to follow.

In the broadest sense, the fundamental question in this field is: How do we replace a receptor of the human body? This perspective of the field dictates a broad-based multidisciplinary foundation. That foundation must be built with structural components from learning theory, anatomy, otopathology, bio-engineering and signal processing, psychophysics, developmental biology, neurophysiology, and biophysics, as well as the emerging contributory fields of signal detection theory, artificial intelligence, and neural networks. Strategies from these areas should provide adaptive systems to meet the changing needs of a plastic nervous system under the varied conditions in which we expect the cochlear prosthesis to operate. For the long-term development of this field, a well-defined basic and theoretical infrastructure is essential to define future programs and goals and to evaluate research activities against credible scientific standards. An appropriate basic foundation will underlie long-term objectives, which provide stability and direction for the field. It will encourage and provide ready means for clinicians and scientists to draw upon the vast knowledge base available in the neurosciences. Moreover, with a clearly defined, basic foundation, a program of research on the cochlear prosthesis becomes an important and useful model for the development of other neuroprostheses.

By addressing questions of the mechanisms that underlie prostheses function, we may begin to form a structure for this theoretical base and define some of its important characteristics. The last two decades of research have provided a body of information concerning the fundamental response characteristics of the peripheral and central auditory system to electrical stimulation. This information has developed from studies of the response characteristics of the auditory system to acoustic stimulation and, more recently, from observations with electrical stimulation. Biophysical and physiological studies now yield insights into the effects of electrical stimulation on excitable tissues of the inner ear. Electrophysiological and 2-deoxyglucose studies now provide information on the distribution of central evoked activity, yielding a better understanding of the spatial limits for independent channels of activation. Physiological studies now provide information about the temporal response characteristics of auditory nerve and central auditory cells to direct electrical stimulation. Psychophysical studies are providing information on the sensitivity and discriminative capabilities provided by cochlear implants; perceptual tests now provide the means to define and assess biophysical and neural models of system function. Together all of these studies yield insights into the form and limits of the encoding of sensory information with electrical stimulation.

These studies provide a database for the formulation of models of peripheral auditory function with electrical stimulation. The models range from those dealing with characteristics of cochlear tissues describing the temporal and spatial excitation patterns of neural elements with electrical stimulation, to those describing the processing and analysis of electrically evoked activity in the central nervous system. The models demonstrate the growing maturity of this field of study. They also establish more realistic expectations of the behavior of cochlear implants in patients. Models will permit specification of rigorous experimental questions, organized within a theoretical framework, and provide a plan which will guide efficiently the development of knowledge and technology in this field.

It is timely to evaluate the state of these models and the database upon which they are being founded. A critical review of recently executed and planned studies is most appropriate. The development of new, more comprehensive models, and the extension of existing models to incorporate a broader base of data, can benefit the field greatly. Identification of weaknesses in the database, as well as out, analysis and interpretation of the existing database at this relatively early stage of development, may avoid costly delays and eliminate early inappropriate or fruitless avenues of investigation.

On the basis of such considerations, a symposium was organized to discuss models of the electrically stimulated ear, on October 3–5, 1988, at the Kresge Hearing Research Institute, The University of Michigan. The purpose of the symposium was to evaluate critically the state of knowledge and current approaches for the development of models of functional electrical stimulation of the auditory nervous system. The purpose of the workshop was to (1) collect the current knowledge in this field, (2) evaluate this knowledge critically, (3) specify research questions of highest priority for the future development of this field, and (4) make this information available to basic scientists and clinical investigators.

We have attempted to meet this final goal in this book. The book assembles the papers presented at the symposium and records edited versions of the timely discussions that took place. The papers are grouped together under three topic areas: (1) Tissue Characteristics, (2) Neural and Behavioral Models, and (3) Encoding Schemes. Clearly, the papers in each area overlap each other in content, as do the questions and the discussion. In some cases the authors propose strategies of study appropriate to this field, in others the authors introduce new concepts that might drive future research and development, and in yet others the authors present rigorous databased investigations. This diversity reflects the state of this vital field of research.

In the following chapters the results of current research on fundamental aspects of prosthetic function are reviewed and discussed. As in any vital field, the discussions are at least as informative as the papers presented. Importantly, these discussions define a number of specific controversies and fundamental questions for the field. They lead to a proposal for a multifacet, basic research program for cochlear prostheses that can now be specified more rigorously than it could previously. This program is outlined in the closing chapter of this book.

References

Hopkinson et al. (1986).
NIH Consensus Meeting (1988).

Part I Tissue Characteristics

C. DANIEL GEISLER, MODERATOR
BRIAN M. JOHNSTONE, DISCUSSION LEADER

2 Electrical Characteristics of Cochlear Tissues

C. DANIEL GEISLER

Introduction

In the normal cochlea, the physical dimensions of the inner hair cell itself largely determine the degree of localization of sensory excitation. That is, with a few notable exceptions, the discharge patterns evoked on a primary auditory-nerve fiber by a wide range of sounds, including speech syllables, can be satisfactorily accounted for using only the mechanical vibrations thought to exist at the location of the single hair cell with which the fiber synapses, and the transducing and synaptic mechanisms of that cell (e.g., Deng and Geisler, 1987). Possible exceptions to this generality are the double-peaked discharge patterns sometimes evoked by low-frequency sinusoids (e.g., Sellick, Patuzzi, and Johnstone, 1982, but see Mountain and Cody, 1988, for an opposing view) and the effects of efferent stimulation (e.g., Guinan and Guifford, 1988).

There are a number of implications of this fine localization that are relevant to the design of cochlear implants. Perhaps the most obvious arises when one adopts the strategy (only one among many) that the implant should reproduce, as closely as possible, natural discharge patterns on the remaining afferent fibers. Such a strategy requires that the same high degree of excitation localization which exists in the normal cochlea be aimed for in the implanted cochlea. A related implication, which is not quite so obvious, is that the cochlea contains built-in isolation mechanisms which very effectively decouple neighboring segments. With appropriate implant design, some of these decoupling mechanisms can be harnessed (see below).

Macroelectrical Phenomena

Regardless of whether or not fine localization is desired, the electrical characteristics of the cochlea are of fundamental importance in implant design. The modern era in this field of inquiry begins, as it so often does in any area of cochlear research, with the work of Georg von Békésy (1951, reprinted in 1960). Recognizing the resemblance of the cochlear scalae to electrical (as well as hydromechanical) transmission lines, he measured the longitudinal attenuation of an electrical signal applied across scala media near the basal end of the guinea pig cochlea. Over a distance of more than 1 cm, he found that the attenuation approximated 8 dB/mm (Békésy, 1960, Fig. 14–24), just the sort of behavior exhibited by a transmission line with a length constant of about 1.3 mm. Accordingly, he proposed a three-dimensional transmission-line model for the cochlea that assumed one-dimensional perilymphatic spaces (Békésy, 1960, Fig. 14–25). Today, almost 40 years later, we still utilize such models (e.g., Black and Clark, 1980), although these latter investigators needed space constants ranging from 2 to 13 mm to fit their indirectly obtained measures of longitudinal current spread within scala tympani (see below).

Later in the 1950s, Davis, another early giant, proposed his famous variable-resistance model of the cochlear cross section (e.g., 1958). This model, although it incorrectly assumed that excitation of the afferent neurons was directly mediated by cochlear potentials, did capture the essence of the transduction mechanism. Flexing of the cilia *does* vary hair cell resistances (Hudspeth and Corey, 1977), and the endocochlear potential *does* force current through those resistances (Russell, 1983). The concept was so soundly conceived that it still forms the basis of our understanding of cochlear transduction (cf. Dallos, 1983).

The next important step was provided by Johnstone, Johnstone, and Pugsley (1966), who provided a model of the cochlear cross section which explicitly included scala media. They inferred, from published work and from their own electrical measurements taken between the three scalae and "ground" (a remote indifferent electrode), that scala media was electrically decoupled from each of the other scalae and from ground by fairly high interface impedances (>13 kohm). That model, with its high-impedance scala media interfaces, is, with minor modifications, still a standard (cf. Geisler et al., 1977; Dallos, 1983). Like the perilymphatic spaces, scala media was also determined by Johnstone and colleagues to behave like a transmission line, having a length constant of approximately 2 mm.

Variations on the same theme have followed. For example, Strelioff (1973) embedded Davis's variable-resistance model in a 3-scalae transmission-line model. Cannon (1976) added a node to the cross-section model to represent the modiolus and, like Johnstone, Johnstone, and Pugsley (1966), found that the model required large interface resistances (>50 kohm) between scala media and the other cochlear structures. Yet these models, valuable as they are, still are imperfect. For example, unpublished observations made in our laboratory suggest that the connections between the scalae and ground are quite complex and are not distributed uniformly in the longitudinal direction.

Microelectrical Phenomena

Up until this point, the scalae have been treated as if they were basically one-dimensional structures. Potentials at a particular longitudinal point in the cochlea were assumed to be uniform across the entire cross-sectional areas of the respective scalae. With inferred scalar length constants of 1–2 mm, some felt that any cross-sectional potential gradients would be small. Yet the hair cells, which provide the transduction currents, occupy only a small fraction of the cochlear cross section. Thus it seemed to an insightful few that important cross-sectional voltage gradients due to these receptor currents should exist.

In the early 1980s Brownell and his colleagues set about to measure these voltage gradients by moving a microelectrode along a scala tympani track just underneath the basilar membrane, parallel to it. Not only have they demonstrated that transient stimulus-evoked potential gradients exist in scala tympani, but clear evidence for the long-predicted "silent" current was also obtained (Brownell, Zidanic, and Spirou, 1986). Several of their findings are remarkable. The first is the large size of the stimulus-evoked potential gradients: they reached 10 mv/mm, greater than those produced by the dark currents in the eye. Related to this is the finding that while these gradients were strong near the spiral ligament, they virtually disappeared as the wall of the modiolus was approached. Arguing from Ohm's law, it would appear from this arrangement that the receptor currents, both standing and evoked, flow principally through the spiral ligament.

Garcia and Clopton (1987) used an orthogonal approach to the same problem. They inserted a pair of fine wire electrodes, roughly 50 μm apart, at right angles to the basilar membrane, and measured the two-dimensional gradient fields produced by acoustic tone stimulation. The results are somewhat difficult to interpret, due to the uncertainty (± 50 μm) of the precise location of the organ of Corti within their fields, but it appears as if strong gradients exist underneath the bony spiral lamina, at least for some frequencies. This field arrangement implies that appreciable currents do flow into the modiolus, a conclusion in apparent conflict with the findings of Brownell, Zidanic, and Spirou (1986). Also at variance are the magnitudes of the gradients measured in the two studies: they differ by approximately an order of magnitude. Only future experimentation will resolve these differences.

For purposes of this paper, however, both reports agree in showing that important voltage gradients do exist in cochlear cross sections. Anyone who has recorded extracellular potentials from within the organ of Corti with micropipettes also knows this. When recording summating potentials (SP) in the organ of Corti, the position of the electrode is crucial: a movement of only a few microns can change the magnitude of the response manyfold. In fact, the approach of the microelectrode to the immediate vicinity of an inner hair cell is reliably signaled by the appearance of these SP responses.

Extremely sharp localizations were also achieved in a two-dimensional simulation of cochlear cross-sectional potential fields produced by radially oriented bipolar stimulation (Wilson and Finley, 1984). If the simulation represented the surrounding of the electrode assembly as being composed solely of bone, a 140-μm space constant was achieved. If a 100-μm-wide layer of perilymph was inserted between the bone and electrode carrier, the simulation produced an even smaller effective space constant.

Highly localized voltage gradients also appear in the longitudinal direction. SP voltages obtained with a microelectrode located in the organ of Corti just underneath an inner hair cell are shown in Figure 2.1 (small data points). These were obtained at approximately the 20-kHz place in the basal turn of the guinea pig cochlea. Note how sharply the voltage drops off on the high-frequency side. The magnitude of the response at 25 kHz (the last point) is only about 5% of the 20-kHz response. Assuming that the response at the 25-kHz point evoked by its characteristic-frequency (CF) tone is similar in nature to that of the 20-kHz point (and that intermediate hair cells provided no 25-kHz SP responses), this figure implies that the SP response generated at the 25-kHz point was attenuated at least 20-fold over the estimated 0.8 mm existing between the two points [the guinea pig's high-frequency tonotopic scale is about 2.5 mm/octave (Robertson et al., 1980)]. The sharp SP tuning curves, resembling those obtained from auditory-nerve-fiber discharges, that are recorded between scala tympani and scala vestibuli in the first turn of the guinea pig cochlea (Cheatham and Dallos, 1984) also imply a tightly confined spread of SP potentials within those scalae.

The SP responses obtained in scala media of the same animal, at a point just above the recording site in the organ of Corti, are also shown in Figure 2.1 (large circular data points). Notice that this scala media response curve is much broader, on both the low- and high-frequency sides, than that obtained in the organ of Corti. There is also a shift in the frequency of the maximum point, although this is perhaps artifactual (see the figure caption). From this curve, we can estimate that the sensory potentials were attenuated by at least 60% (4.4 dB) over the distance between the 20- and 25-kHz points, implying a space constant of less than 0.8 mm.

All of these data imply that the mode of stimulation makes a large difference in the type of spread exhibited by cochlear potentials. For stimulation which is confined to a fraction of a scalar cross section (e.g., a hair cell), the electrical fields can drop by an order of magnitude over a distance equal to the scala's diameter. Under those conditions, the concept of a one-dimensional transmission line is not really applicable. In this case, a full three-dimensional treatment of the entire cochlea is needed to obtain accurate representations (see below). If, on the other

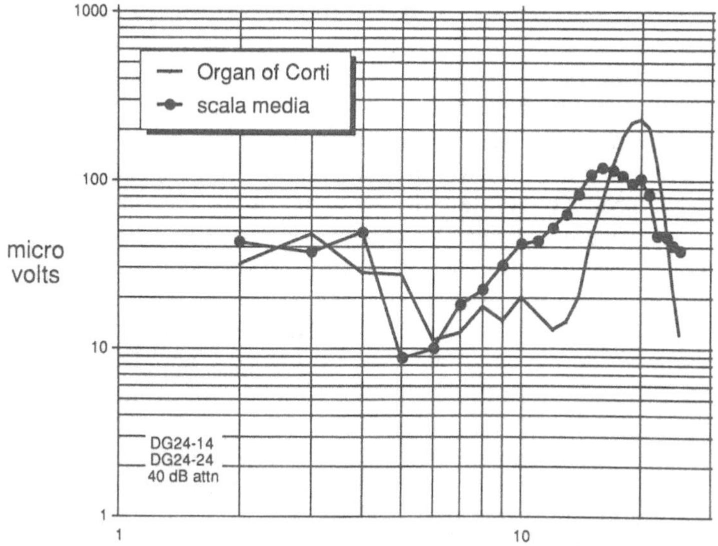

FIGURE 2.1. Extracellular SP responses as a function of stimulus frequency, obtained in the living guinea pig organ of Corti near an inner hair cell (small points) and, shortly after that, from a point just into scala media (filled circles) along the same electrode track (animal DG24). A hyperfine microelectrode was used in experimental procedures very similar to those employed by Sellick, Patuzzi, and Johnstone (1982). After penetrating the reticular lamina (and obtaining an endocochlear potential of 88 mv), the threshold value of the round-window CAP (compound action potential) response to 20-kHz tones (originally about 40-dB SPL) deteriorated by 11 dB (7 dB at 18 kHz). This implies that the magnitudes of the SP responses generated near the 20-kHz region were reduced by the penetration. Pairs of response curves showing the same general characteristics as those shown were obtained in two other experiments (DG17 and DG35), with penetration-induced losses in CAP thresholds at 20 kHz of 5 and 29 dB, respectively.

hand, stimulation by large electrodes produces nearly uniform potentials across a scalar cross section, then transmission-line models may become appropriate. Even in that case, however, care must be exercised in considering the perilymphatic scalae, for their length constants may not be much larger than the scalar dimensions themselves (e.g., Békésy, 1960, Fig. 14–24). Scala media, with its high-impedance walls and a length constant that is long relative to its cross-sectional dimensions (cf. Johnstone, Johnstone, and Pugsley, 1966), appears to be a better candidate for such representation. The appreciable longitudinal spread of sensory potentials shown in the scala-media curve of Figure 2.1 seems consistent with that idea.

Stimulation by Implanted Electrodes

There have been only a few investigations of the voltage fields produced in the cochlea by implanted electrodes. The first made ingenious use of binaural inferior-colliculus neurons (Merzenich and White, 1977). Acoustically stimulating the normal (unoperated) ear allowed determination of a particular neuron's characteristic frequency (CF). This frequency in turn allowed investigators, using the known tonotopicity of the cochlea (e.g., Liberman, 1982), to estimate the location in the acoustically stimulated cochlea from which the neuron's responses arose. More importantly, as binaural inferior-colliculus neurons usually display comparable CFs to monaural stimulation of either ear (Merzenich and Reid, 1974), the location of the region in the implanted cochlea from which the neuron's electrically excited responses arose could also be inferred. Thresholds of these inferior-colliculus neurons, when excited by closely spaced bipolar electrodes, changed as a function of these inferred cochlear locations by about 10–25 dB/octave [about 2.6–6.6 dB/mm, according to the 3.8 mm/octave high-frequency tonotopic scale of the cat cochlea (cf. Liberman, 1982)].

Black and Clark (1980) also used this same binaural technique to show the great localizing advantages of bipolar stimulation. With monopolar stimulation, practically the whole cochlea was excited (a difference of only 10 dB separated the thresholds of neurons coming from locations nearly half a cochlea apart). Interpreting these data in terms of a one-dimensional transmission line led to the unreasonably large estimate of 13 mm for the scala-tympani length constant. With bipolar stimulation, a much more restricted cochlear segment (estimated at 2 mm on either side of the electrodes) was stimulated with currents of the same magnitudes.

Valuable as these inferior-colliculus studies have been, they are indirect and leave many questions unanswered. It remained for van den Honert and Stypulkowski (1987) to make, rather elegantly, direct measurements from auditory-nerve fibers in implanted cat cochleas which also had their acoustic-sensing properties operative. Their findings, some of which were startling, support to a large extent the conclusions reached in the first sections of this paper. One finding, surprising in spite of the inferior-colliculus data, was the extreme spread of excitation that occurred with monopolar stimulation. There was only a weak correlation between excitation threshold and cochlear location (as estimated by CF) for basal excitation: in only 16 out of 31 ears was a correlation found between fiber CF and electrical threshold. This implies such an unreasonably long one-dimensional length constant that one is tempted to think that direct modiolar stimulation was occurring. Possibly at variance with that idea is the previous finding by van den Honert and Stypulkowski (1984) that, in a presumably similar case (round-window excitation), the resulting auditory-nerve-fiber discharge patterns were similar in character to those obtained in other experiments with dendritic, not with axonal, stimulation.

The biggest surprise of their 1987 study, however, was the extremely fine localization that they achieved with radially oriented bipolar electrodes. In several preparations, differences in threshold of more than 30 dB were displayed by neurons whose dendrites were longitudinally separated by approximately 1.9 mm (one-half octave) from each other. Clearly, large longitudinal and radial gradients must exist in these latter cases.

Current Modeling Work

In view of the work cited above, it is not surprising that there is a growing conviction in the field that only detailed multidimensional models will be able to account satisfactorily for the experimental data. One of the most promising of such models to data was recently reported by Finley et al. (1987). Utilizing a finite-element (161 elements) two-dimensional model that included the entire cochlear cross section with its osseous parts as well as fluid scalae, these investigators obtained potential profiles along the simulated neural pathway. Surprising in their results was the relative insensitivity of these potential profiles to large changes in certain model parameters that one would think important. When representations of the nerve fibers are added to such simulations (e.g., Wilson and Finley, 1984), potentially powerful models result. We will be hearing more about this work from Dr. Finley (see Chapter 5).

As the models get more detailed, more electroanatomical information is needed. What, for example, is the impedance of the modiolar wall relative to that of the perilymph? Until recently, such information was just not available, and so estimates based on the impedances of other bones were used. Utilizing a noninvasive reflection technique, the Ann Arbor–Seattle group is now beginning to measure such impedances directly. At a recent conference, Spelman, Clopton, and Suesserman (1987) reported that the average resistivity of the modiolar wall in the first turn averages 3.9 times that of normal saline. Surprising was their estimate of the impedance of the bony spiral lamina: 9.0 times that of saline. With its perforated zone, one would expect the impedance of the lamina to be less than that of the modiolar wall, not greater. Dr. Spelman will report further on that work (see Chapter 4).

Conclusion

The cochlea is complex, electrically as well as anatomically. From animal experiments, it is clear that sharply localized excitatory voltage fields as well as widely spread ones can be achieved with intracochlear electrodes.

In order to account theoretically for these localizations, and in order to take full advantage of them in future implant design, detailed multidimensional models, and the information about cochlear structures on which they depend, will be necessary.

Acknowledgments. This review was supported in part by NIH-NINCDS Grant NS-12732. It is a pleasure to acknowledge that the data in Figure 2.1 were obtained in the laboratory of Professor Brian Johnstone (University of Western Australia, Perth), in collaboration with Drs. Robert Patuzzi and Graeme Yates.

References

Békésy, G. von (1951). The coarse pattern of the electrical resistance in the cochlea of the guinea pig (electro-anatomy of the cochlea). *J. Acoust. Soc. Am.* 23:18–28. Reprinted in *Experiments in Hearing,* by G. von Békésy (McGraw-Hill, New York), 1960, pp. 654–672.

Black, R.C., and Clark, G.M. (1980). Differential electrical excitation of the auditory nerve. *J. Acoust. Soc. Am.* 67:868–874.

Brownell, W.E., Zidanic, M., and Spirou, G.A. (1986). Standing currents and their modulation in the cochlea. In *Neurobiology of Hearing: The Cochlea,* edited by R.A. Altschuler, D.W. Hoffman, and R.P. Bobbin (Raven Press, New York), pp. 91–107.

Cannon, M.W., Jr. (1976). Electrical impedances, current pathways and voltage sources in the guinea pig cochlea. Institute for Sensory Research Report ISR-S-14, Syracuse University, Syracuse, N.Y.

Cheatham, M.A., and Dallos, P. (1984). Summating potential (SP) tuning curves. *Hearing Res.* 16:189–200.

Dallos, P. (1983). Some electrical circuit properties of the organ of Corti. I. Analysis without reactive elements. *Hearing Res.* 12:89–119.

Davis, H. (1958). A mechano-electrical theory of cochlear action. *Ann. Otol. Rhinol. Laryngol.* 67:789–801.

Deng, L., and Geisler, C.D. (1987). A composite auditory model for processing speech sounds. *J. Acoust. Soc. Am.* 82:2001–2012.

Finley, C.C., Wilson, B.S., and White, M.W. (1987). A finite-element model of bipolar field patterns in the electrically stimulated cochlea—A two-dimensional approximation. *Proceedings of the Ninth Annual Conference of the IEEE Engineering in Medicine and Biology Society,* Boston, pp. 1901–1903.

Garcia, P., and Clopton, B.M. (1987). Radial current flow and source density in the basal scala tympani. *Hearing Res.* 31:55–64.

Geisler, C.D., Mountain, D.C., Hubbard, A.E., Adrian, H.O., and Ravindran, A. (1977). Alternating electrical-resistance changes in the guinea-pig cochlea caused by acoustic stimulation. *J. Acoust. Soc. Am.* 61:1557–1566.

Guinan, J.J., Jr., and Gifford, M.L. (1988). Effects of electrical stimulation of efferent olivocochlear neurons on cat auditory-nerve fibers. II. Spontaneous rate. *Hearing Res.* 33:115–128.

Hudspeth, A.J., and Corey, D.P. (1977). Sensitivity, polarity, and conductance change in the response of vertebrate hair cells to controlled mechanical stimuli. *Proc. Natl. Acad. Sci.* 74:2407–2411.

Johnstone, B.M., Johnstone, J.R., and Pugsley, I.O. (1966). Membrane resistance in endolymphatic walls of the first turn of the guinea pig cochlea. *J. Acoust. Soc. Am.* 40:1398–1404.

Liberman, M.C. (1982). The cochlear frequency map for the cat: Labeling auditory-nerve fibers of known characteristic frequency. *J. Acoust. Soc. Am.* 72:1441–1449.

Merzenich, M.M., and Reid, M.D. (1974). Representation of the cochlea within the inferior colliculus of the cat. *Brain Res.* 77:397–416.

Merzenich, M.M., and White, M.W. (1977). Cochlear implant: The interface problem. In *Functional Electrical Stimulation,* edited by J. Resnick and T. Hambrecht (Marcel Dekker, New York), pp. 321–340.

Mountain, D.C., and Cody, A.R. (1988). Mechanical coupling between inner and outer hair cells in the mammalian cochlea. In *Cochlear Mechanisms-Structure, Function and Models,* edited by J.P. Wilson and D.T. Kemp (Plenum, London, in press).

Robertson, D., Cody, A.R., Bredberg, G., and Johnstone, B.M. (1980). Response properties of spiral ganglion neurons in cochleas damaged by direct mechanical trauma. *J. Acoust. Soc. Am.* 67:1295–1303.

Russell, I.J. (1983). Origin of the receptor potential in inner hair cells of the mammalian cochlea—Evidence for Davis' theory. *Nature* 301:334–336.

Sellick, P.M., Patuzzi, R., and Johnstone, B.M. (1982). Modulation of responses of spiral ganglion cells in the guinea pig cochlea by low frequency sound. *Hearing Res.* 7:199–221.

Spelman, F.A., Clopton, B.M., and Suesserman, M.F. (1987). Measurements of the resistivity of bony tissues of the cochlea. *Proceedings of the Ninth Annual Conference of the IEEE Engineering in Medicine and Biology Society,* pp. 1911–1912.

Strelioff, D. (1973). A computer simulation of the generation and distribution of cochlear potentials. *J. Acoust. Soc. Am.* 54:620–629.

van den Honert, C., and Stypulkowski, P.H. (1984). Physiological properties of the electrically stimulated auditory nerve II. Single fiber recordings. *Hearing Res.* 14:225–243.

van den Honert, C., and Stypulkowski, P.H. (1987). Single fiber mapping of spatial excitation patterns in the electrically stimulated auditory nerve. *Hearing Res.* 29:195–206.

Wilson, B.S., and Finley, C.C. (1984). Fifth Quarterly Progress Report, NIH Contract N01-NS-2356, Research Triangle Institute, North Carolina.

3
Selective Stimulation of Peripheral Axons

MOSHE SOLOMONOW

Introduction

Electrical nerve stimulation may be a highly useful tool for the in vivo study of skeletal muscle contractile properties in experimental animals. Unfortunately, currently available stimulation techniques fail to provide contraction under conditions which are similar to the known recruitment properties of various muscles. A frequently used technique delivers to the nerve brief rectangular pulses of suprathreshold amplitude while varying the pulse frequency (rate coding). In essence, all the motor units are always active, which is a significant deviation from the "size principle" mode (Henneman, Somjen, and Carpenter, 1965) under which units are recruited according to their size, small ones first and then progressively larger ones. Attempts to elicit a more favorable condition by increasing the stimulus pulse amplitude from subthreshold to suprathreshold are also deficient, since the larger axons have lower excitation thresholds (Blair and Erlanger, 1933) and are always activated first in a "reverse recruitment" mode. Such an approach yields large initial force increments and results in fast setting fatigue which is characteristic of large motor units. The problem, therefore, is the lack of a method which can allow excitation of small units first and progressively larger ones with capabilities to modify simultaneously the firing rate of the action potentials of the active units at various strategies similar to that observed in various skeletal muscles (Basmajian and DeLuca, 1985; Clamann 1970; Grimby and Hannerz, 1977).

The early work of Wedensky (1884) showed that high-frequency (20 KHz) nerve stimulation inhibits the muscle from contracting. Tanner (1962), who studied Wedensky's high-frequency stimulation technique, demonstrated that inhibition of motor units was dependent on their size as the stimulus amplitude varied. Lowering the stimulus amplitude allowed axons of small size, which have high excitation thresholds to electrical stimulus, to escape the inhibition and conduct action potentials elicited by a proximal stimulus. Further reduction of the high-frequency stimulus amplitude allowed progressively larger axons to escape the inhibition and conduct action potentials to the muscle. Tanner's convincing demonstration was not surprising since it only confirmed Erlanger's Nobel Prize–winning work (Blair and Erlanger, 1933; the prize was won in 1944), in which Erlanger showed, with single-axon recordings from a whole nerve trunk, that the excitation threshold to electrical stimulus was dependent on the axon diameter (or its conduction velocity). Large-diameter axons were shown to have low excitation thresholds, while progressively smaller axons had progressively higher thresholds. Erlanger's work is recognized today in the well-known strength-duration curves for axons of various diameters. Tanner, therefore, extended Erlanger's findings to stimuli of high repetition rates, which inhibit muscular activity. Our previous work (Solomonow, 1984) with high-frequency stimulation demonstrated that rates of 600 Hz provided the most efficient block (i.e., requiring the lowest stimulus amplitude), and that the stimulus could consist of short rectangular pulses of 100 μs duration, instead of a sinusoidal waveform.

The objective of this study is to describe and validate a new method, employing high-frequency stimulation, which can recruit motor units according to their size, while maintaining fully independent control of the firing rate. The technique is based on dual stimuli applied to the nerve with a cuff electrode, and may serve as a useful tool to study various electrophysiological and biomechanical properties of muscles under more favorable physiological conditions than currently employed stimulation techniques.

Method

Preparation

Six adult cats anesthetized with chloralose (60 mg/kg) were used. The hind limb muscles were denervated except for the muscle nerves to the soleus and m. gastrocnemius. Later, the muscle nerve to one of the muscles above was cut in order to study the response of a single muscle. The calcaneal tendon was cut at its insertion and connected to a force transducer. Pins were inserted in the distal femur and mid tibia, and attached to a rigid frame including a pelvic clamp to provide isometric conditions to the muscles under study (with hip, knee, and ankle at 90° to each other).

Instrumentation

A tripolar cuff electrode (1-cm-long cuff and 3-mm spacing between the stainless-steel poles) was mounted on the sciatic nerve, as shown in Figure 3.1. The center pole was used as common to two stimulators, while the stimuli were delivered to the distal and proximal poles.

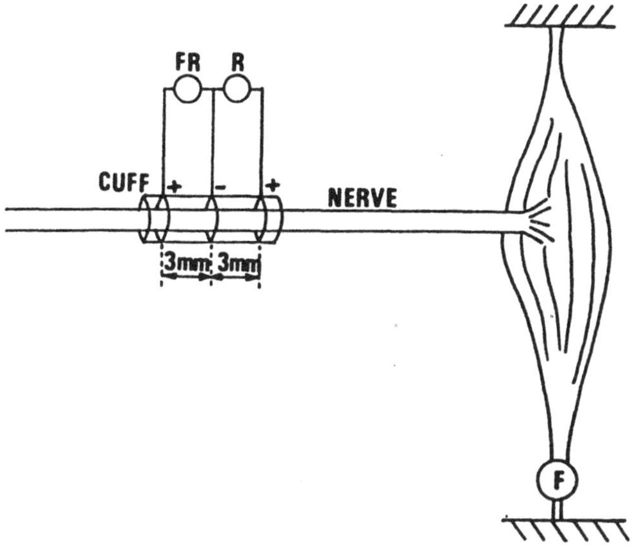

FIGURE 3.1. Schematic of the tripolar electrode mounted on the nerve-muscle preparation, showing the setup of the two stimulators. (FR—firing rate. R—recruitment. F—the force transducer.)

The instrumentation of the stimulation system was described in detail elsewhere (Zhou, Baratta, and Solomonow, 1987). Briefly, an IBM-XT computer delivered two voltage envelopes. The first envelope served as the input to a voltage-controlled oscillator (VCO), the output of which yielded 100-μs rectangular pulses at suprathreshold amplitude with rate corresponding to the input voltage to the VCO. Rates from 0 to 100 pulses per second (pps) were available. This constituted the firing rate (FR) stimulus.

The second voltage envelope was modulated by 100-μS rectangular pulses at 600 pps. The pulse amplitude was governed by the voltage envelope input and normally decreased linearly from the just-above-threshold of the smallest axon to the just-below-threshold of the largest axon. This constituted the recruitment (R) stimulus. Since suprathreshold high-frequency (600 pps) stimulation inhibits the muscle from contracting as a response to the FR stimulus (Solomonow, 1984; Tanner, 1962; Wedensky, 1884; Zhou, Baratta, and Solomonow, 1987), gradual reduction of the pulse amplitude (as shown in Figure 3.2) allows the smallest motor axon (which has a high excitation threshold) to escape the inhibitory effect of the R stimulus first, and conduct the action potentials generated by the FR stimulus. Progressively larger axons escape the R stimulus as its pulse amplitude decreases and allows orderly recruitment similar to that in voluntary contraction (Henneman, Somjen, and Carpenter, 1965).

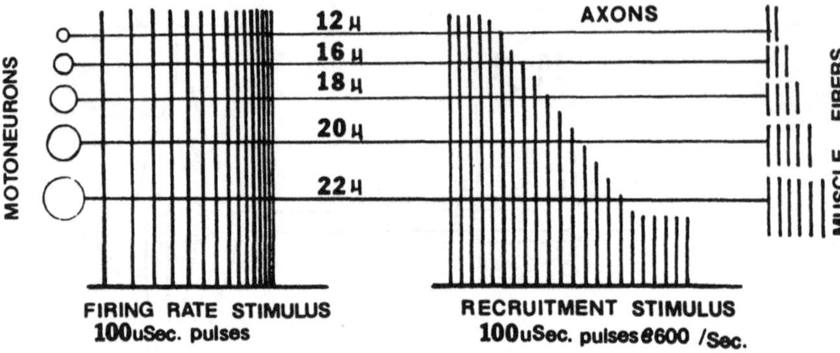

FIGURE 3.2. Schematic of a sample of motor units of increasing size, their increasing axon diameter and innervation ratio, and the two stimuli. Each stimulus spike represents a 100-μs pulse, and both stimuli have a common time base. Note the increase of firing rate with time and the simultaneous decrease of pulse amplitude in the recruitment stimulus, which allows progressively larger axons to escape the blocking effect and conduct the FR action potentials.

EMG was recorded with two fine, insulated stainless-steel wires with 1-mm exposed tip inserted with hypodermic needles in each muscle one-half the distance between its motor point and the distal tendon. The EMG was amplified differentially with 110-dB CMRR and bandpass-filtered (10–500 Hz). Force was recorded with a Grass FT-10 transducer. Force and EMG were recorded by an IBM-AT computer at a 6000-Hz sampling rate.

Protocol

Three test categories were applied once the FR stimulus was calibrated at 1.5× suprathreshold and the R stimulus values were set at the just-above-threshold of the smallest axon and the just-below-threshold of the largest axon. All threshold values were determined experimentally.

In the first test, with both soleus and m. gastrocnemius muscle nerves intact, the R stimulus pulse amplitude was linearly decreased, while the FR stimulus rate was fixed at 45 pps. Since the soleus predominantly consists of small motor units (Eccles and Sherington, 1930; McPhedran, Wuerker, and Henneman, 1965), while the m. gastrocnemius has primarily large motor units (Burke and Tsairis, 1975; Wuerker, McPhedran, and Henneman, 1965), as shown in Figure 3.3, M-wave activity should be evident from the soleus well in advance of any M waves in the m. gastrocnemius, if recruitment of motor units was accomplished according to the size principle. Conversely, applying a stimulus of linearly increasing pulse amplitude at constant rate (shown schematically in Figure 3.5*b*) via two poles of the electrode with the FR stimulus set at

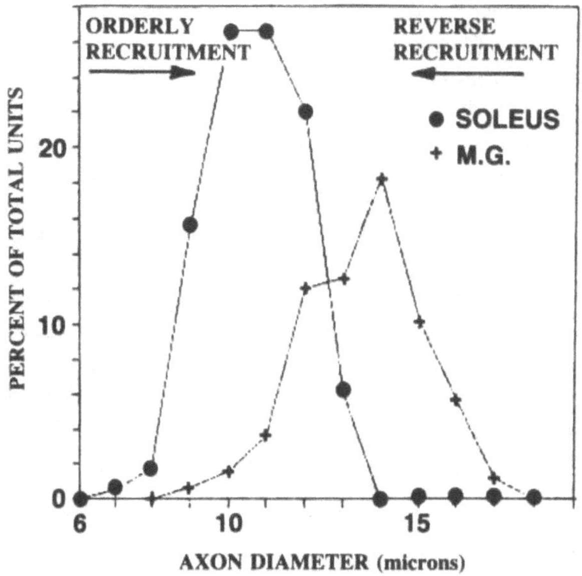

FIGURE 3.3. The distribution of soleus and m. gastrocnemius motor units versus their axon diameter (compounded data from Burke and Tsairis, 1975; Eccles and Sherington, 1930; McPhedran, Wuerker, and Henneman, 1965; Wuerker, McPhedran, and Henneman, 1965). Note that an orderly recruitment stimulus will excite axons from left to right (as shown by the arrow), activating the soleus first. A reverse recruitment (shown by a right-to-left arrow) will, however, excite the m. gastrocnemius first.

zero should induce *reverse recruitment,* exciting the large axons first and smaller ones later, as the pulse amplitude increases (Blair and Erlanger, 1933). Under such conditions, the EMG from the m. gastrocnemius should be evident well in advance of any M waves in the soleus, if reverse recruitment indeed occurred.

The second test category was performed on a single muscle, having the nerve branch to the soleus or m. gastrocnemius cut. The FR was fixed at a constant value while the R stimulus was applied. FR values of 5, 10, 20, 30, 40, and 50 pps were used, each in a separate trial. Since the M wave is the response to each single pulse of the FR stimulus, the number and rate of the recorded M waves for any time period should be identical to the constant FR stimulus frequency applied in that trial. This should validate the independence of the FR stimulus from the R stimulus, if there is no interaction between the two stimuli.

Furthermore, if recruitment is indeed orderly, the force trace should exhibit the gradual appearance and then increase of unfused force late in the recruitment phase (i.e., late in the force rise phase), as the larger motor units are recruited in trials when the firing rate is fixed below their frequency of fusion (5–20 pps).

The third test category consisted of validating the orderly recruitment from the fatigue standpoint. With the FR set constant, the R stimulus was adjusted to decrease slightly such that only a few small motor units were recruited within 1 s and then remained active for 10 s. Since small motor units are fatigue-resistant compared with larger motor units, they were expected to demonstrate relatively little reduction of force at the end of the trial. In consecutive trials, the R stimulus was adjusted to recruit larger motor units, with the expectation of a larger decrease of force at the end of 10 s of activity due to the gradual decrease in resistance to fatigue, which is characteristic of larger units. The percent fatigue was calculated, representing the amount of force reduction at the end of 10 s, as compared with the peak force.

Results

M Waves during Orderly and Reversed Recruitment

Figure 3.4 shows the force, soleus EMG, and m. gastrocnemius EMG recorded during orderly recruitment of motor units while the FR was constant at 45 pps. It is evident that initiation and increase in the M-wave amplitude was seen in the soleus nearly 1 s before any activity in the m. gastrocnemius was detected, attesting to the fact that the soleus's small motor units became active first. Furthermore, M-wave initiation in the m. gastrocnemius was evident shortly before the M-wave amplitude of the soleus saturated (once all its motor units were recruited), confirming the partial overlap of some motor units in both muscles, as reported by Burke and Tsairis (1975) and also shown in Figure 3.3.

A similar response pattern was obtained from all six preparations in which EMG discharge from the soleus was seen well in advance of any discharge in the m. gastrocnemius. The lead time of the soleus discharge over that of the m. gastrocnemius ranged from 0.92 s to 1.04 s, and the average lead time of all preparations was 0.98 s. The minor variability of the lead time was attributed to minor anatomical variations which exist from animal to animal.

Figure 3.5*a* shows the force, soleus EMG, and m. gastrocnemius EMG during *reverse recruitment* (shown schematically in Figure 3.5*b*) applied via two poles of the electrode (common and positive) at a fixed rate of 55 pps (the FR stimulus was set at zero). It is evident from the traces that M-wave activity in the m. gastrocnemius is seen nearly 1.2 s prior to any M-wave activity in the soleus, confirming that the larger motor units were excited first in this reverse recruitment stimulation paradigm, as was first described by Erlanger (Blair and Erlanger, 1933). It can be concluded,

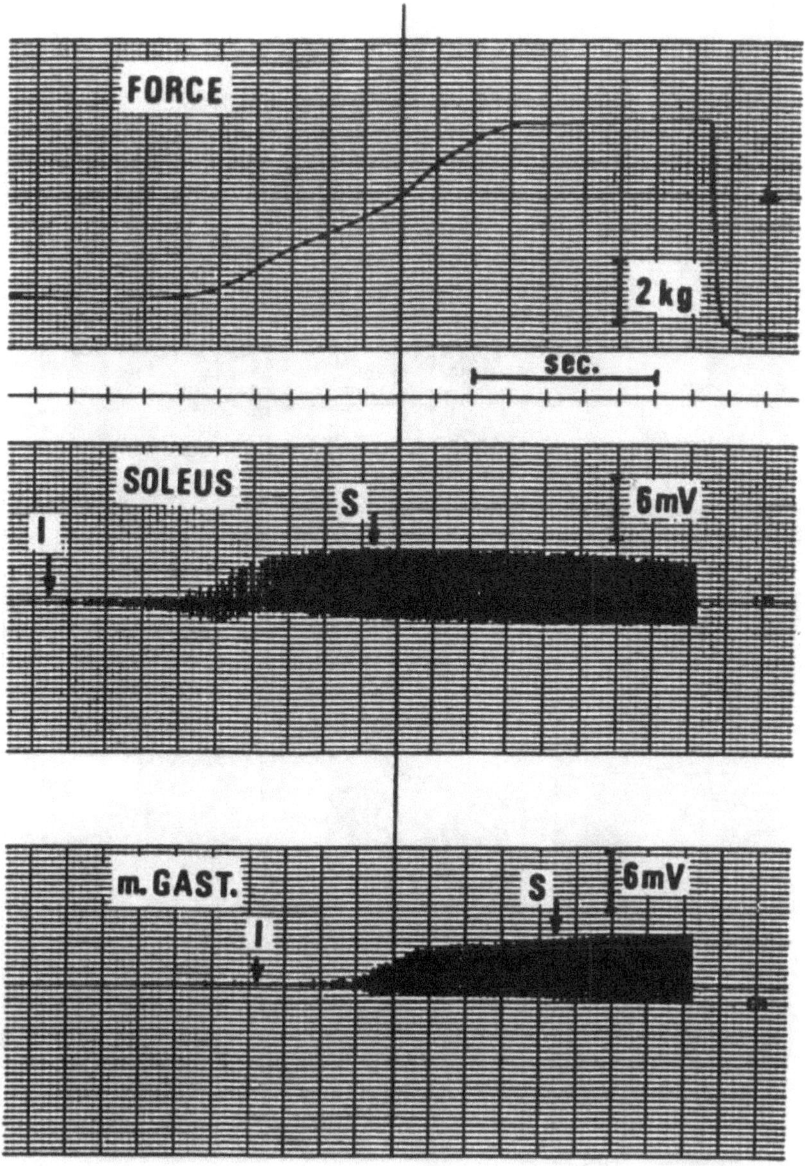

FIGURE 3.4. The force, soleus EMG, and m. gastrocnemius EMG responses to the orderly recruitment stimulus of Figure 3.2. The EMG (M-wave train) from the soleus was seen first, about 1 s before any EMG in the m. gastrocnemius, confirming the ability of the stimulus to excite small units first and progressively larger ones later. (I—initiation of the M wave. S—saturation of the M wave.)

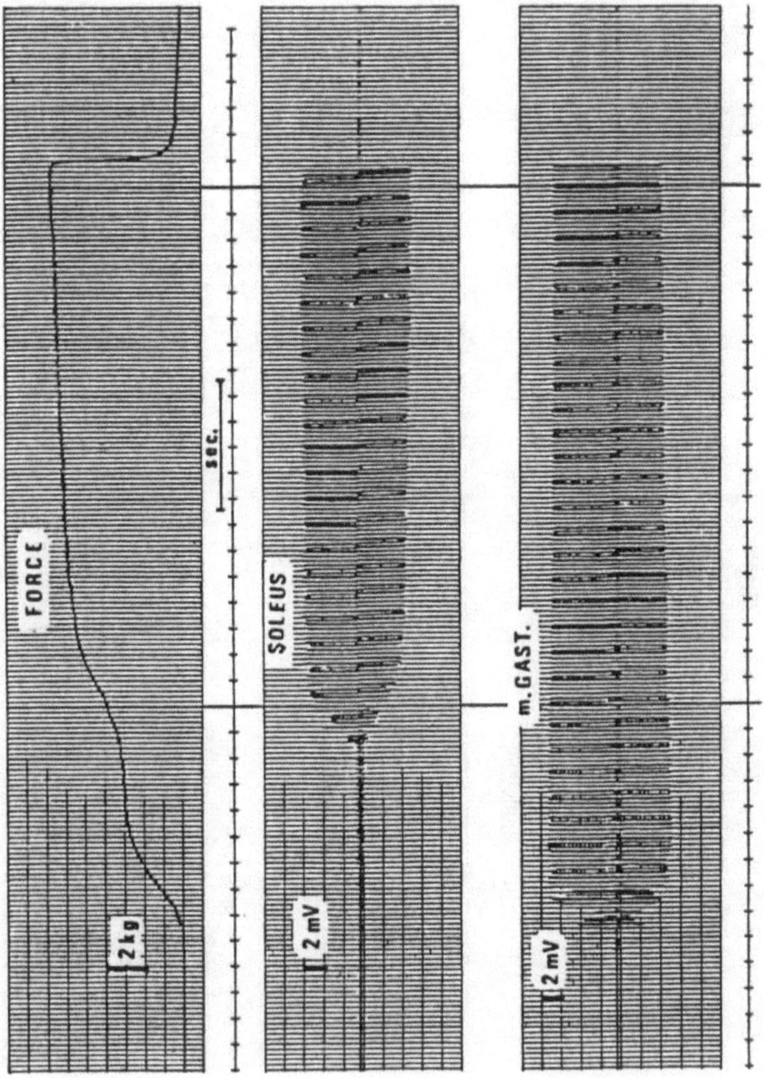

(a)

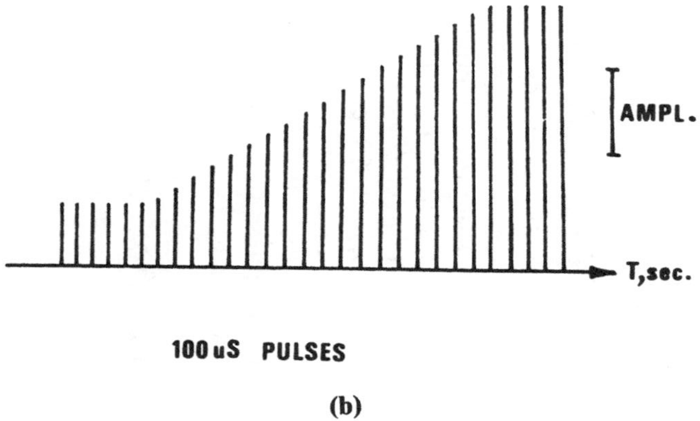

FIGURE 3.5. In this figure, part (*a*) shows the force, soleus EMG, and m. gastrocnemius EMG responses to the reversed recruitment stimulus shown schematically in part (*b*). Note that the m. gastrocnemius initiated EMG discharge 1.1 s before any EMG discharge was seen in the soleus, confirming Erlanger's strength-duration curves for axons of different diameter—or the reverse recruitment properties of pulses of increasing amplitude. In part (*b*), each vertical spike represents a 100-μs pulse, and the pulses are increasing in intensity to recruit large-diameter axons first and smaller ones later. The rate of the pulses was set at 55 pps.

then, that the control paradigm shown in Figure 3.2 indeed recruited small motor units first and larger ones later, in an orderly manner, as was confirmed by the consistently reproduced response in the six preparations.

Force Response during Orderly Recruitment

Figure 3.6 shows force traces which are the response to orderly recruitment applied while the FR was constant at various rates during each trial. Two important facts are evident from the traces: the gradual appearance and then increase of unfused force in the final segment of the force rise for trials in which low rates were applied (5, 10, and 20 pps), and the progressive reduction of the maximal force as the FR was reduced. The gradual appearance and increase of the unfused force in the terminal phase of the force rise are the manifestation of the late recruitment of large motor units at rates much below their rate of force fusion. This observation is in agreement with the well-founded firing rate behavior of motor units in voluntary contraction, with large units (which are normally recruited later in the force generation phase) having higher initial, as well as higher maximal, firing rates than small-sized units (Basmajian and DeLuca, 1985; Clamann, 1970; Grimby and Hannerz, 1977). Since the firing rate was kept constant, below the initial activation rate of such large units, the units responded with unfused force upon their recruitment. The important fact is that the initial force rise was smooth, indicating that small motor units (of low initial firing rate) were recruited first. The gradual appearance of twitches, as well as the gradual increase of their amplitude, indicates the progressive recruitment of larger motor units which require progressively higher initial firing rates to yield fused force. Since the FR stimulus was held constant, at low rates (5, 10, and 20 pps), the medium-size motor units contributed their force in a partially fused manner while the larger ones, recruited later, responded with pure twitches. The unfused force seen only at the late phase of the force rise confirmed that motor units were recruited according to the size principle.

The Independence of the Firing Rate from the Recruitment Stimulus

Figure 3.7 shows six traces (corresponding to the force traces of Figure 3.6 but in reverse order) of EMG (M-wave trains) recordings from the M. gastrocnemius during orderly recruitment, while the FR stimulus was set constant at 5, 10, 20, 30, 40, and 50 pps, respectively. It is evident from the figure that the rate of the M waves is identical to the FR stimulus rate, demonstrating total independence of the R from the FR stimulus. Furthermore, the amplitude of the M wave demonstrated a gradual

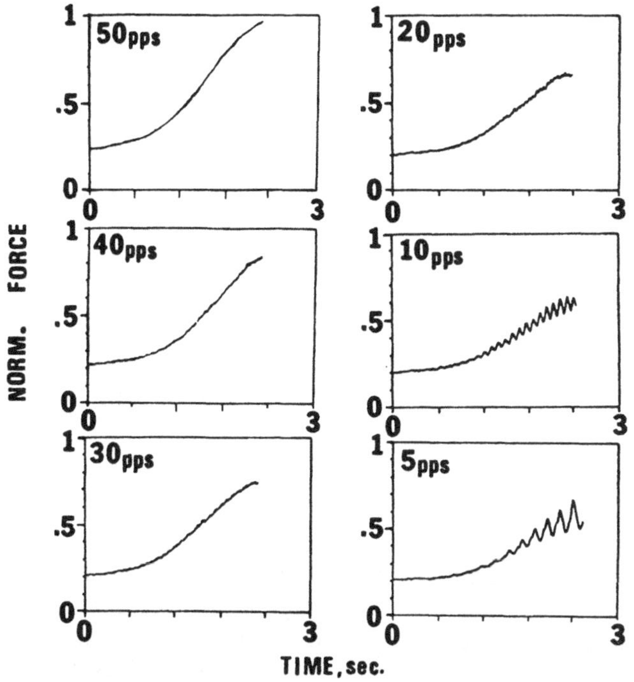

FIGURE 3.6. Normalized force versus time traces from an m. gastrocnemius preparation subjected to the orderly recruitment stimulus, while the firing rate was constant at several values. Note that in the traces where the firing rate was fixed at 5, 10, and 20 pps throughout the recruitment cycle, the initial increase of force was smooth, but as larger units (which require a higher initial firing rate) were recruited, the force shows gradual appearance and increase of unfused twitches, clearly demonstrating that orderly recruitment took place. (Force was normalized with respect to the maximal tetanic force at 50 pps.)

increase as larger motor units were recruited and their corresponding MUAPs spatially added to those of the previously active motor units.

Figure 3.8*a* shows the M-wave train recorded from a trial in which motor units were orderly recruited while the firing rate was simultaneously increased. In this trial, the last motor unit was recruited as the FR just reached the highest rate. Such control strategy is similar to that employed by the biceps and deltoid (Basmajian and DeLuca, 1985). Careful evaluation of the figure confirms that the inter-M-wave interval was indeed shorter and its rate identical to the firing rate as it increased, while each consecutive M-wave amplitude was larger as newly recruited MUAPs were spatially adding. The last few M waves, two of which are shown, were of the largest amplitude, indicating that all units were fully recruited.

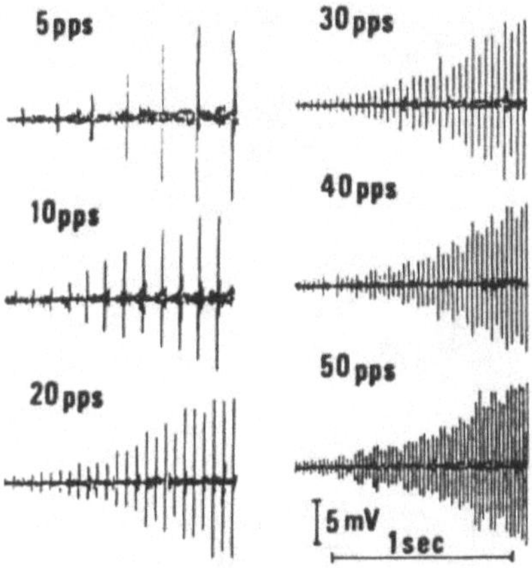

FIGURE 3.7. M-wave trains recorded from an m. gastrocnemius preparation during the application of orderly recruitment, while the firing rate held constant at various frequencies. Note that the number of M waves per second is identical to the FR frequency, confirming the independence of the two stimuli. Also note the gradual increase of the M-wave amplitude due to the spatial addition of the muscle action potentials from the newly recruited units.

Figure 3.8*b* was recorded from a trial in which all the motor units were fully recruited according to the size principle to generate 50% of the muscle's maximal force, while the firing rate was simultaneously increasing throughout the full force generation cycle, a control strategy similar to that employed by the FDI muscle (Basmajian and DeLuca, 1933). It is evident from the figure that the M-wave amplitude was indeed increasing during the initial period and then was saturated and remained constant in the final force generation period. The inter-M-wave interval, however, was progressively shorter throughout the trial, a manifestation of the simultaneously increasing firing rate.

In summary, Figures 3.7 and 3.8 demonstrate the independence of the firing rate from the recruitment stimulus, as well as the ability of the control scheme to increase the firing rate simultaneously with recruitment and at various control strategies, in which all the motor units are fully recruited to generate any portion of the initial force increase (Zhou, Baratta, and Solomonow, 1987).

Fatigue

Figure 3.9 shows typical force traces from an isolated soleus preparation in which motor units were recruited over 1 s and then left active for a 10-s duration. The figure clearly shows that when only a few small motor units are recruited (trace *a*), the force displays minimal fatigue (12% decrease from the peak force), confirming the fatigue resistance capabilities of such small units. As larger units (which are more susceptible to fatigue) are recruited, the forces display a gradual increase in fatigue. The fatigue calculated for force traces *b, c, d,* and *e* indicates a 36%, 46%, 51%, and

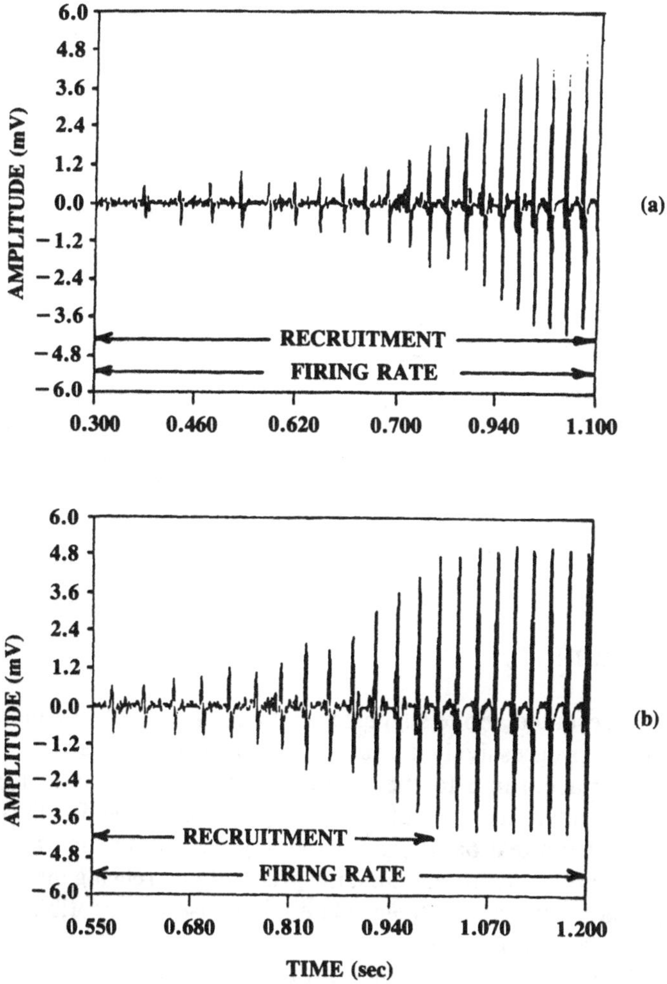

FIGURE 3.8. The M-wave train during an increase in the firing rate throughout the orderly recruitment cycle (*a*) and an increase in the firing rate during and after all the motor units were fully recruited (*b*). Note the constant amplitude of the M wave after the completion of the recruitment cycle in (*b*), which attests that no further addition of MUAPs occurred.

56% reduction of force, respectively. The traces, therefore, demonstrate the gradual decrease in resistance to fatigue associated with the increasing size of motor units. This, in turn, further confirms that recruitment was accomplished according to the size principle, exciting the small, fatigue-resistant units first and the fast-to-fatigue, larger units later.

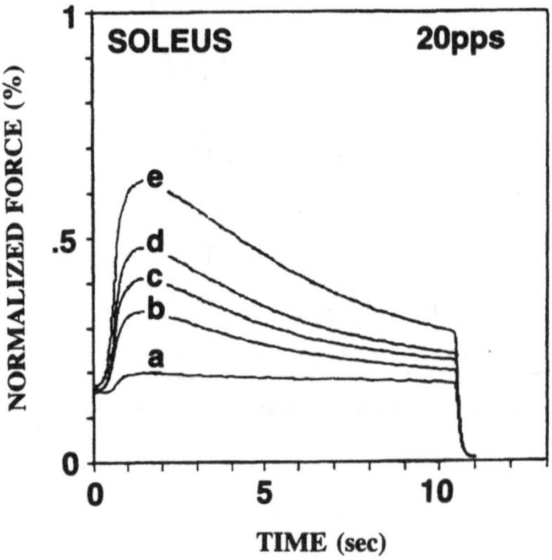

FIGURE 3.9. Force traces recorded from a soleus preparation at various recruitment levels. In trace *a*, only a few small fatigue-resistant units were recruited, demonstrating little fatigue, while in traces *b*, *c*, *d*, and *e* progressively larger motor units, which are more susceptible to fatigue, were recruited. The force traces corroborate that orderly recruitment occurred by the gradual increase in fatigue as larger units were recruited. (The force of each trial was normalized with respect to the maximal tetanic force of the muscle at 47 pps.)

Conclusions

The data presented above suggest that the high-frequency stimulus whose amplitude is progressively decreased in time has the capabilities to recruit motor units according to their size, small ones first and progressively larger ones later (as the pulse amplitude is decreased). This fact was established from test paradigms, including the motor unit architecture of the soleus and m. gastrocnemius, the gradually increasing initial firing rate of larger motor units, and the gradually increased susceptibility to fatigue of such larger motor units.

Combining the above evidence with the time-proven classical strength-duration curves established by the single-fiber recordings of Erlanger (Blair and Erlanger, 1933), it could be concluded that the technique presented in this study allows one to recruit motor units according to the size principle.

On the basis of the M-wave recordings presented in this study, it is clear that complete independence in the control of the motor units' firing rate and their orderly recruitment is available when using the described technique. Furthermore, the technique developed here allows the activation of a muscle with a large choice of firing rate and recruitment control strategies, similar to that of various skeletal muscles by proper adjustment of the two stimuli.

The reader should recognize, however, that in the technique described here, all the motor units fired synchronously, while under voluntary control, asynchronous discharge is evident. Unfortunately, attempts to induce asynchronous discharge may require improvements in technology which are not currently available, but are well worth looking forward to.

In summary, the technique described here, using single tripolar electrodes, allows recruitment of motor units according to their size independently and simultaneously with changes of firing rate at various control strategies similar to the voluntary control of various muscles. Such a technique provides a highly useful tool for basic and applied investigations into the biomechanics and electrophysiology of skeletal muscles.

Acknowledgment. This work was supported by the National Science Foundation with Grant EET 8613807. Figures are reproduced with permission of Butterworth Scientific & Co.© (publishers).

References

Basmajian, J., and DeLuca, C. (1985). *Muscles Alive* (Williams and Wilkins, Baltimore), pp. 138–149.

Blair, E., and Erlanger, J. (1933). A comparison of the characteristics of axons through their individual electrical responses. *Am. J. Physiology* 106:524–564.

Burke, R., and Tsairis, P. (1975). Anatomy and innervation ratios in motor units of the cat's gastrocnemius. *J. Physiol.* (*London*) 234:749–765.

Clamann, P. (1970). Activity of single motor units during isometric tension. *Neurology* 20:254–260.

Eccles, J., and Sherington, C. (1930). Numbers and contraction values of individual motor units examined in some muscles of the limbs. *Proc. Royal Society* B106:326–357.

Grimby, L., and Hannerz, J. (1977). Firing rates and recruitment order of toe extensor motor units in different modes of voluntary contraction. *J. Physiology* (*London*) 264:865–879.

Henneman, E., Somjen, G., and Carpenter, D. (1965). Functional significance of cell size in spinal motor neurons. *J. Neurophysiology* 28:560–580.

McPhedran, A., Wuerker, R., and Henneman, E. (1965). Properties of motor units in a homogeneous red muscle (soleus) of the cat. *J. Neurophysiology* 28:71–84.

Solomonow, M. (1984). External control of the neuromuscular system. *IEEE—Trans. Biomed. Eng.* 31:752–763.

Tanner, J. (1962). Reversible blocking of nerve conduction by alternating current excitation. *Nature* 195:712–713.

Wedensky, N. (1884). Wise Rasch Ermudet der Nerv. *ZBL. Med.* Wiss., 65–68.

Wuerker, R., McPhedran, A., and Henneman, E. (1965). Properties of motor units in heterogeneous pale muscle (m. gastrocnemius) of the cat. *J. Neurophysiology* 28:85–99.

Zhou, B., Baratta, R., and Solomonow, M. (1987). Manipulation of muscle force with various firing rates and recruitment control strategies. *IEEE—Trans. Biomed. Eng.* 34:128–139.

Moshe Solomonow: Discussion

Dr. Spelman: One of the advantages that you have, that we do not, is that you can apply your electrodes directly to nerves. Do you think your strategy might work at a distance, let's say with surface-mounted electrodes, or have you or your colleagues tried that method?

Dr. Solomonow: You mean put electrodes on the skin and try?

Dr. Spelman: Yes, so that you are a distance from the nerve trunk. Are you still able to assert the kind of fine control that you had with your strategy?

Dr. Solomonow: Yes, we've tried that. It was a total failure. The reason for that finding is very simple. The skin has the characteristics of a low-pass filter, and all high-frequency stimuli are attenuated to the point where the nerve is passing all the information to the muscle as a contraction rather than as an inhibition. However, we tried it in a different way. You can take a wire electrode insulated only with 1 mm or so of exposed conductor, put it in a hypodermic needle, insert that into the point in which the nerve separates into the muscle, and then apply the 600 pps and see what happens. This inhibits the muscle. So this tells us the skin is the culprit here when you use surface stimulation. Originally we thought the technique worked with surface electrodes. We were so excited we thought we can do so many things immediately, like reduce spasticity in patients or maybe control the link to the muscle without surgery. It didn't work; what a disappointment!

Dr. Spelman: With that system, have you tried to stimulate with the driving electrode and then with the inhibitor electrodes to control, within a population, those that are activated. One might be able to use it in a way to modulate the recruitment of fibers within a group.

Dr. Solomonow: Are you referring to stimulating only a specific fascicle in a mixed nerve?

Dr. Spelman: Yes. I am thinking about spatial control and spatial restriction, which is of course a primary problem for the cochlear prosthesis.

Dr. Solomonow: No, I have not tried that. There are several complex factors involved that I do not know how to control. If you use bipolar electrodes in the sciatic nerve, not tightly coupled, it is easy to show that axons get stimulated according to the size of the axon, that is, the diameter of the axon, and not according to what is closer to the electrode. On the other hand, I have read several reports, from other groups, saying it is possible if one were to use unipolar electrodes. I still have not sorted out in my mind why this happens this way and not the other way. Obviously you restrict the current when you use the bipolar electrodes, and you get larger spread with monopolar stimulation. I recently served as an external examiner for an electrical engineering Ph.D. in the University of Twente, Holland, where the student did a theoretical analysis of a nerve model and showed very convincingly from a theoretical standpoint that a bipolar electrode would always recruit fibers according to their diameter, not their location in the nerve. If he used intramascular electrodes or unipolar electrodes, he would recruit fibers according to their distance from the electrode, rather than their diameter.

Dr. Spelman: I wonder what happens if you apply only high-frequency stimuli to the nerve. Does it activate the muscle? If you apply the high-frequency stimuli to the auditory nerve, it does produce a sensation.

Dr. Solomonow: If you apply only high-frequency stimuli, you will get a very fast response; it is a spike that will immediately decay to about 5 or 6% of the maximum force of the muscle and will remain that way. This tells me there are some fatigue-resistant fibers that do not care what the frequency of stimulation is. A colleague of mine at UCLA just sent me a paper in which he speculates that there are some fatigue-resistant units in the ventral root.

Dr. Spelman: You mentioned that 600 Hz was optimal for recruitment of central fibers. What was the shape of that response function?

Dr. Solomonow: I didn't bring the curve. As I recall, from 50 Hz up to 600, it increases almost linearly. Then after 600 it decreases. So we assume you can use a reduced amplitude in the 600–900-Hz range, because the frequency would make it more efficient.

4
Determination of Tissue Impedances of the Inner Ear: Models and Measurements

FRANCIS A. SPELMAN

Introduction

Electrical Properties of the Inner Ear

Investigators have studied the passive electrical properties of the inner ear to provide information about transduction processes (Asakuma, Snow, and Murakami, 1978; Davis, 1965; Geisler et al., 1977; Johnstone, Johnstone, and Pugsley, 1966). Others have observed the inner ear in order to learn how better to apply improved cochlear implants (Ifukube and White, 1987; Spelman, Clopton, and Pfingst, 1982; Spelman, Clopton, and Suesserman, 1987). The techniques employed by these investigators have a common basis in their use of lumped-element circuit models for the interpretation of data. Such models can be one-dimensional (Geisler et al., 1977), two-dimensional (Johnstone, Johnstone, and Pugsley, 1966; Suesserman, 1988), or three-dimensional (Honrubia, Strelioff, and Sitko, 1976). More recently, the distributed character of the volume conductors in the cochlea has been considered when tissue properties have been measured (Ifukube and White, 1987; Spelman, Clopton, and Suesserman, 1987).

Techniques of Measurement

The models that were used profoundly influence not only the interpretation of the experimental data but also the techniques of measurement. The techniques can be placed in three categories: (1) the use of a chamber to estimate the properties of a sample of tissue; (2) estimation of lumped tissue parameters in situ; and (3) estimation of distributed tissue parameters in situ. Each technique presents unique strengths and weaknesses.

Limitations of Measurements

The Sample Chamber

Tissue is excised from an animal and placed in a chamber of known geometry. The geometry of the tissue is also known, and the resistivity, either real or complex, can be measured with great precision. Given the resistivity, the impedance of the tissue can be estimated for any geometry (Wait, 1982). While this technique accounts for the geometry of tissue by measuring tissue resistivity, a constant that is independent of geometry, it suffers from severe limitations.

The nature of the measurement requires that the tissue sample be taken from a living animal and, at best, preserved in artificial biological media at body temperature, maintained at room temperature or below in preservatives such as formalin, or dessicated. Singh and Saha (1984) pointed out that techniques of preservation certainly cause variations in the estimates of resistivity made in bone—hence the descriptions of measurements in "fresh," "wet," or "dry" bone samples. In cochlear tissues, differential effects of postmortem measurements have been observed (Spelman, Clopton, and Pfingst, 1982). Hence, the data from preserved tissue samples are probably different from those obtained in vivo and will lead to incorrect models of current flow in the inner ear.

The design of the sample chamber and of its electrodes also contributes to the estimates of resistivity. Figure 4.1 is a schematic drawing of a chamber used in our laboratory to estimate the resistivity of fluids. The simple design employs two electrodes to deliver constant-density current and two electrodes to measure potential difference. Given the dimensions of the chamber, the measurement of resistivity is trivial. Some investiga-

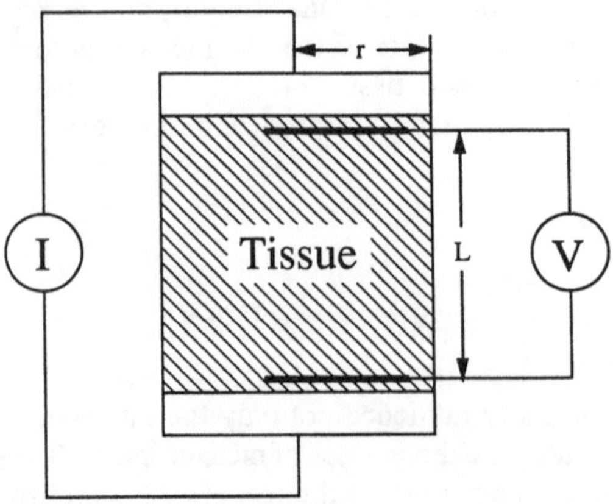

*For a Cylindrical Plug - $\rho = \left(\frac{V}{I}\right)\left[\frac{\pi r^2}{L}\right]$

FIGURE 4.1. Measuring impedance with a sample chamber. Resistivity of the tissue is given for a cylindrical chamber.

tors employ two-electrode measurements (Figure 1 in Singh and Saha, 1984), but those measurements are confounded by the influences of electrode impedance.

The sample chamber technique suffers primarily from its destructive nature and secondarily from the effects of chamber and electrode design. The design of sample chambers for cochlear tissues is difficult at best, imprecise and difficult to interpret at worst (Ifukube and White, 1987). Obtaining representative samples from the tissues of the inner ear is both difficult and tedious.

Lumped and Distributed Parameter Estimates

Measurement of the electrical properties of lumped tissue parameters in situ guarantees that, with proper treatment of the animal, the tissues will not be influenced by the measurement. Hence, the concerns raised about the sample chamber technique do not hold. However, there are biological, instrumental, and theoretical difficulties inherent in this technique.

Biological Problems

The biological problems are related to electrode materials, electrode size, energy transfer, and tissue destruction. Electrodes that inject electric current into tissues and record resultant potentials (Figure 4.2) must be

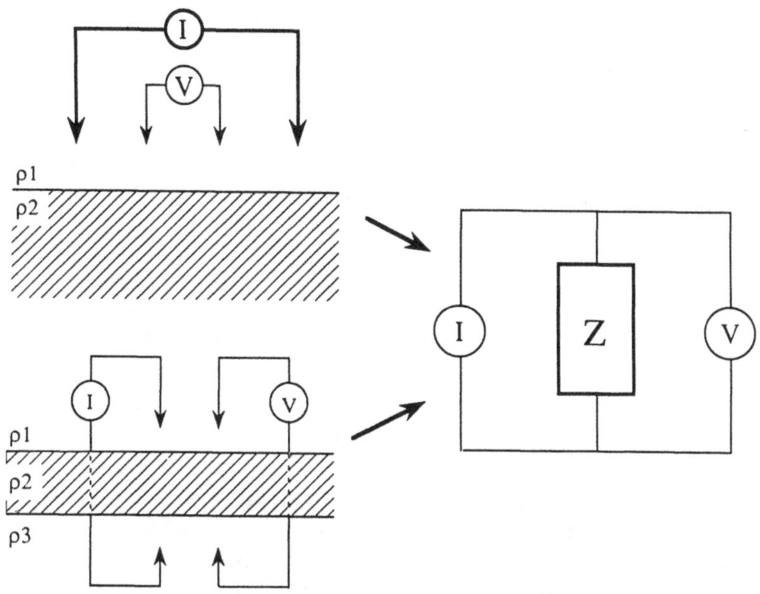

FIGURE 4.2. Tissue impedance estimated with a four-electrode technique. Impedance can be estimated in one medium or in two media with a third intervening. In both cases a single impedance is modeled.

made of materials that minimize the generation of toxic by-products. The use of micropipettes (Geisler et al., 1977) offers one solution; the use of noble metals (Spelman, Clopton, and Pfingst, 1982) offers another. Care must be taken to avoid current densities that produce toxic by-products (Brummer and Turner, 1977).

Electrode arrays must be small to minimize tissue damage and to permit investigators to obtain appropriate numbers of spatial samples from the cochlear tissues. Small size requires small stimulating currents, since the current densities at the surfaces of the stimulating electrodes must be held at safe levels to avoid disturbance of the chemical environment of the tissues (Brummer and Turner, 1977).

Theoretical and experimental studies have also shown that the shape of the electrode must be designed to prevent current densities from being unacceptably high (Rubinstein et al., 1987).

Instrumental Problems

Instrumental problems for the measurement of tissue impedance in small volumes are formidable and are related to the microscopic size of the electrodes. Small electrodes have large impedances, often on the order of megohms. Hence the design of current generators and recording amplifiers that can operate reliably at frequencies in the 10-kHz range requires care. We currently employ amplifiers whose input impedances exceed 10^{15} ohms in parallel with 0.4 pF.

The coupling between current sources and recording amplifiers must be small, <1 pF in some cases (Geisler et al., 1977) and even less in others (<0.5 pF; Spelman, unpublished results). In the former case, measurements were based on a lumped-element model; in the latter, they were based on a distributed model, which required small, battery-powered current generators whose signal generators were built on the same circuit board. Shielded transformers did not provide sufficient decoupling between the input and the output circuitries.

Theoretical Problems

In the two sections above, measurements of tissue impedance using lumped-element models and distributed models were discussed together. This section cites the differences between the two techniques and illustrates potential problems that can arise with each.

Measurements of tissue impedance and the models that are used to interpret the measurements are shown schematically in Figures 4.2 and 4.3. Figure 4.2 illustrates a lumped-element model which consists of a single element. If current is applied to a volume of tissue, and if voltage is measured at two points near the current sources, an estimate of an impedance can be made using Ohm's law. Figure 4.3 illustrates a more complicated, three-element model. If current is applied at each pair of

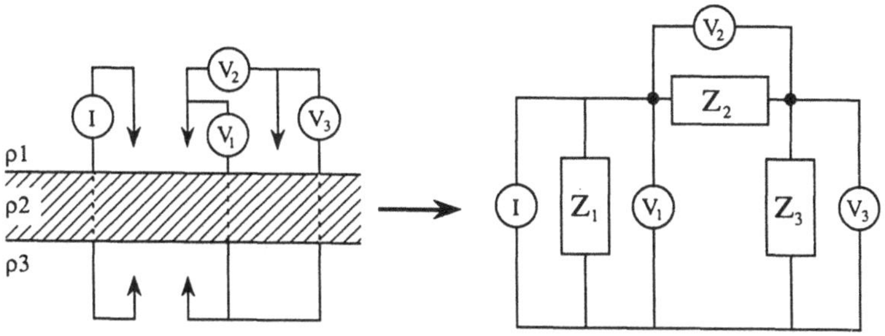

FIGURE 4.3. Lumped-element model used to estimate three impedances. In this case, two media are separated by a third. All have different resistivities.

terminals and voltage is measured at the other pairs, the impedances of the model can be determined. This is the technique that has been used commonly to measure the electrical properties of the inner ear (Geisler et al., 1977; Johnstone, Johnstone, and Pugsley, 1966; Spelman, Clopton, and Pfingst, 1982).

The primary difficulty with this approach to measurement lies in its geometrical interpretation. Measurements of the impedances are influenced by the separation between electrode pairs, the separation between current sources and voltage sensors, and the proximity of the arrays to tissue boundaries. Asakuma, Snow, and Murakami (1978) discussed the effects of electrode separation on impedance measurement, obtaining a series of measurements with electrodes placed across the cochlear partition of the guinea pig. They found that electrode separation had a direct influence on their estimates of resistance in the membranous tissues of the partition in the first turn of the cochlea. As they varied the distance between their voltage-sensing electrodes from 200 to 1000 μm, potential difference and estimated impedance decreased by a factor of 2.

The effects of the distance between electrodes and tissues can be shown with a simple model. Figure 4.4 shows a medium composed of three conducting layers of resistivities, ρ_1, ρ_2, and ρ_3. A current source I_0 is placed at $r=0$, $z=-z_0$, with voltage sensors placed at $r=r_1$, $z=-z_1$ and at $r=r_2$, $z=z_2$. The current source produces an infinite number of images whose positions are functions of the location of the source and the medium in which observations are made. The drawing shows the images for the measurement in medium 1, in which $z<0$.

The general case of the three-layer medium is reduced to the specific case shown in Figure 4.5. The resistivities of the first and third media are equal, 70 ohm-cm, while that of the intervening medium is set to 1000 ohm-cm. The middle medium has a thickness of 70 μm. The current source lies at $r=0$ and has altitudes of -50 and -100 μm. The voltage sources are laced at 50 and 100 μm from their respective boundaries, and have positions that vary together from 100 to 200 μm from $r=0$, the

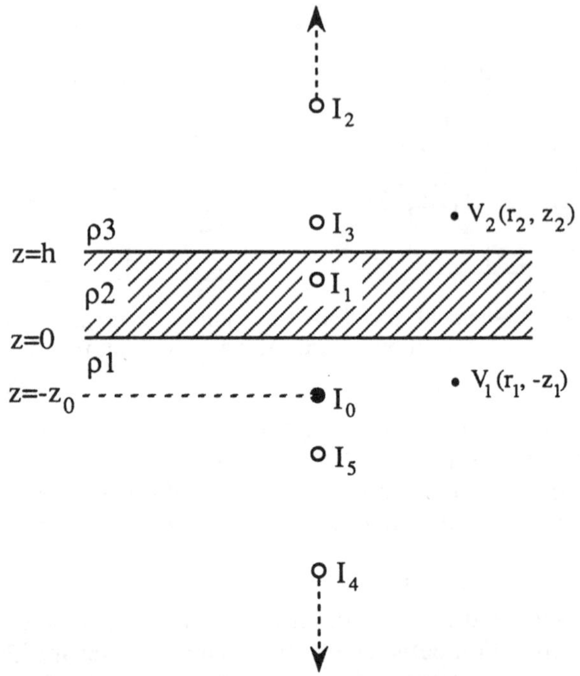

FIGURE 4.4. Current source in a three-layered volume conductor. Reflections of the source from the boundaries produce an infinite number of image sources whose intensities vary as functions of the resistivities of the media.

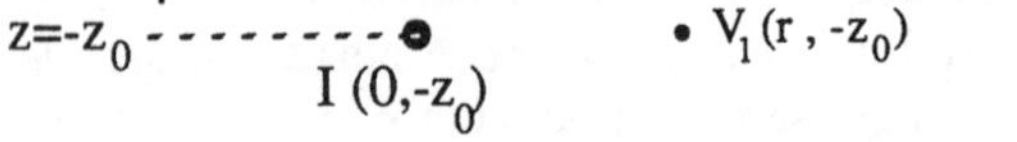

$I = 100\ \mu A$

$\rho 1 = \rho 3 = 70\ \Omega\text{-cm}$

$\rho 2 = 1000\ \Omega\text{-cm}$

$h = 70\ \mu m$

$z_0 = \begin{Bmatrix} 50 \\ 100 \end{Bmatrix}\ \mu m$

$100\ \mu m \leq r \leq 200\ \mu m$

$$R = (2/I)[V_1(r, -z_0) - V_2(r, h + z_0)]$$

FIGURE 4.5. Specific source and volume conductor: Dimensions and the current delivered are shown in the figure.

position of the current source. The current source has a magnitude of 100 μA. The choice of a symmetrical pair of media above and below the central medium simplifies the calculation of apparent resistance, which is

$$R=(2/I)[V_1(r,-z_0)-V_2(r,h+z_0)]$$

where

$$V_1(r,z) = \frac{I\rho_1\rho_2\rho_3}{2\pi(\rho_2+\rho_1)(\rho_3+\rho_2)}\left[\frac{1}{[r^2+(z+z_0)^2]^{1/2}} + \sum_{i=1}^{\infty}\left\{\frac{(-1)^{i+1}(\Gamma_{12}\Gamma_{23})^i}{[r^2+(z+z_0-2ih)^2]^{1/2}} + \frac{(-1)^{i+1}(\Gamma_{12}\Gamma_{23})^i}{[r^2+(z+z_0-2ih)^2]^{1/2}}\right\}\right]$$

$$V_2(r,z) = \frac{\rho_1 I}{4\pi}\left[\sum_{i=0}^{\infty}\Gamma_{23}{}^i\Gamma_{21}{}^i\left\{\frac{1}{[r^2+(z+2ih+z_0)^2]^{1/2}} + \frac{\Gamma_{12}}{[r^2+(z+2ih-z_0)^2]^{1/2}}\right\} + \sum_{j=1}^{\infty}\Gamma_{23}{}^j\Gamma_{21}{}^{j-1}\left\{\frac{1}{[r^2+(z-2jh+z_0)^2]^{1/2}} + \frac{\Gamma_{12}}{[r^2+(z-2jh-z_0)^2]^{1/2}}\right\}\right]$$

and

$$\Gamma_{12} = \frac{\rho_2-\rho_1}{\rho_2+\rho_1} = -\Gamma_{21}$$

$$\Gamma_{23} = \frac{\rho_3-\rho_2}{\rho_3+\rho_2} = -\Gamma_{32}$$

The values of r, h, z_0, ρ_1, ρ_2, ρ_3, and I are given in Figure 4.5.

The results of varying the altitude of the electrodes and the distance between the source and the measuring electrodes are shown in Figure 4.6. The apparent resistance decreases when the electrodes are closer to the middle medium, as it would in any medium in which constant current is applied to electrodes that are closer together. The apparent resistance decreases as well when the voltage-sensing electrodes are placed at greater distances from the current source. In this example, apparent resistance decreases by a factor of 2 as the distance varies from 100 to 200 μm.

The example above illustrates the importance of maintaining strict control over the placement of electrodes in living tissues when precise impedances are to be measured. That control is required whether lumped-element or distributed models are used to define the measurements.

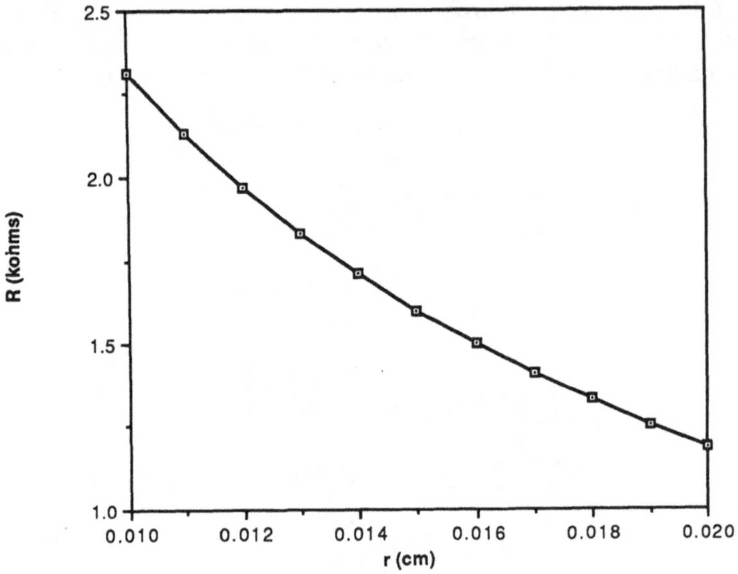

(a)

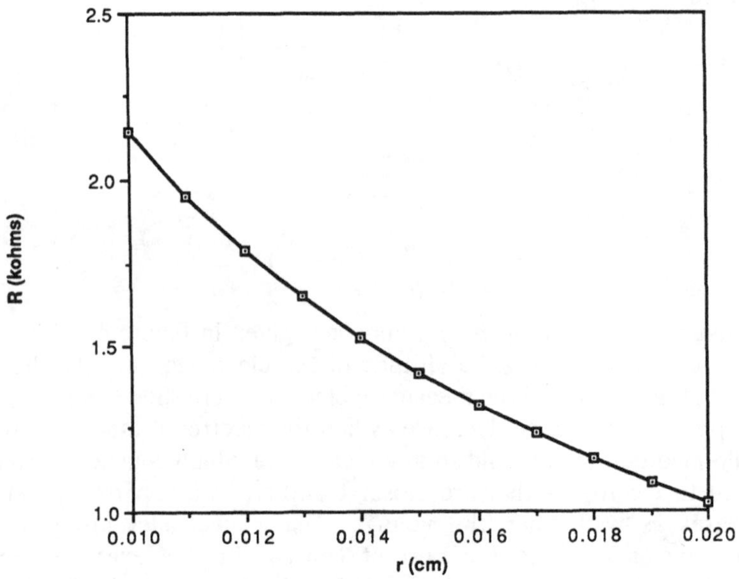

(b)

FIGURE 4.6. Effects of varying sample position. Apparent resistance is larger when the electrodes are further from the boundaries (*a*) and smaller when they are closer (*b*). Variation of the spacing between sample and source electrodes has profound effects on the apparent resistance.

A distributed model uses the theoretical ideas above to estimate tissue resistivity, real or complex, by using a four-electrode reflection-coefficient technique (Figure 4.7; Spelman, Clopton, and Suesserman, 1987). This technique employs a pair of electrodes to deliver current to the tissues of interest, and a pair to record potential. The array is advanced through one tissue to its boundary with a second tissue. Potential varies as a function of distance from the boundary and the resistivities of the two tissues (Spelman, Clopton, and Suesserman, 1987). The technique is analogous to that used to define the electrical impedance of an antenna with a slotted transmission line (Terman, 1955). Ideally, one could estimate resistivity of a two-layered medium with two measurements, one far from the boundary and one at the boundary. Practically, one must make a series of position-dependent measurements to define the shape of the potential curve and, from the shape, to estimate the composition of the tissues and the angle of approach to the boundary (Spelman, unpublished results). Estimates of the position of each electrode are critical to the technique, since it requires measurements of potential difference that are accurate to 1%. Figure 4.8 shows a theoretical curve and the measured potential-distance curve for an array that was driven until it contacted a glass plate.

The reflection coefficient technique can be applied to media with planar or curved boundaries and to multilayered media as well as to media with single boundaries. At this time, the tissues of the ear have been assumed to be planar and thick with respect to electrode spacing. Those assumptions are valid if the radii of tissue curvatures and the thicknesses of the tissue layers are at least five times greater than the distances between electrodes.

The position of electrode arrays is important, as is the character of the underlying tissues. In the example above, the model is composed of discrete, isotropic layers. Biological tissues may have boundaries whose resistivities vary continuously. The tissues may be antisotropic (Singh

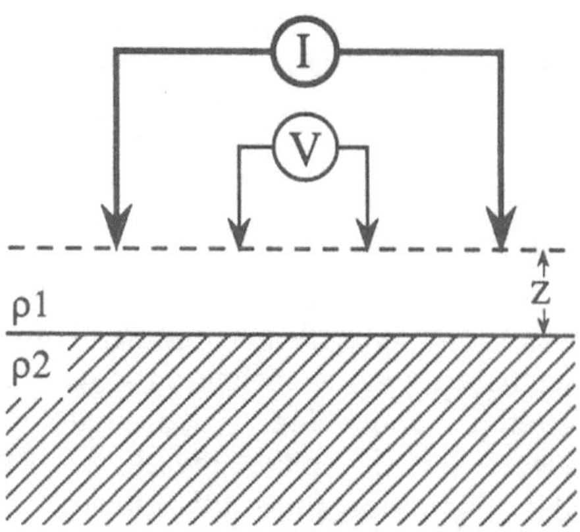

FIGURE 4.7. Reflection coefficent method: A schematic representation of the electrodes in a two-layered medium. Potential varies as the distance z is varied.

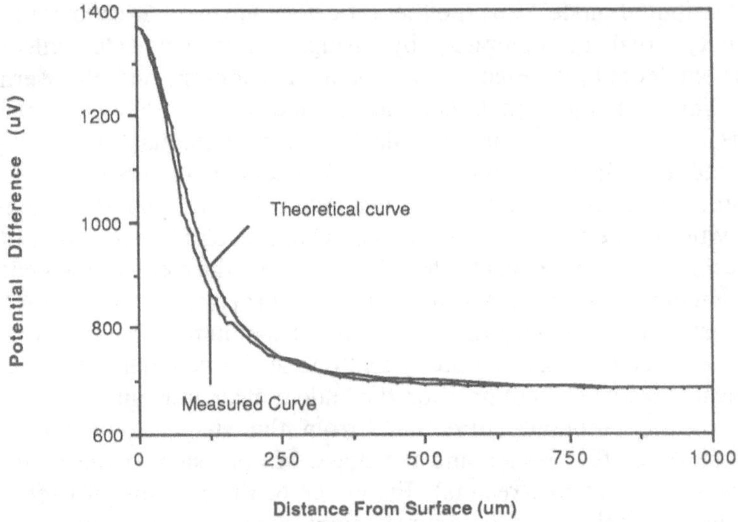

FIGURE 4.8. Reflection coefficient method: Theory and measurement for a four-electrode array moved through normal saline until it touches a glass surface.

and Saha, 1984). The model above consists of parallel boundaries; cochlear tissues are neither planar nor parallel. Clearly, the theoretical underpinnings of impedance measurements must account for these variations.

Future Measurements

Estimates of Distributed Properties

Future measurements of tissue impedance will account for the difficulties cited above. Briefly, measurements must include independent, precise measurements of electrode locations; knowledge of the quantitative anatomy of the inner ear; careful mechanical and electronic design of the measurement apparatus; and a theoretical basis of measurement that accounts for the anatomy, chemistry, and physiology of the tissues.

Electrode Location and Anatomy of the Inner Ear

Electrode location and quantitative anatomy are directly coupled to precise impedance measurement. In a series of studies in the guinea pig, we have begun to measure the quantitative anatomy of the cochlea in an attempt to develop a coordinate system within which to locate our electrodes. In the first measurements we used the classical technique of determining anatomy quantitatively from serial sections of the tissues

(Santos, Spelman, and Sutton, 1987). More recently we developed a technique that eliminates the need for serial sections. Figure 4.9 shows an image obtained from a cochlea whose bony capsule was rendered clear by soaking it in Spalteholtz fluid and staining it with procion blue dye (Haq, 1988). A cochlea prepared in this way can be mounted in a precise rotator, illuminated, and imaged as a series of sections through the modiolar axis rotated at different angles. With this technique, one can, for example, rotate the cochlea about the centerline of the basilar membrane and thereby obtain data that are more detailed and less noisy than those obtained with the classical technique (Figure 4.10).

Data thus obtained can be used to model the locus of points that defines a particular structure, and to define the locus in three-dimensional space (Arts, Soma, and Spelman, 1988). The model consists of a series of three-dimensional spirals constructed of Fresnel integrals. Those integrals were fit after noting that (*a*) no defined "cochlear axis" can be found for real ears and (*b*) curvature varies as a function of distance along the cochlear spiral. The technique fits the cochlear spiral without the hook region. To define the cochlear geometry completely, it will be necessary to include the hook region. Figure 4.11*a* shows the fit of the model to the cochlear spiral for two Cartesian coordinates as a function of the arc length of the centerline of the basilar membrane; Figure 4.11*b* shows the fit of the model to the data in three dimensions.

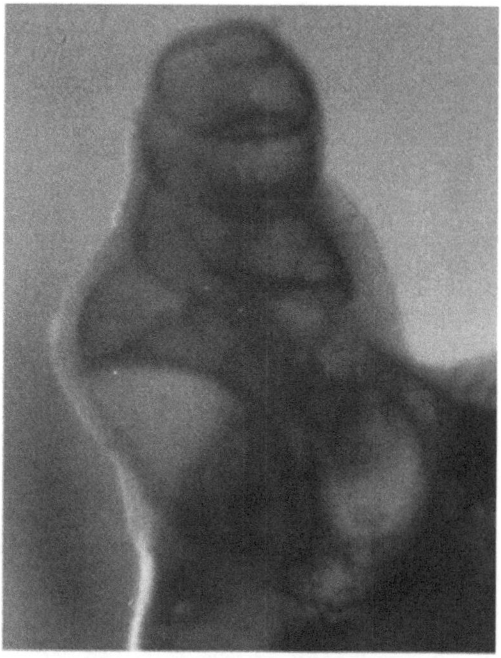

FIGURE 4.9. An entire cochlea stained with procion blue and rendered translucent in Spalteholtz fluid; magnification 25×.

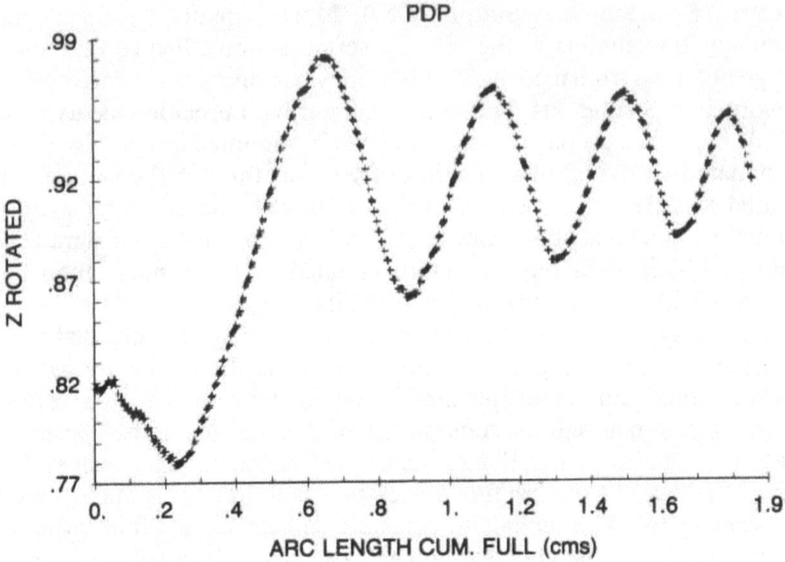

(a) + Z ROTATED

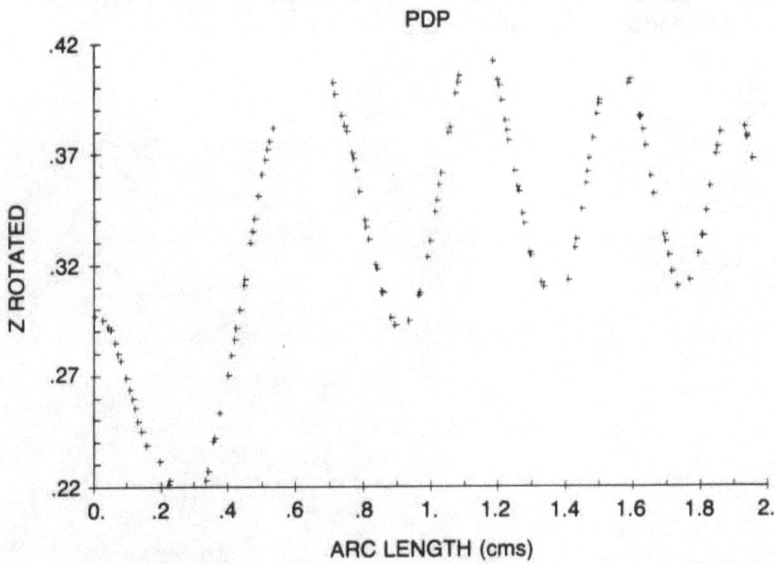

(b) + Z ROTATED

FIGURE 4.10. Data obtained from a single cochlea with (*a*) the imaging technique (Haq, 1988) and (*b*) the classical sectioning technique.

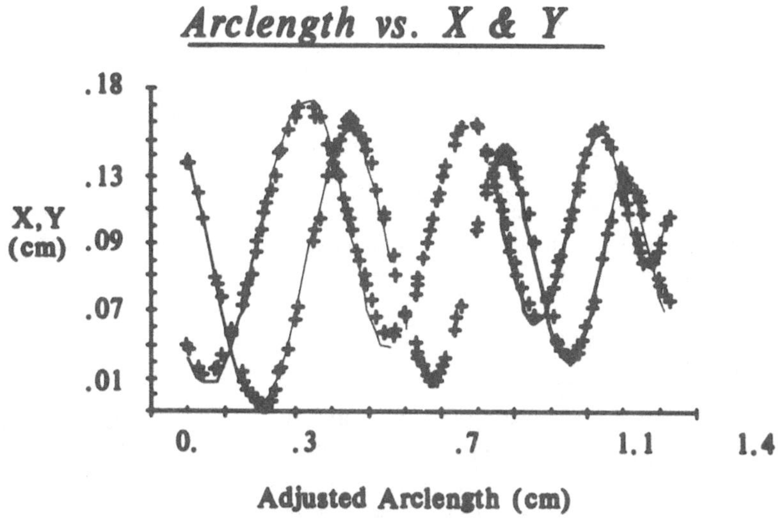

(a)

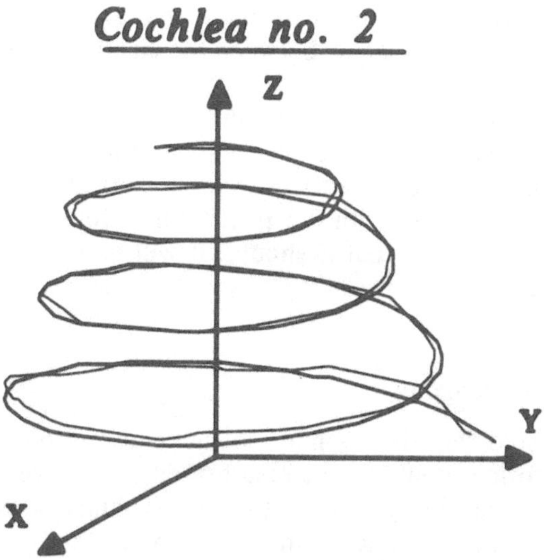

(b)

FIGURE 4.11. Three-dimensional model of the basilar membrane produced with Fresnel integrals. The upper image (*a*) shows two dimensions as functions of arc length; the dots are the data, and the lines are the model. The lower image (*b*) shows the cochlear spiral in three dimensions.

Given a defined geometry and coordinate system, one must determine the exact position of the electrode within the coordinates. We are working on two techniques: well-defined stereotaxy, in which position is known within a volume 4 μm on a side, and a means by which we can detect contact with cochlear tissues by the electrode array. Determining contact is difficult, but we think it will be possible to measure the point at which the array contacts the tissues by using a force transducer that is sensitive to 0.1 gm and whose deflection at that force is 0.1 μm. We are currently testing such a transducer.

Instrument Design

Instrument design consists of a current generator, voltage monitor, electrode array, and micromanipulator to move the array through space. The characteristics of the generator and the micromanipulator were discussed in foregoing sections. The electrode array and its voltage monitor are worthy of mention here. The array should be both precise and small, suggesting the use of microcircuit fabrication. We are currently having such arrays manufactured and will test three types: two end-fire arrays (Figure 4.12, upper) and one planar rectangular broadside array (Figure 4.12, lower). The spacing between the electrodes in the upper part of the figure is 10 μm.

Electrodes as small as those in Figure 4.12 require that the current source and recording amplifier be designed carefully. We are now having a monolithic amplifier fabricated whose input impedance will be greater than 10^{15} ohms in parallel with 0.2 pF. If this circuit works as well as computer models indicate that it should, it will be used with the arrays shown in Figure 4.12.

Theoretical Improvements

Earlier I suggested that tissues may not have abrupt boundaries nor be isotropic. The former could be the result of diffusion layers which bound the margins between bony tissues and scalar fluids or between scalar fluids and membranes (Goodisman, 1987). Singh and Saha (1984) described anisotropy in bone in their review about the impedance of bone. The theory underlying the reflection coefficient technique will have to be modified to account for those complications. Techniques have been suggested in the geophysical literature to analyze media with continuously varying resistivity and anisotropic resistivity (Wait, 1982). Bioengineers have already described methods to measure anisotropic tissues in the heart (Plonsey and Barr, 1982).

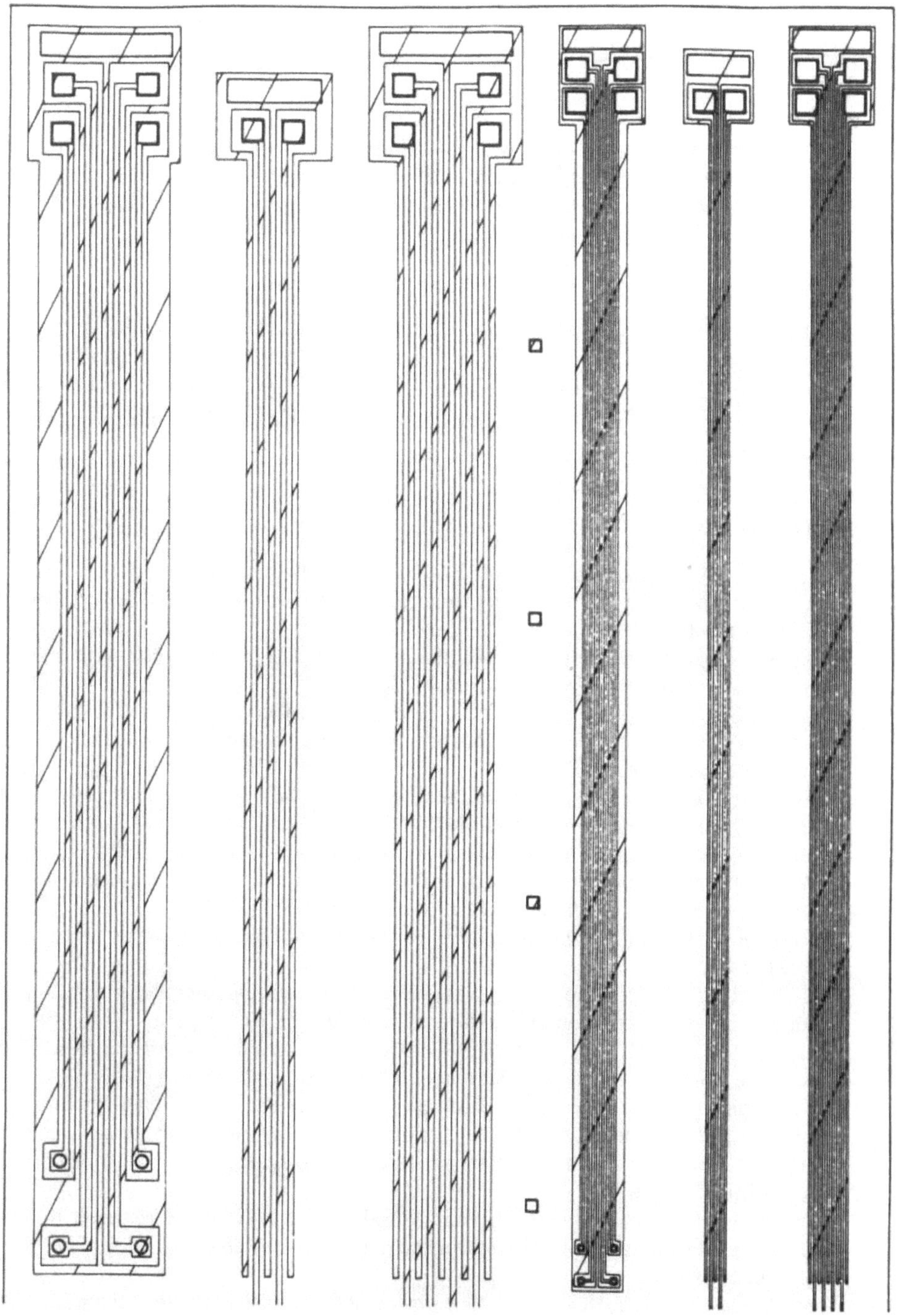

FIGURE 4.12. Masks for monolithic electrode arrays to be used to measure resistivities in the cochlea. The small lines are 10 μm apart.

Conclusion

Measurement of the electrical properties of cochlear tissues is challenging both theoretically and practically. It requires a clear definition of anatomy of the tissues and the boundaries between tissues, and an understanding of the physical properties of the tissues and of the measurement system. Care spent in defining and understanding the problem should yield data that will advance basic understanding of cochlear physiology and lead to improvement of cochlear implants.

Acknowledgments. This work was supported by NIH Grants RR00166, NS21440, and NS23930, and by a grant from the Deafness Research Foundation. The work of Michael Suesserman, Perry Santos, Alex Arts, and Nadeem Haq is gratefully acknowledged. Kate Elias edited the manuscript.

References

Arts, H.A., Soma, M., and Spelman, F.A. (1988). A mathematical model of the cochlear spiral in three dimensions. Abstracts of the 11th Midwinter Research Meeting, Abstr. 206.

Asakuma, S., Snow, J.B., Jr., and Murakami, Y. (1978). Electrical resistance of the cochlear partition. *Hearing Res*. 1:25–30.

Brummer, S.B., and Turner, J.J. (1977). Electrochemical considerations for safe electrical stimulations of the nervous system with platinum electrodes. *IEEE Trans. Biomed. Eng*. BME24:59–68.

Davis, H. (1965). A model for transducer action in the cochlea. *Cold Spring Harbor Symp. Quant. Biol*. 30:181–195.

Geisler, C.D., Mountain, D.C., Hubbard, A.E., Adrian, H.O., and Ravindran, A. (1977). Alternating electrical-resistance changes in the guinea-pig cochlea caused by acoustic stimuli. *J. Acoust. Soc. Am*. 61:1557–1566.

Goodisman, J. (1987). *Electrochemistry: Theoretical Foundations* (Wiley, New York), 1987.

Haq, N. (1988). Application and evaluation of an imaging technique for 3-dimensional reconstruction. M.S. thesis, University of Washington.

Honrubia, V., Strelioff, D., and Sitko, S. (1976). Electroanatomy of the cochlea: Its role in cochlear potential measurements. In *Electrocochleography*, edited by R.J. Ruben, C. Eberling, and G. Salomon (University Park Press, Baltimore).

Ifukube, T., and White, R.L. (1987). Current distributions produced inside and outside the cochlea from a scala tympani electrode array. *IEEE Trans. Biomed. Eng*. BME34:876–890.

Johnstone, B.M., Johnstone, J.R., and Pugsley, I.D. (1966). Resistance in endolymphatic walls of the first turn of the guinea pig cochlea. *J. Acoust. Soc. Am*. 40:1398–1404.

Plonsey, R., and Barr, R. (1982). The four-electrode resistivity technique as applied to cardiac muscle. *IEEE Trans. Biomed. Eng*. BME29:541–546.

Rubinstein, J.T., Spelman, F.A., Soma, M., and Suesserman, M.F. (1987). Current density profiles of surface mounted and recessed electrodes for neural prostheses. *IEEE Trans. Biomed. Eng.* BME34:864–875.

Santos, P.M., Spelman, F.A., and Sutton, D. (1987). A computer-assisted method to determine cochlear spiral differential geometry. *Head Neck Surg.* 97:164.

Singh, S., and Saha, S. (1984). Electrical properties of bone, A review. *Clin. Orthop.* 186:249–271.

Spelman, F.A., Clopton, B.M., and Pfingst, B.E. (1982). Tissue impedance and current flow in the implanted ear: Implications for the cochlear prosthesis. *Ann. Otol. Rhinol. Laryngol. Suppl.* 98, 91:3–8.

Spelman, F.A., Clopton, B.M., and Suesserman, M.F. (1987). Measurements of the resistivity of bony tissues of the cochlea. *Proceedings of the 9th Annual Conference IEEE EMBS,* pp 191–192.

Suesserman, M.F. (1988). Lumped parameter models for simulating the electrical properties of in vivo cochlear stimulation. M.S. thesis, University of Washington.

Terman, F.E. (1955). *Electronic and Radio Engineering* (McGraw-Hill, New York).

Wait, J.R. (1982). *Geo-electromagnetism* (Academic Press, New York).

Francis A. Spelman: Discussion

Dr. Eddington: The carriers of those electrodes have a substantial mass that is very close to the electrodes. How does that affect your model? It looks as if your conceptual model has two very tiny electrodes in an infinite space. There are large amounts of carriers very close to those electrodes.

Dr. Spelman: Unless there is a substantial part of the conductor which is exposed, the data seem to fit the theoretical model very well. This holds as long as the conductors are less than one-fifth that of the spacing. Now that's going to be a problem with the monolithic electrodes, and what we intend to do there, to overcome the problem, is a series of calibrations. The calibrations that we can do are, obviously, simple. One can run the electrode up against an insulator, or one can run the electrode up against a good conductor like a silver, silver chloride electrode, and get reasonable estimates of the boundary limits. We also are using intermediate calibration standards, e.g., blocks of alumina oxide. Alumina oxide has a resistivity of about 300 ohm-cm and can be used as a calibration standard as well, so we should be able to develop calibration curves for each electrode array as we use it.

Dr. Eddington: Are those calibration curves a function of the geometry of the surface you're trying to measure?

Dr. Spelman: Yes, they certainly are.

Dr. Eddington: Your model assumes a really large, flat surface, but you are applying it to a very small curve, a radial structure. What's the likelihood that the calibration in terms of the flat surface will be incorrect?

Dr. Spelman: Well, once again, as long as the radii of curvature are greater than about five times the dimensions of the electrode array, we can assume that we are dealing with a planar structure, and that's the kind of measurement that we will make at first. We will also look at molded calibration standards. Those are easy to obtain in insulators and get in conductors. They'll be much more difficult to obtain in material like alumina oxide.

Dr. Finley: Your descriptions of the reflection model predict a homogeneous structure. I was hoping you would address also the heterogeneous nature of the cochlea, particularly in regard to the perforated region of the osseous spiral lamina. I wonder if you would also address some of the issues about in vivo versus in vitro measurement techniques and Ifukube's work.

Dr. Spelman: The first issues I'm going to sidestep and say that we have not modeled heterogeneous media, media with pockets or with holes in them. One of my students right now has the task to determine the heterogeneity of the material. Once we get detailed information about that, we're going to try to model it. That's at least 2 or 3 years away, because that's not going to be a simple modeling task for us.

But in regard to the Ifukube and White data, I had some concerns. There were a number of technical details omitted from the paper. Their impedance values would suggest that the bony tissues of the cochlea have very high resistivities. One of the problems with that is that they were using fixed bone, and when one fixes the tissue, the resistivity changes. It increases, and so I'm not sure that those in vitro measurements are representative, other than in a most general way, of the characteristics of living bone.

Dr. Josef Miller: In looking at the tissue that you showed us, it looked as though one could see a lot more details than just the curvature of the osseous spiral lamina that you report. Can you see it well enough to take depth measurements of the structures in the cochlea? Can you see through it enough to see whether you have pathological tissue? Whether there are myelinated nerve fibers running in the osseous spiral lamina? Are details like that available?

Dr. Spelman: I can't answer that directly. I can say we certainly can see the hair cells, and we certainly can see spiral ganglion cells. Whether the technique is going to preserve the myelin, I can't say for certain. I have a student using a technique called fluorescence microtomography, and what we have developed is an ultraviolet beam which is 40 μm thick—it's a fan beam—and we have fluorescently dyed the tissue so that we can basically take a slice through at the level of our axis of rotation; then we rotate the cochlea known amounts, and we can get the dimensions of the bony tissues fairly precisely. Going back to Charlie's question, we're also developing a confocal microscope, and we're using that to look at the fine structure of the bone. We should be able to get submicron resolution with that, so we should be able to say something about the random nature of the bone.

5
Models of Neural Responsiveness to Electrical Stimulation

CHARLES C. FINLEY, BLAKE S. WILSON, AND MARK W. WHITE

Introduction

In principle, electrical stimulation of the cochlea is a simple process. Intracochlear electrodes, when stimulated, create electrical field patterns within the cochlea. In the vicinity of the neural elements, these fields appear as extracellular voltage gradients or profiles that are continuous along the entire length of the neurons. These extracellular voltage fields produce current flow into and out of the neural elements depending on the local impedances of the neural membranes. If the neural elements are sufficiently depolarized, action potentials are generated that propagate along each cell's axon to the cochlear nucleus. Globally these events occur simultaneously, but in varying degree, across a population of nerve cells, producing a group or ensemble of neural responses to the stimulation.

In practice, however, the details of the stimulation process are governed by a number of complex physical, anatomical, and physiological factors. These include the configuration and placement of electrodes; the type, shape, and magnitude of the stimulus waveform; the impedance of the cochlear tissue; the location and fine-detailed anatomy of surviving neural elements; and the deterministic and stochastic characteristics of stimulated neural membranes. There is evidence that each of these factors plays a significant role in determining both the specific response properties of neural elements individually and the global characteristics of the neural ensemble response in general. At present the specific details of these mechanisms are not well understood.

This paper describes an *integrated field-neuron model* that combines all aspects of the interface problem into a single structure. The model predicts, assuming a given electrode configuration, the extracellular electrical field patterns in the vicinity of the target neural elements and then computes the resultant response from the fibers. The integrated field-neuron model is composed of two complementary models that treat each step of the stimulation process separately. The first model describes the extracellular fields for scala tympani electrode configurations of arbitrary geometry and scalar placement using three-dimensional finite-element modeling techniques. The extracellular field estimates are then fed to a lumped-element, electrical-analog, neural response model that describes the response of a single fiber to external electrical stimulation. Two neural models are discussed. One is an estimator of the initial site of stimulation based on the second spatial derivative of the extracellular fields. This model assumes a uniform myelinated fiber lying in the electrical field. The other is a lumped-element, electrical-analog model that addresses specific anatomical and physiological features of the neurons that significantly affect the elements' responsiveness to external electrical fields.

The objective of the integrated field-neuron modeling approach is to better define the events and controlling factors involved in the interface between the electrode and neural elements and to create testable hypotheses that may be further evaluated in human and animal experimentation. In the following sections, the field and neural models are discussed separately. First, finite-element field calculations for several experimentally and clinically applied bipolar electrode systems are presented. Then initial stimulation sites for myelinated neurons are estimated using second spatial derivatives for each computed electrical field condition. Next an expanded, anatomically and physiologically based neural model is used to show the significance of the ganglion cell body in electrical stimulation. Finally, the limitations of these models are discussed, and future model refinements are outlined.

Three-Dimensional Finite-Element Field Model

A variety of electrical field models has been proposed for the electrically stimulated cochlea. These models include lumped-element transmission-line models (Békésy, 1951; Black and Clark, 1980; Cannon, 1976; Honrubia, Strelioff, and Sitko, 1974; Johnstone, Johnstone, and Pugsley, 1966; Misrahy et al., 1958; Sitko, 1976; Strelioff, 1973), closed-form analytical models (Rubinstein, Soma, and Spelman; Soma, Spelman, and Rubinstein, 1984), and numerical finite-difference models (Grizon, 1987; Wilson and Finley, 1984). To further our understanding of the electrical-to-neural interface problem involved in the electrically stimulated cochlea, a field model must describe the electrical stimulus in the immediate vicinity of the target neural fibers. Most models have focused primarily on describing potential patterns within scala tympani. Existing field models are limited in their abilities to account for fine details of cochlear anatomy and electrode structure. The analytical approach must assume simplifying geometries to obtain closed-form solutions, and the finite-difference method is limited in spatial resolution for reasonable problem size. This paper describes the use of a three-dimensional, finite-element model of intracochlear electrical fields that alleviates these limitations. A two-dimensional version of this model has been published previously (Finley, Wilson, and White, 1987).

The present model assumes that impedances within the cochlea are purely resistive. This assumption is based on the experimental finding that measured scala tympani field potentials are frequency-independent for frequencies below 12.5 kHz (Spelman, Clopton, and Pfingst, 1982). This assumption allows the field calculation to be treated as a static field problem. Simple scaling of electrode input potentials produces appropriately scaled field estimates. Time-varying stimuli also may be evaluated readily without consideration of capacitive, charge-storage effects of tissue. The assumption of a purely resistive system for the present model should be considered as a first approximation only. The cited experimental work on field frequency dependence applies only to fields within scala tympani. Still open is the question of frequency dependence of fields in other parts of the cochlea, in particular in the habenula and along tracts containing myelinated axonal processes. Similarly, significant capacitive effects may appear in the case of cross-turn stimulation due to the myelinated neural fibers filling the core of the modiolus. Consideration of capacitive effects is left to later refinements of the model.

In its simplest form, the finite-element approach is a piecewise approximation method in which the field region to be modeled is divided into small discrete elements. Here solid elements are used, with each element being defined by the interconnection of six or eight vertices or nodes. Any one node may define the corner of any number of elements. Potentials within each element are described by planar functions based on the potentials at the element's nodes. Boundary potentials for each side of an element are interpolations of the potentials at the nodes which define each side. Regional resistivities are defined for each element, and node potentials either are fixed to preset values or are allowed to vary freely. Iterative minimization of the energy in each element of the model system produces a field description based on the final potentials at the nodes. The general finite-element method as applied to biological problems has been reviewed recently (Miller and Henriquez, 1988). Coburn (1980) applied the technique to study two-dimensional field patterns during electrical stimulation of the spinal cord.

Figure 5.1 shows a two-dimensional, finite-element description of the cross section of a human cochlea. A bipolar electrode pair is mounted in a support insulator within scala tympani. Figure 5.1*a* shows a drawing of the histological section represented in the model shown in Figure 5.1*b*. This two-dimensional plane contains 152 nodes and 204 triangular and quadrilateral element profiles. Note that elements are smaller and more numerous in the central region of the plane, thus increasing the spatial resolution of the model in that area. This plane is then expanded into a

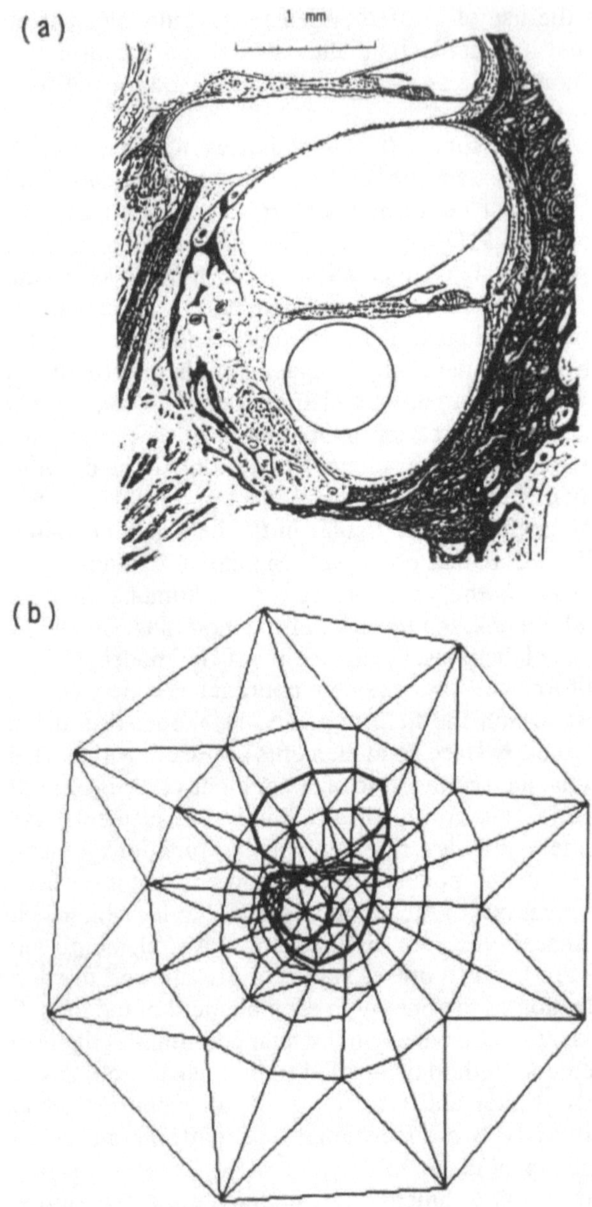

FIGURE 5.1. Two-dimensional, finite-element description of a cross section of a human cochlea. Panel (*a*) (reproduced with permission from Pernkopf [1960]) shows a drawing of the histological section from Ranck (1975) that is modeled in panel (*b*). A bipolar electrode pair mounted in a support insulator is included in the finite-element model representation. Note the higher spatial resolution in the central region of the cross section.

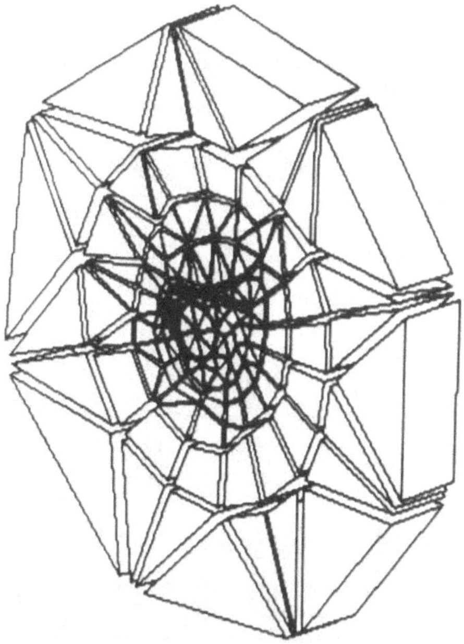

FIGURE 5.2. Single three-dimensional, finite-element model layer of the cross section of Figure 5.1. Each element is shown in its original position but shrunk 15% geometrically to emphasize the element structure.

three-dimensional layer, shown in Figure 5.2, by replicating the original node positions in a plane parallel to the original. A layer or slab consisting of five-sided prisms and six-sided solids is produced by defining three-dimensional elements that bridge these planes of nodes. Figure 5.3 shows an enlarged view of the scala region of the layer of Figure 5.2, with each element located in its original position in the layer but shrunk 10% geometrically. Here discrete anatomical regions that are modeled with different electrical resistivities are observable.

The model is further expanded by adding multiple parallel layers of varying thicknesses. Twelve layers constitute the final model as shown in Figure 5.4. This three-dimensional model represents a short straight section of the cochlear cross section projected linearly along an axis perpendicular to the plane of the section. No curvature of the cochlear spiral is modeled. Layer thicknesses, described in Figure 5.5, are graded to provide maximal spatial resolution in the center of the model.

Resistivities are defined regionally to characterize the electrodes, the carrier insulator, the endolymph, the perilymph, Reisner's membrane, the basilar membrane, the anisotropic neural tissue leading down from the habenula to the spiral ganglion, the spiral ganglion itself, and bone. Table 5.1 describes the resistivities used in the model calculations presented in this paper. All regions are assumed to be isotropic with the exception of the tract of the peripheral axonal processes between the habenula and ganglion. Regions outside of the model are treated as insulators, thus allowing node potentials along the outer periphery to vary.

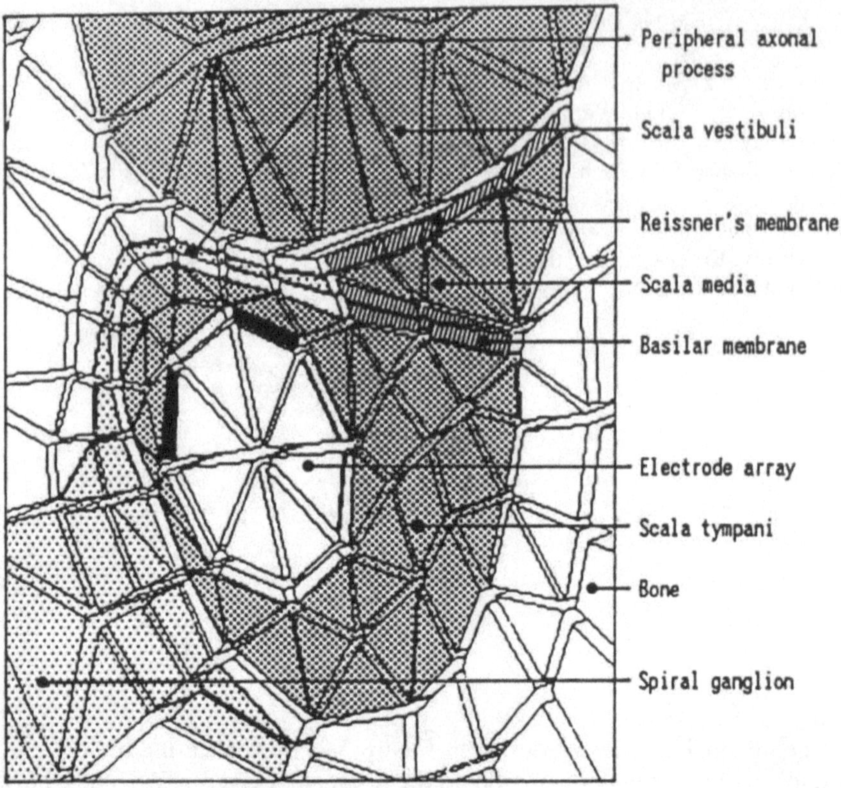

FIGURE 5.3. Enlarged view of the central region of the layer of Figure 5.2, showing the electrode array in scala tympani. Discrete anatomical regions with different resistivities are indicated. Table 5.1 summarizes the resistivities.

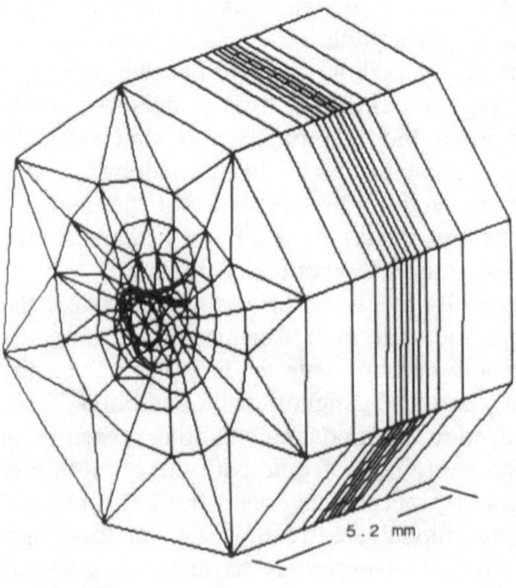

FIGURE 5.4. Full three-dimensional model of a straight section of the cochlea. Twelve layers, each similar to the layer shown in Figure 5.2 but differing in thickness, are assembled along a straight longitudinal axis. Note the higher spatial resolution in the center of the model denoted by smaller element sizes in the cross-sectional view and thinner layers centrally along the longitudinal axis. Figure 5.5 describes the layer thicknesses.

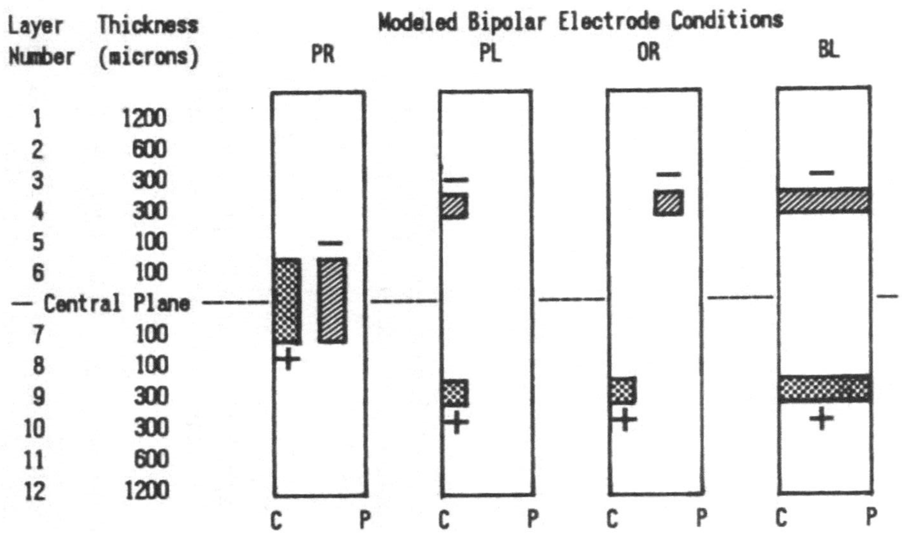

FIGURE 5.5. Layer thicknesses and electrode assignments for modeled bipolar electrode conditions. Pure radial (PR), pure longitudinal (PL), offset radial (OR), and banded longitudinal (BL) bipolar electrode configurations are shown as viewed looking down on the electrode assemblies from scala media. Polarity symbols (+ and −) indicate the assigned layers and relative element positions on the electrode insulator assemblies for the positive and negative electrode elements, respectively. Letters C and P beneath the electrode assembly outlines indicate the central and peripheral sides of the assemblies, respectively. Layer numbers and thicknesses in microns are indicated. Layer thicknesses are symmetrical about the central plane of the model.

TABLE 5.1. Regional resistivities for finite-element field model.

Region	Resistivity*
Insulator	10^9
Electrode	0.1
Perilymph	70
Endolymph	60
Bone	630†
Spiral ganglion	300
Peripheral axonal process	300 axial (anisotropic) 1,500 transverse
Reisner's membrane	60,480 (27 kOhm/mm SV to SM)‡
Basilar membrane	1,800 (2 kOhm/mm SM to ST)‡

* All resistivities are in ohm-cm and are assumed to be isotropic unless otherwise noted.
† Based on Spelman and Clopton, 1987.
‡ Resistivity selection based on membrane thickness of FE model to provide intercompartmental resistivities between scala media (SM), scala vestibuli (SV), and scala tympani (ST) as measured by Strelioff, 1973.

The modeling of specific electrode geometries requires slight modifications of the detailed element structure within scala tympani. Figure 5.6*a* shows the electrode array assembly as it would appear if removed from scala tympani. In cross section the electrode array shows an octagonally shaped core of eight prism elements arranged about a central axis. This central core is specified to be an insulator in all conditions. The outer planes of the prisms are capped with thin, solid, platelike elements that form the outer surface of the electrode assembly. An electrode configuration is specified by setting resistivities of these surface plate elements to be either insulators or electrode conductors. Node potentials at nodes bordering the conductive electrode surfaces are fixed arbitrarily at +100 or −100 mv prior to computation.

Figures 5.6*b* through 5.6*e* illustrate the selection of surface elements for four different electrode configurations. All views are drawn as if looking toward the right from the modiolus into scala tympani. Figure 5.6*b* and 5.6*c* represent pure radial bipolar and pure longitudinal bipolar electrode configurations, respectively. Figure 5.6*d* is an offset radial configuration that represents the bipolar configuration implemented in the University of California at San Francisco (UCSF) electrode array (Loeb et al., 1983). Figure 5.6*e* shows a banded longitudinal bipolar configuration that represents the adjacent band configuration of the University of Melbourne electrode array (Patrick et al., 1985). Note that the surface elements selected for the electrodes of the banded longitudinal configuration are selected around the full circumference of the core insulator. The

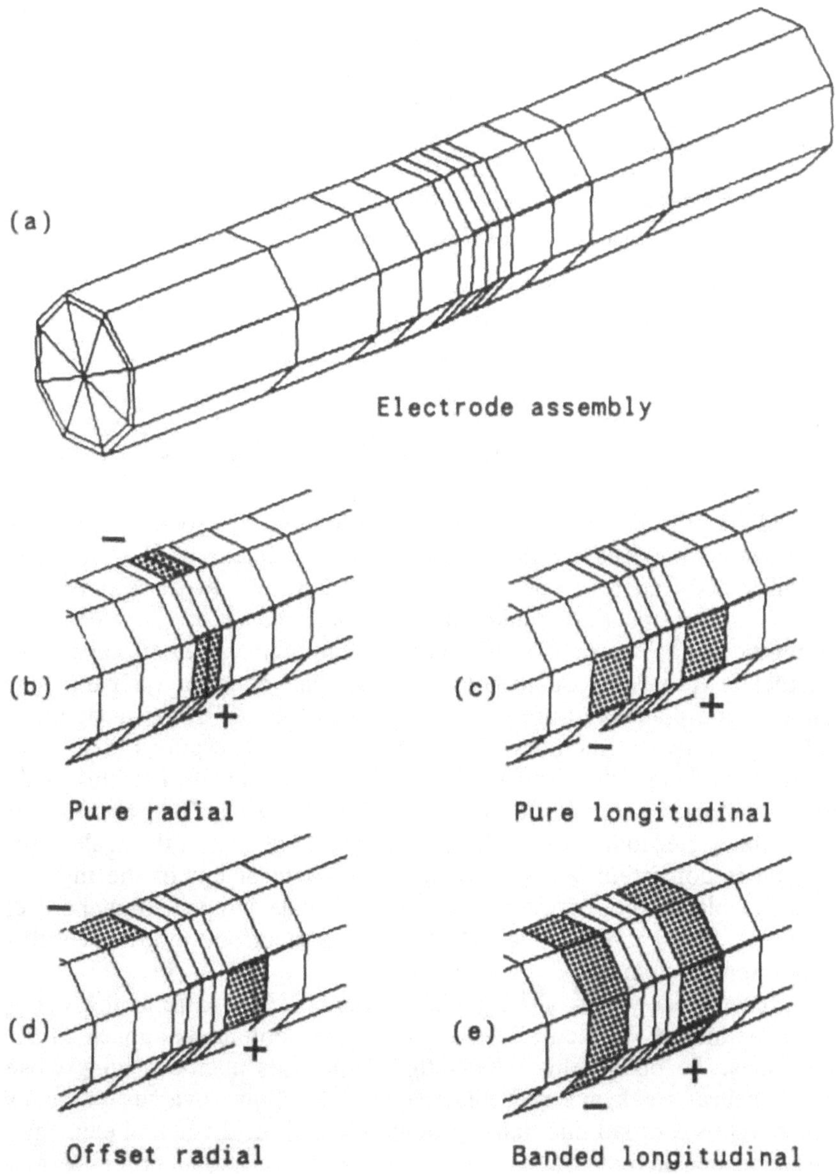

FIGURE 5.6. Finite-element model of scala tympani electrode assembly. Panel (*a*) shows the electrode carrier insulator removed from full model of Figure 5.4. Panels (*b*), (*c*), (*d*), and (*e*) indicate the element selection and polarity conventions used for the pure radial, pure longitudinal, offset radial, and banded longitudinal bipolar electrode configurations, respectively. Table 5.2 summarizes the dimensions of these configurations.

TABLE 5.2. Electrode-pair dimensions for pure radial (PR), pure longitudial (PL), offset radial (OR), and banded longitudinal (BL) configurations.

	Modeled bipolar electrode conditons			
	PR	PL	OR	BL
Single-electrode width, μm	200	300	300	300
Electrode carrier diameter, μm*	800	800	800	500
Interelectrode distance, μm†	604	700	924	700

* Electrode carrier diameters are the maximum diameters of the carrier cross sections shown in Figure 5.6.

† Interelectrode distance is measured between the centers of the electrodes along the surface of the electrode carrier.

electrode configurations and polarity assignments are summarized in Figures 5.5 and 5.6. Table 5.2 summarizes the electrode widths, electrode assembly diameter, and interelectrode distances.

In addition to the surface configuration of the electrode structure as described above, the diameter and scalar placement of the electrode assembly also must be specified. Figure 5.7 shows two scala tympani element structures that model different placements of the electrodes within the scala. Figure 5.7*a* shows an 800-μm-diameter electrode assembly that is located close to the modiolar wall of scala tympani. The diameter and placement are similar to that of the UCSF electrode array with its mechanical memory (Loeb et al., 1983). The pure radial, pure longitudinal, and offset radial bipolar electrode models use this scala tympani element configuration. Figure 5.7*b* shows a 500-μm-diameter electrode carrier that is located close to the lateral wall of the scala. This position is consistent with the diameter and placement of the thinner, more flexible Melbourne electrode array in scala tympani (Shepherd et al., 1985). The banded, longitudinal, bipolar electrode model uses this scala tympani element configuration.

The principal outputs of the model are the potential patterns that occur in the vicinity of the neural elements for fixed potentials applied to the electrodes. To obtain this information, potentials at nodes lying close to the neural track are reported. Figure 5.7 shows a locus of nodes connected by a broad line that lies along the path of the neural elements. This locus lies on the modiolar side of the peripheral axonal processes and extends from the center of the ganglion region to the habenula. The node locus extends beyond the habenula laterally across the basilar membrane into the bony lateral wall, as shown by the dotted line. Node potentials in this region provide insight into field patterns along the wall of scala tympani. This locus of nodes, as shown in Figure 5.7, is defined across all layers of the full three-dimensional model, thus forming a generalized locus resembling a curved *neural sheet*. The spatial dimensions of the neural sheet are thus *radial* (central to peripheral) along the axes of single

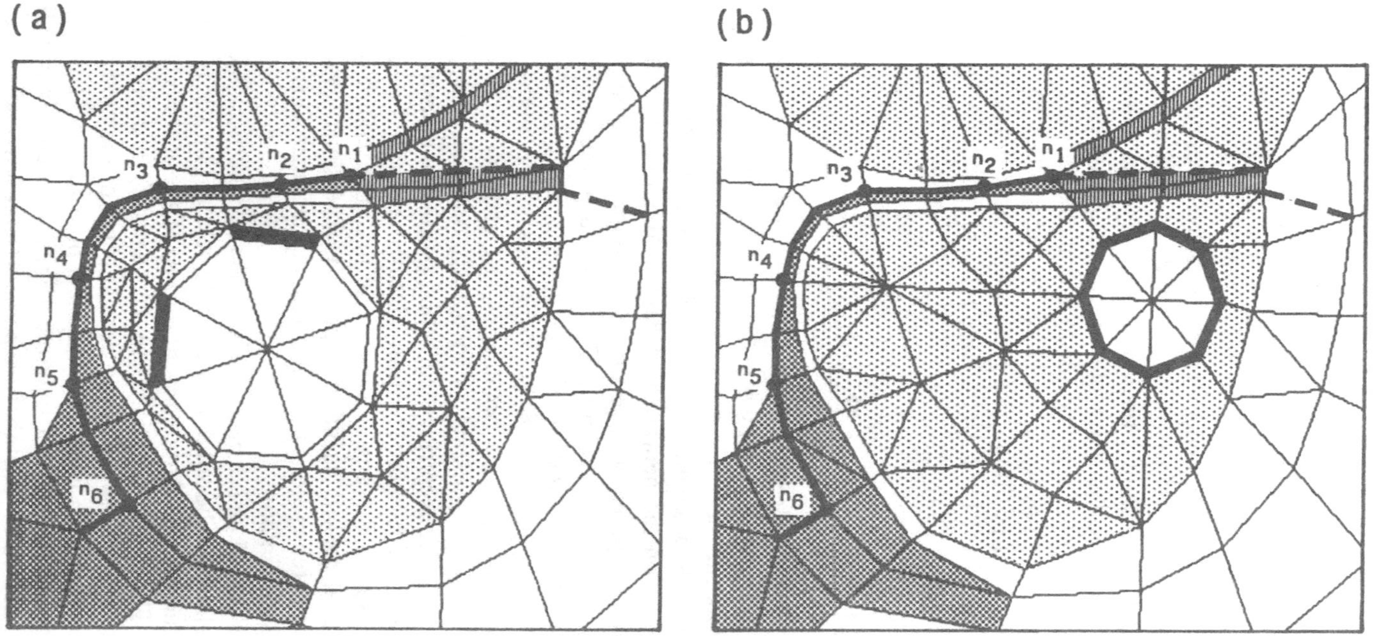

FIGURE 5.7. Detailed cross-sectional element structures for the electrode assembly in scala tympani. Panel (*a*) shows the elements used for the pure radial, pure longitudinal, and offset radial electrode configurations. Panel (*b*) shows the elements used for the banded longitudinal electrode configuration. The edge of the neural sheet locus is indicated by the broad line. Node positions n_1–n_6 are shown along this locus also. See text for full description.

individual fibers and *longitudinal* (basal to apical) across the ensemble of many fibers. Field potential estimates from the model are reported by flattening this neural sheet and examining potential distributions on its surface. Potentials along edges of elements are linear interpolations of the node potentials that define each edge. Three discrete representations are used to display the potential distribution on the neural sheet. First, isopotential contours are shown on a flattened representation of the neural sheet. Second, specific extracellular potential profiles along the radially oriented trajectory of selected single neural elements are graphed as a function of position along the fiber. Third, spread function plots show potentials at fixed radial positions along each fiber as a function of the longitudinal location of the fiber, to indicate relative rates of field decay away from the electrode pair.

Potential Field Calculation Results

Model predictions for the electrical field patterns of the pure radial bipolar electrode configuration are shown in Figure 5.8. This calculation is conducted assuming the electrode configuration of Figure 5.6*b* with the scala tympani electrode placement of Figure 5.7*a*. Figure 5.8*a* shows the isopotential contours on the neural sheet described above. Isopotential contours are drawn for potential levels at 5% increments (10 mv) of the fixed electrode potentials (± 100 mv). The abscissa is the longitudinal (basal to apical) location along the basilar membrane, and the ordinate is the radial (central to peripheral) position along neural fibers in the sheet. Node locations, defining element boundaries, are shown on the neural sheet by crosses. Figure 5.8*a* shows two radially oriented peaks, each indicated by patterns of concentric isocontours, positioned midway along the longitudinal axis. The more centrally located peak is positive in polarity, being closer to the positive electrode near the modiolus. The more radially located peak is negative in polarity. The single, gradually arcing contour that extends along the full extent of the longitudinal axis is the zero potential isocontour.

Also shown in Figure 5.8*a* is a grid consisting of solid, vertical lines and dashed, horizontal lines. The solid lines indicate selected locations along the model's longitudinal axis that represent the loci of seven fibers lying in the neural sheet. These fiber locations are designated f_1 through f_7 from basal to apical-most. Fiber f_4 lies in the central plane of the model. The symbol associated with each line is used to label plots of data associated with that fiber locus. The dashed horizontal lines indicate six radially positioned loci in the neural sheet that are parallel to the longitudinal axis. These are labeled n_1 through n_6. Position n_1 defines the locus of the habenula. Positions n_2 through n_5 define node positions along the peripheral axonal processes of the fibers with approximately 300-μm internodal spacing. Position n_5 lies adjacent to the fiber's cell body on the peripheral side. Position n_6 lies in the center of the ganglion region. Again the symbol associated with each position locus is used to label plots of associated data.

Potentials profiles for fibers (f_1 through f_7) are plotted as a function of radial position along the fiber in Figure 5.8*b*. The greatest peak potential levels and steepest gradients occur along the fibers located closest to the electrode pair (f_3 through f_5). Decreasing peak levels and shallower gradients are seen along fibers located at progressively more distant longitudinal locations (f_1 and f_7). Regardless of its location, each fiber is exposed locally to both positive and negative potentials along its length. The potential spread functions, showing potentials along the longitudinal fiber position loci (n_1 through n_6), are shown in Figure 5.8*c* for this condition. High absolute peak levels are observed at the midpoint longitudinal location f_4 for both the peripheral-most node (n_2) and the node (n_5) adjacent to the cell body. The fields diminish rapidly in the vicinity of the potential peaks. For instance, at the peripheral-most node position (n_2), the potential on f_7 is approximately 17 dB below the peak level at the same position on f_4, 800 μm away along the longitudinal axis. At greater longitudinal distances beyond the f_4 location, the potential levels continue to decline.

Field patterns for the pure longitudinal configuration are shown in Figure 5.9. Figures 5.6*c* and 5.7*a* indicate the electrode configuration and the scala tympani electrode placement used in this calculation. The isopotential contour plot of Figure 5.9*a* shows two relative potential peaks of opposite polarity oriented parallel to the longitudinal axis of the model. The maximum potential levels are at node positions n_4 and n_5 along fibers closest to each electrode (f_2 and f_6). The potential profiles of Figure 5.9*b* indicate that each fiber, depending on its location, is exposed to either wholly positive or negative potentials along its length. Potential gradients are small along the fiber length as compared with the patterns seen for the pure radial configuration. The geometrical symmetry of the longitudinal electrode configuration means that fibers located midway between the electrode positions (near f_4) receive little or no stimulation. The spread functions of Figure 5.9*c* show substantial potential spread along the longitudinal axis. At a location 800 μm longitudinally from the central plane of the model (f_7), potential levels along node position n_5 are at most 5 dB below peak levels and are decreasing toward more distant locations.

The offset radial bipolar configuration is a combination of the pure longitudinal and pure radial bipolar configurations. Figure 5.10 shows the model field predictions based on the electrode configuration of Figure 5.6*d* and the scala tympani placement shown in Figure 5.7*a*. The isopotential contour plot shows a more complicated pattern than seen before. Again two relative potential peaks are observed that are offset in

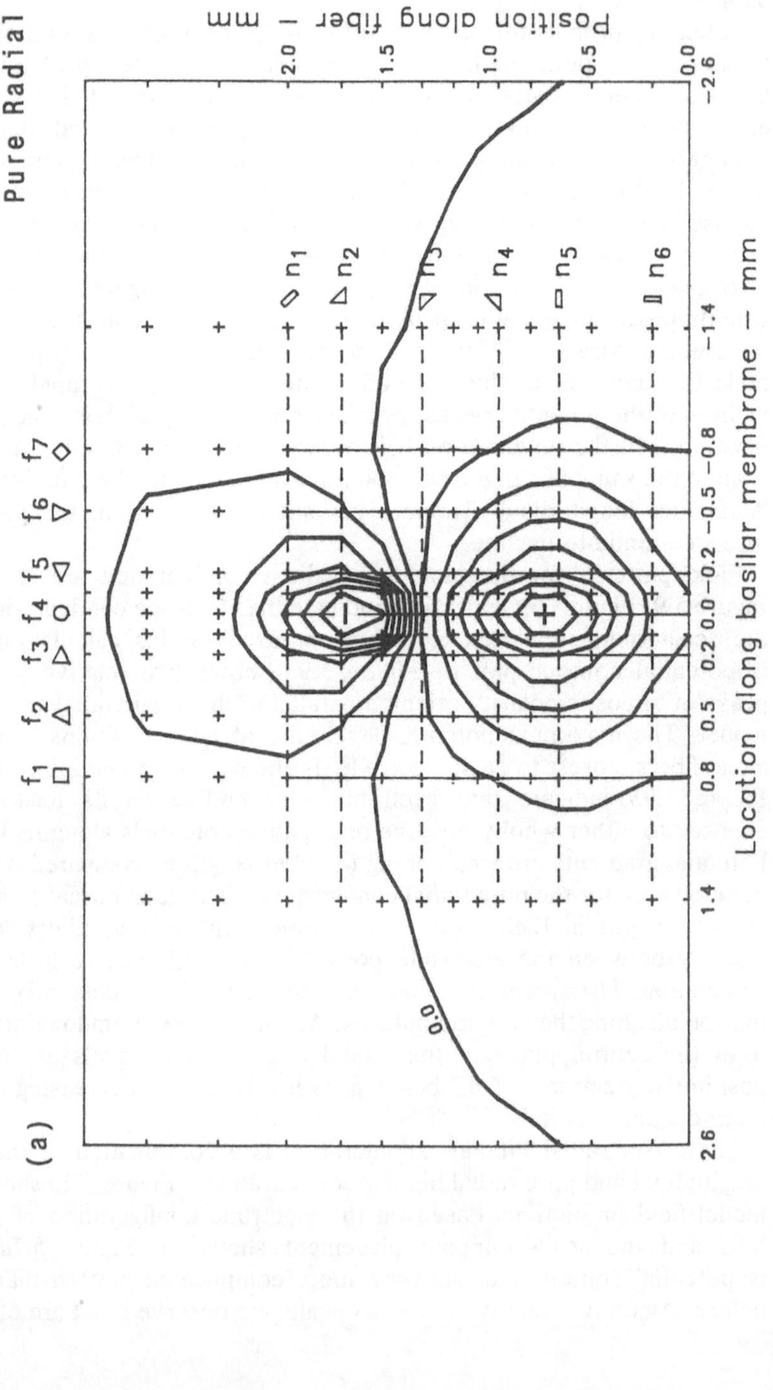
(a)
Pure Radial
f_1 f_2 f_3 f_4 f_5 f_6 f_7
n_1
n_2
n_3
n_4
n_5
n_6
0.0
Position along fiber — mm
2.0
1.5
1.0
0.5
0.0
Location along basilar membrane — mm
2.6
1.4
0.8
0.5
0.2
0.0
−0.2
−0.5
−0.8
−1.4
−2.6

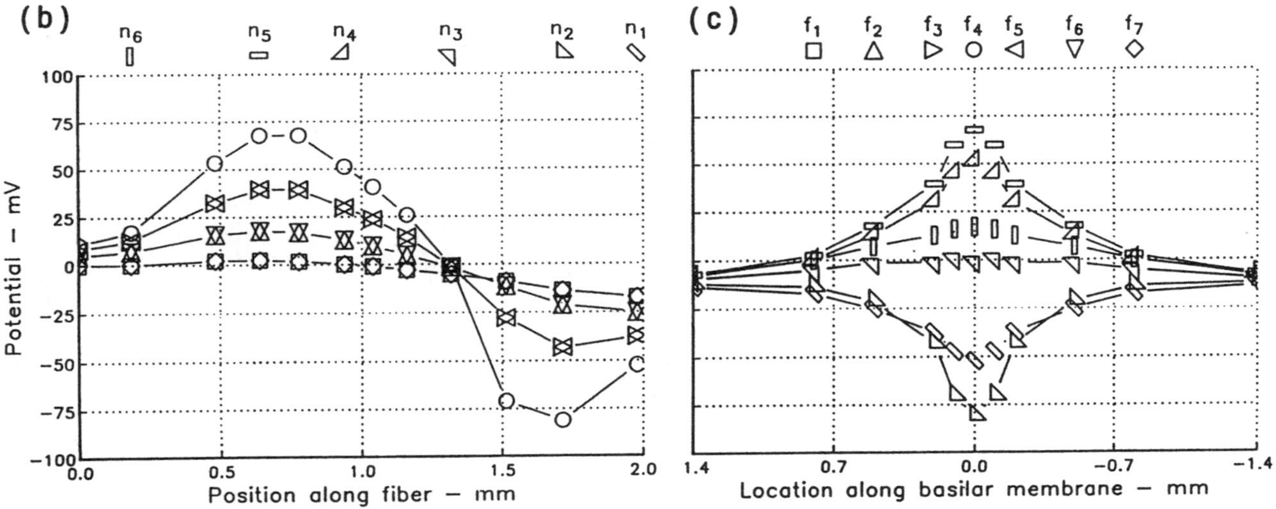

FIGURE 5.8. Neural sheet potential patterns for the pure radial bipolar electrode configuration. Panel (*a*) shows isopotential contours at 10-mv intervals for potentials lying on the sheet. The zero potential isocontour is explicitly labeled. Symbols (+ and −) indicate the polarities and the locations of peak potential levels. Panel (*b*) indicates potential profiles along selected fibers lying in the sheet. Panel (*c*) indicates the spread of potentials along the longitudinal axis at fixed fiber node positions. See text for full discussion.

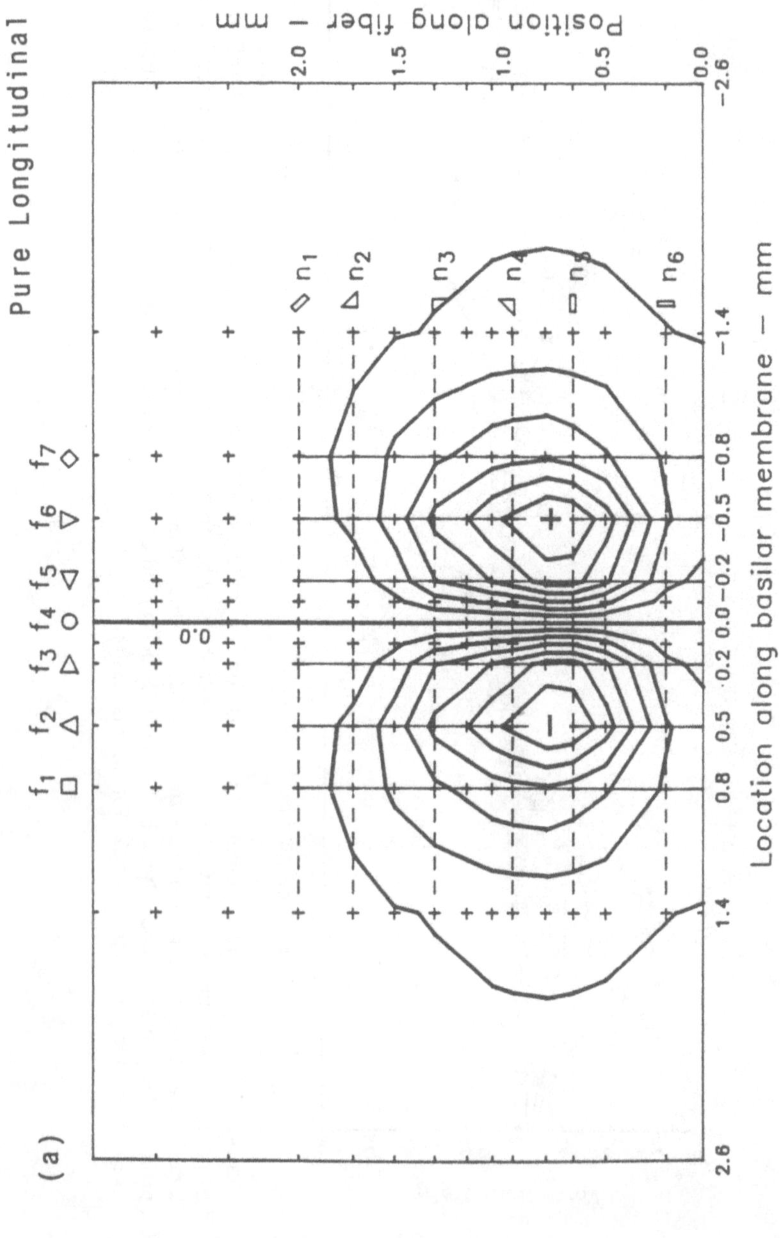
(a)
Pure Longitudinal
Position along fiber — mm
Location along basilar membrane — mm

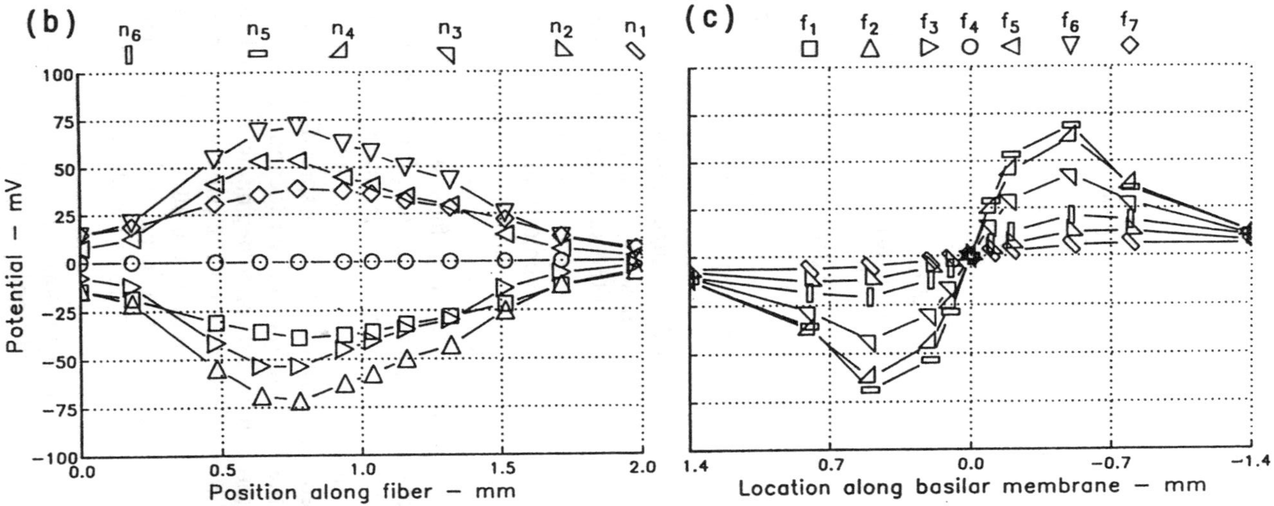

FIGURE 5.9. Neural sheet potential patterns for the pure longitudinal bipolar electrode configuration. Panel (*a*) shows isopotential contours at 10-mv intervals for potentials lying on the sheet. The zero potential isocontour is explicitly labeled. Symbols (+ and −) indicate the polarities and the locations of peak potential levels. Panel (*b*) indicates potential profiles along selected fibers lying in the sheet. Panel (*c*) indicates the spread of potentials along the longitudinal axis at fixed fiber node positions. See text for full discussion.

radial position and longitudinal location (Figure 5.10*a*). The fiber potential profiles of Figure 5.10*b* reveal a heterogeneous pattern of stimulation that varies dramatically as a function of fiber longitudinal location. Fibers located near the positive, apical electrode (f_5 and f_6) have profiles almost identical to those seen with the pure longitudinal configuration. High peak values with relatively small gradients are observed with positive potentials along almost the entirety of the peripheral fiber process. Peak levels for these fibers are near the cell body at node position n_5. In contrast, potential profiles for fibers located near the negative, basal electrode (f_2 and f_3) have high peak negative potentials with steep gradients occurring at the more peripheral end of the fiber (n_2). At more central positions along these fibers (n_4 through n_6), the extracellular potentials approach zero. Fibers located near the central plane of the model (near f_4) are exposed to low peak stimulus levels of both polarities with relatively shallow gradients. The spread function (Figure 5.10*c*) for the offset radial longitudinal configuration shows a pattern of field decay similar to that of the pure longitudinal configuration. On fiber f_7, 800 μm longitudinally from the central plane, potential levels at node positions n_5 are about 7 dB below peak levels. Potentials at this node position continue to decline at most distant longitudinal locations.

The banded longitudinal bipolar electrode configuration produces a fundamentally different field pattern from those previously discussed. The electrode configuration of Figure 5.6*e* and the scala tympani placement of Figure 5.7*b* are used. Figure 5.11*a* shows the isopotential contours. Two longitudinally oriented peaks are present in the region of the basilar membrane, radially beyond the most peripheral extent of the fibers (n_1). This is a consequence of the radial placement of the electrode carrier within scala tympani. The fiber potential profiles of Figure 5.11*b* reveal a field pattern of single-polarity, almost-constant, low-amplitude potential levels along the fibers. Only at the most peripheral ends (n_1) of some of the fibers are significant gradients present. The spread functions show a remarkably homogeneous pattern of a broadly spreading field of potential (Figure 5.11*c*). At the 800-μm longitudinal location (f_7), field levels at node positions n_3 through n_5 are only beginning to reach a maximum, indicative of a broadly spreading field pattern. The one exception to this pattern is the spread function computed for the most peripheral fiber positions (n_1). Here a relative peak is observed near 500 μm longitudinally on f_6, decreasing by 3.2 dB at the 800-μm location of f_7.

Two limitations of the present field model emerge from examination of the neural sheet potential patterns. First, the model is spatially limited in total length and element resolution along the longitudinal axis. This is particularly evident in the case of the banded longitudinal electrode configuration. One design goal of the model was to provide a model structure with fine spatial resolution in the central region surrounded by progressively larger elements (hence lower resolution) toward the model boundary. This structural organization minimizes the model's node and element count and leads to more efficient calculations with smaller memory requirements. Generally, such a configuration would be adequate for modeling the spatially constrained field patterns of bipolar electrode pairs located in the central region of the model. The broadly spreading fields of monopolar electrodes (Grizon, 1987) cannot be accurately calculated in the present model and are thus not addressed in this paper. For the present model the pure radial, pure longitudinal, and offset radial electrode-pair field patterns are reasonably modeled. However, in the case of the banded longitudinal configuration, the spread of the electrical fields is unexpectedly large. Here the total length and relatively coarse resolution of the elements along the longitudinal axis of the model may produce distorted longitudinal field estimates. The relative degree of distortion is not presently known but may be examined by adding elements to expand the model longitudinally and then computing the fields again. Lengthening the model, however, will further distort the field estimates from those existing in an intact cochlea, since cochlear spiral curvature is not addressed in the present model. The second limitation of the field model is that additional anatomical detail needs to be modeled in particular regions of the cochlea. One region is the lateral wall of scala tympani, which should be described as the soft tissue structure of the stria vascularis and the spiral ligament, instead of the presently modeled bone. Another region requiring refinement is the modiolus. Here anisotropic tracts of fibers from higher cochlear turns are missing, as well as details of the axons coursing centrally from neuronal cell bodies lying in the spiral ganglion near the electrodes. Detailing the modiolus is particularly important since the calculated potential indicates that axons of fibers projecting centrally off the edge of the *neural sheet* are still in the presence of significant extracellular fields. To model the response of a neuron to electrical stimulation, it is most important to model all surfaces of the neuron that are exposed to nonzero extracellular fields and are thus passing current. For instance, anodic currents entering a fiber near an anode stimulate a neuron by activation of sites remote to the anode as current passes out of the cell (Ranck, 1975).

To explore how the predicted extracellular potential fields influence the firing probability of the neural fibers, we turn to the neural component of the integrated field-neuron model.

Neural Responsiveness to Extracellular Fields

A variety of lumped-element models have been proposed to describe the response of myelinated nerve fibers to extracellular potential fields. All of these models are extensions of the original work of McNeal (1976) for

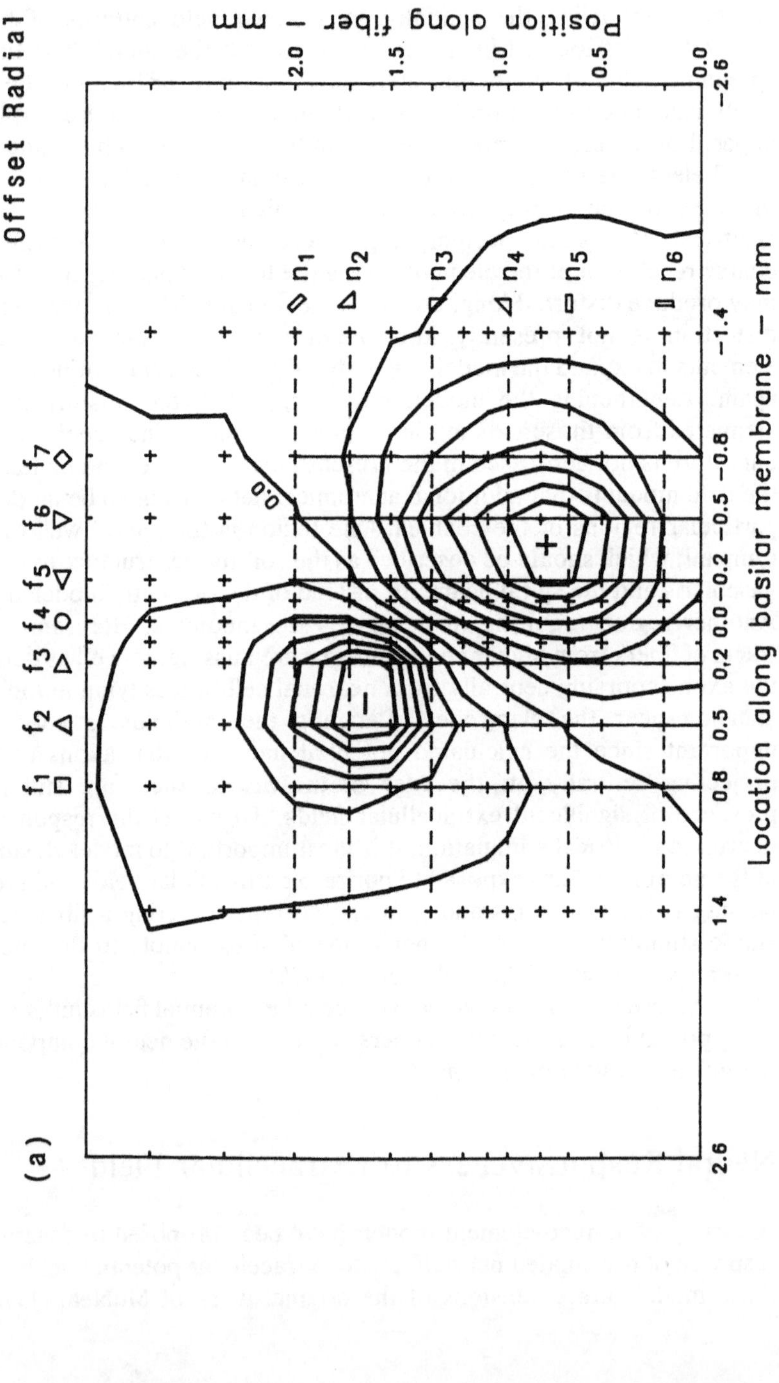
(a)
Offset Radial
Position along fiber – mm
Location along basilar membrane – mm
0.0
f_1 f_2 f_3 f_4 f_5 f_6 f_7
n_1 n_2 n_3 n_4 n_5 n_6

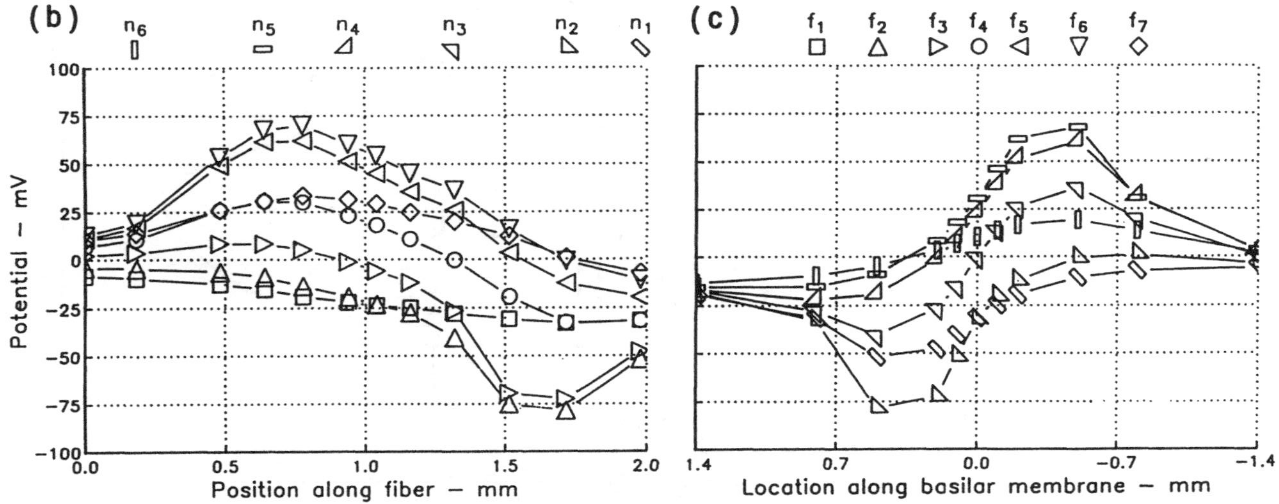

FIGURE 5.10. Neural sheet potential patterns for the offset radial bipolar electrode configuration. Panel (*a*) shows isopotential contours at 10-mv intervals for potentials lying on the sheet. The zero potential isocontour is explicitly labeled. Symbols (+ and −) indicate the polarities and the locations of peak potential levels. Panel (*b*) indicates potential profiles along selected fibers lying in the sheet. Panel (*c*) indicates the spread of potentials along the longitudinal axis at fixed fiber node positions. See text for full discussion.

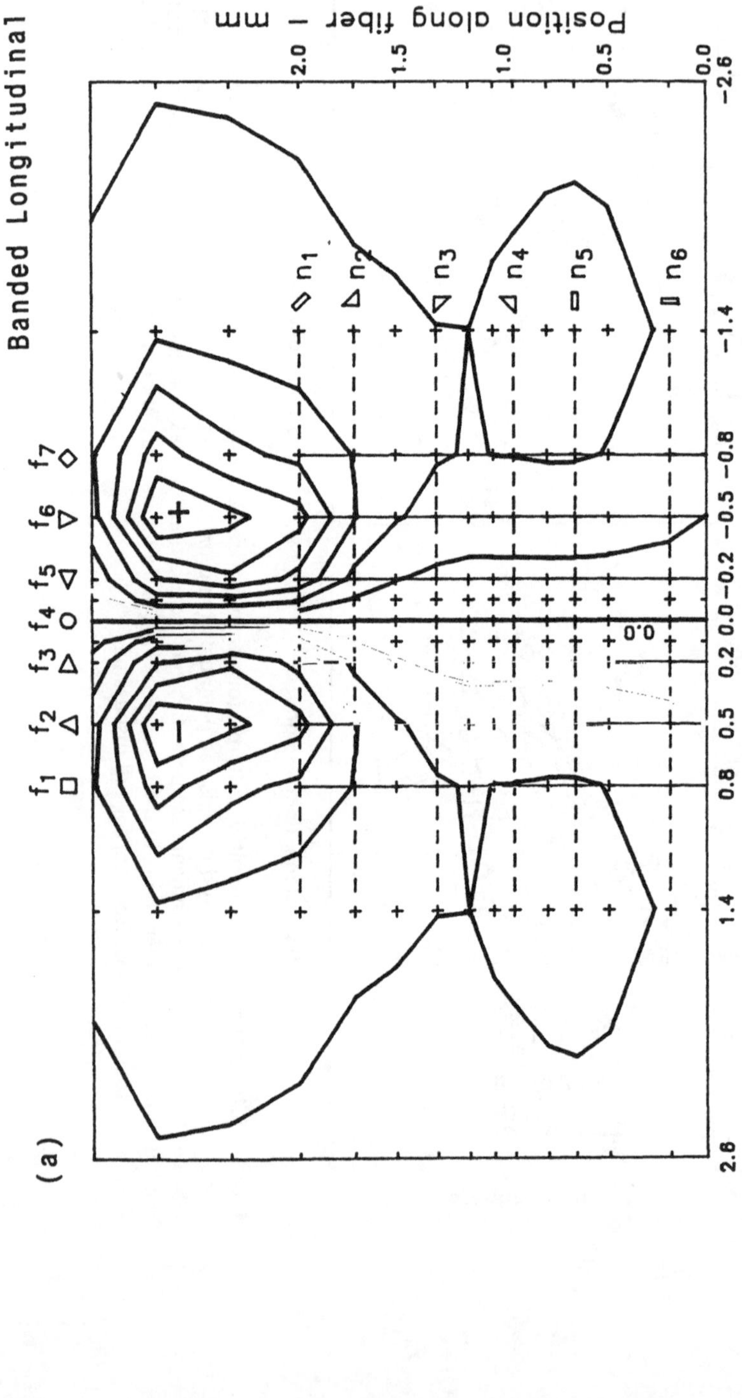
(a)
Banded Longitudinal
f1 f2 f3 f4 f5 f6 f7
n1 n2 n3 n4 n5 n6
Position along fiber — mm
2.0
1.5
1.0
0.5
0.0
2.6 1.4 0.8 0.5 0.2 0.0 −0.2 −0.5 −0.8 −1.4 −2.6
Location along basilar membrane — mm

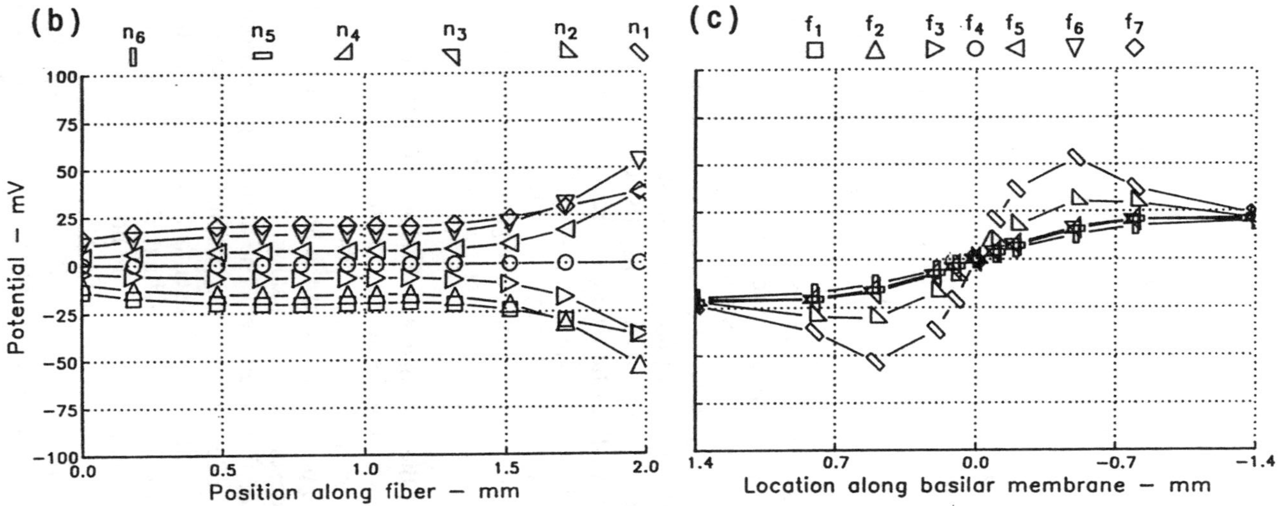

FIGURE 5.11. Neural sheet potential patterns for the banded longitudinal bipolar electrode configuration. Panel (*a*) shows isopotential contours at 10-mv intervals for potentials lying on the sheet. The zero potential isocontour is explicitly labeled. Symbols (+ and −) indicate the polarities and the locations of peak potential levels. Panel (*b*) indicates potential profiles along selected fibers lying in the sheet. Panel (*c*) indicates the spread of potentials along the longitudinal axis at fixed fiber node positions. See text for full discussion.

predicting the subthreshold behavior of a myelinated neuron in an electrical field. McNeal's model describes an electrical network of the distributed myelin and nodal membrane characteristics of an infinitely long myelinated fiber. Node behavior is described by the Frankenhaeuser-Huxley equations (1964). Such a model is capable of predicting the occurrence of an initial spike from a resting state. Enhanced versions of this model have been described for computing suprathreshold and repeated spiking behavior (Finley and Wilson, 1985; Reilly, Freeman, and Larkin, 1985). Similar models have been developed to describe the behavior of intracochlear fibers during electrical stimulation (Colombo and Parkins, 1987; Finley and Wilson, 1985).

Rattay (1986, 1987) has shown that the responsiveness from a resting state of both myelinated and unmyelinated infinitely long fibers in electrical fields depends on the second spatial derivative of the field in the extracellular medium. He defines an *activating function,* which for myelinated fibers is the second difference quotient of the extracellular potential field when sampled at node positions along the fiber. Biophysically, the activating function at a particular node is proportional to the summation of intraaxonal longitudinal currents at the node position. At rest this current summation is zero; however, during exposure to extracellular fields, the net longitudinal current flow may be either positive or negative. This field-induced net summation current flows across the nodal membrane in addition to the resting-state nodal currents. A positive activating function value correlates with a positive outward current at the node, leading to nodal depolarization. A negative activation function value corresponds to nodal hyperpolarization. The greater the absolute magnitude of the activating function, the greater the local effect at the node.

As an initial examination of the responsiveness of neural fibers to the predicted electrical fields, we compute the activating functions for the set of neurons whose potential profiles were described above. Here we assume that no cell bodies are present and that the fibers are of uniform diameter with the previously described node spacing. Activating function predictions are independent of fiber diameter. The activating functions are computed for the four node positions (n_2 through n_5) along the peripheral axonal process from the edge of Rosenthal's canal (n_5) to the node position (n_2) adjacent to, but not including, the habenula. End effects due to fibers terminating at the habenula are not specially treated. Fiber termination regions are probably specific stimulation sites for neurons in electrical fields (Reilly and Bauer, 1987), a result that would not appreciably change the neuronal behavior predicted by this present analysis. In Figures 5.12–5.15, activating function values are plotted for each of the modeled electrode configurations for each node both as a function of node position along the fiber (panel *a* of each figure) and as a function of fiber location along the basilar membrane (panel *b* of each

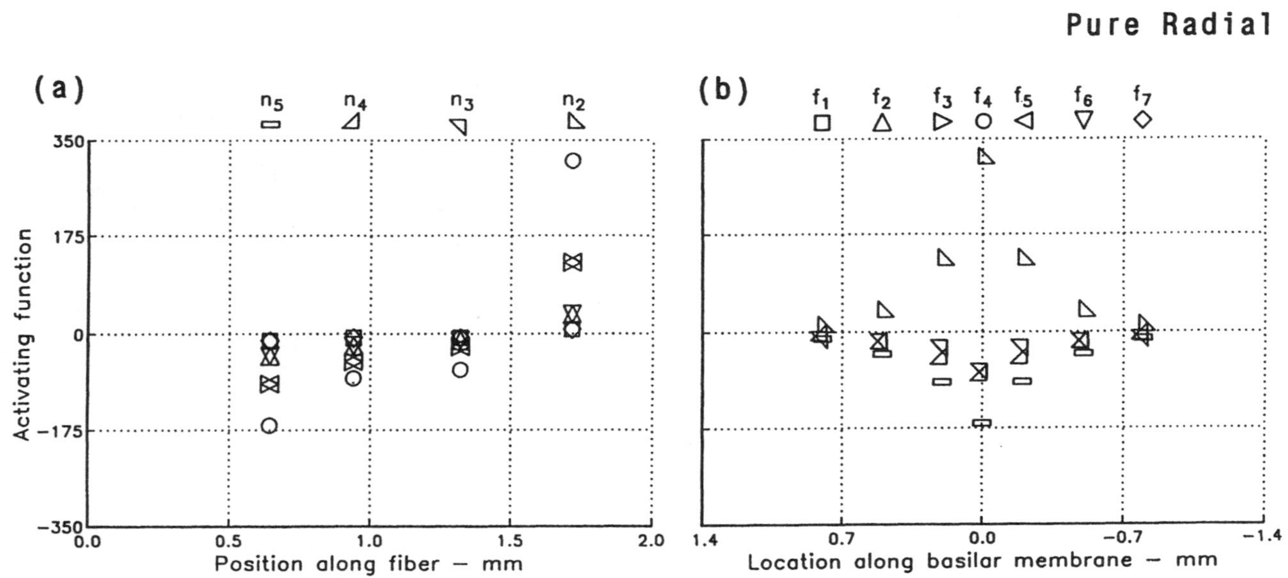

FIGURE 5.12. Fiber activating function plots for the pure radial bipolar electrode configuration as a function of nodal position along fibers (*a*) and of location of a fiber along the basilar membrane (*b*).

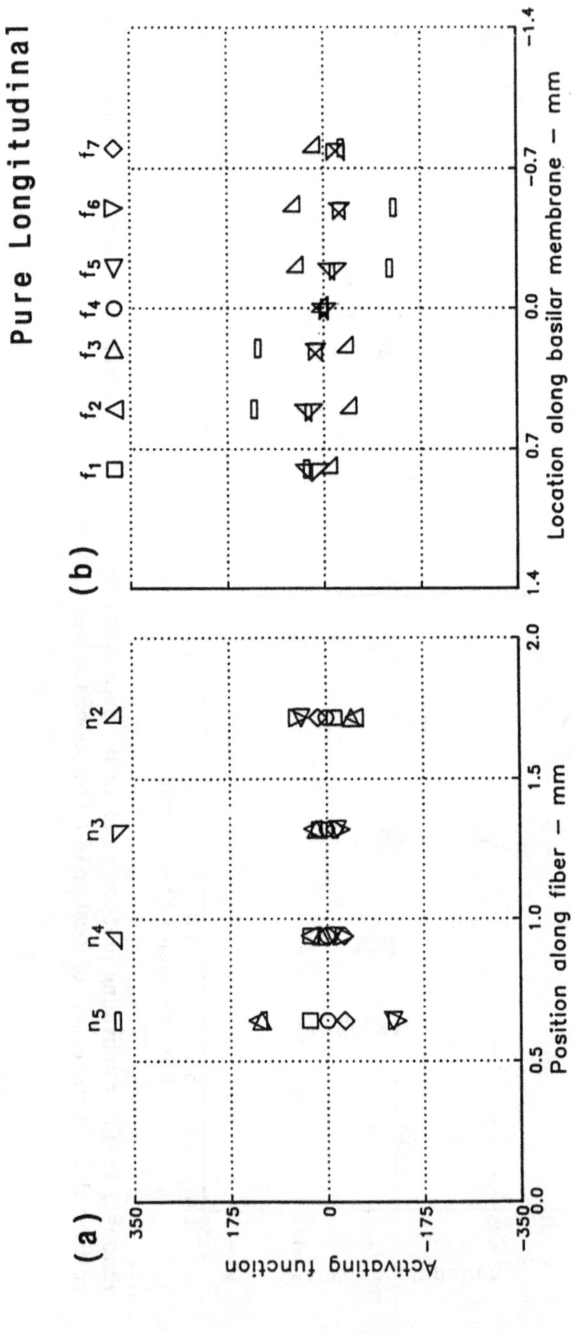

FIGURE 5.13. Fiber activating function plots for the pure longitudinal bipolar electrode configuration as a function of nodal position along fibers (*a*) and of location of a fiber along the basilar membrane (*b*).

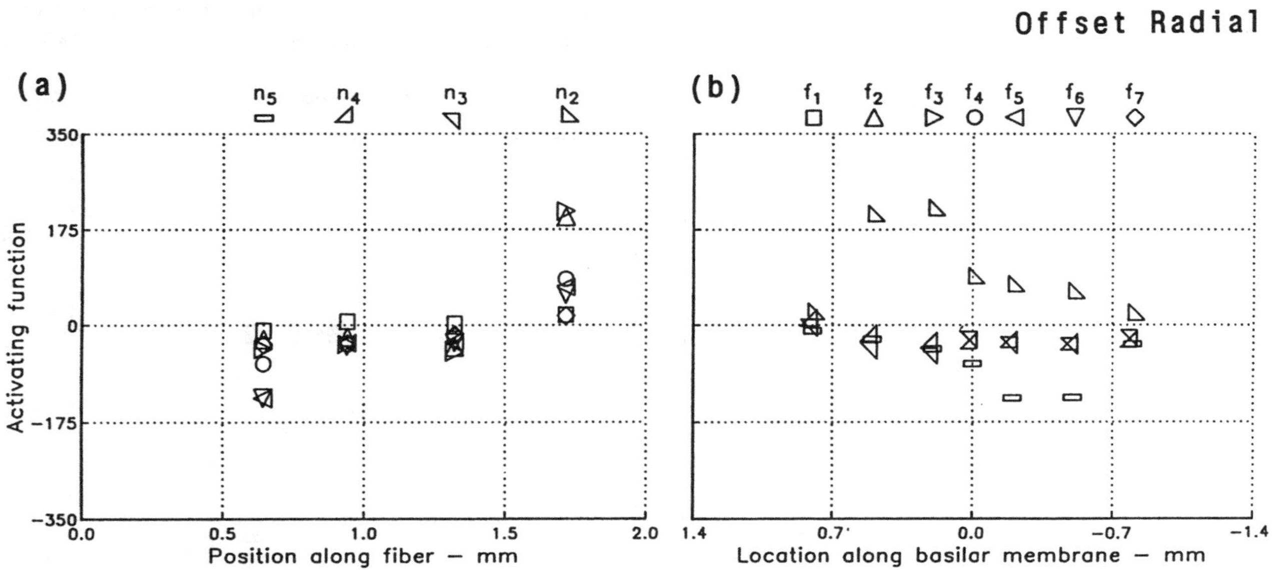

FIGURE 5.14. Fiber activating function plots for the offset radial bipolar electrode configuration as a function of nodal position along fibers (*a*) and of location of a fiber along the basilar membrane (*b*).

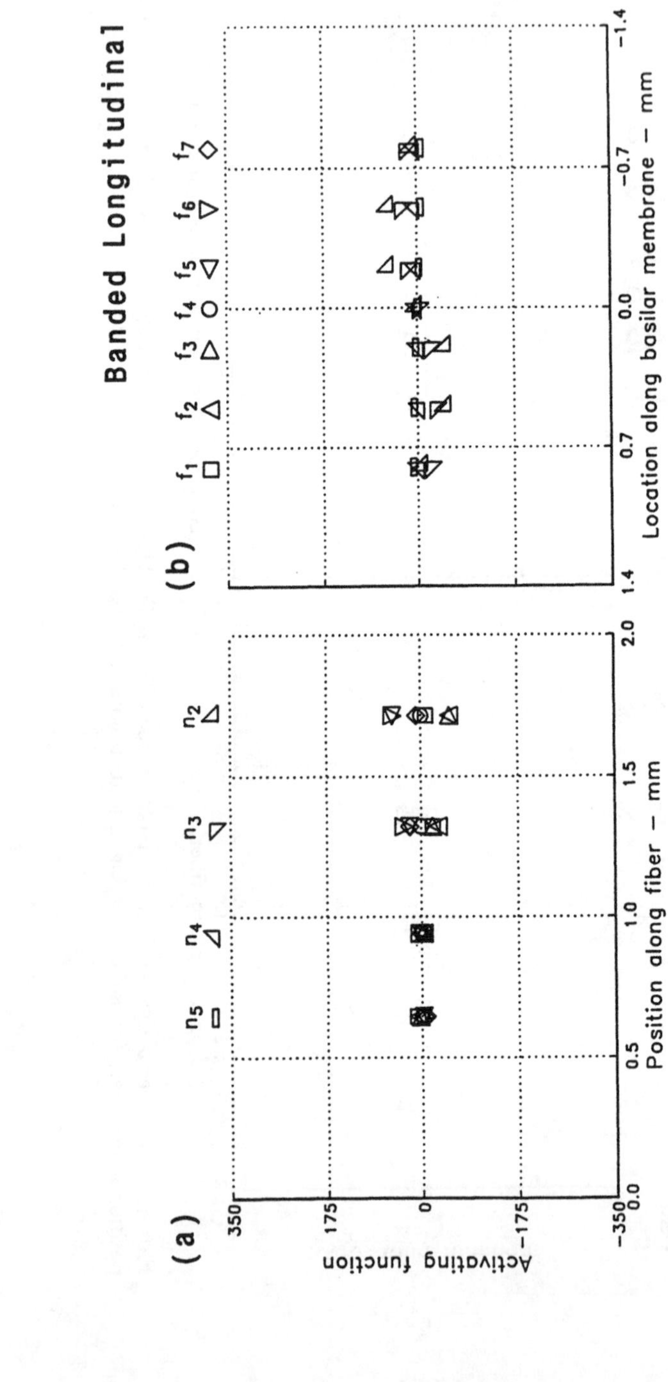

FIGURE 5.15. Fiber activating function plots for the banded longitudinal bipolar electrode configuration as a function of nodal position along fibers (*a*) and of location of a fiber along the basilar membrane (*b*).

figure). The functions are calculated assuming a positive current stimulus applied to the modeled electrode configurations and using the polarity conventions described in Figures 5.8–5.11. A reversal of stimulus polarity at the electrodes reverses the field polarity but conserves its shape; hence, with a negative stimulus applied, a negative activating function value signifies depolarization of the node.

This analysis of neuronal responsiveness is useful only for identifying the probability that a node will or will not initiate a neural spike in response to a monophasic pulsatile stimulus. By definition the activation function assumes the neuron is at resting state, so the measure indicates only the direction and degree of tendency of the node to change from quiescence. No temporal integration behavior is included. Similarly, anodic blocking phenomena cannot be demonstrated; however, the possibility of their occurrence can be noted.

It is important to emphasize that the present analysis assumes the presence of myelinated fibers extending from the habenula centrally. This is more often not the case in the implanted, deafened cochlea (Hinojosa and Marion, 1983; Laurence, 1980; Leake-Jones and Rebscher, 1983). Extensive loss of complete auditory afferents often occurs. When the fiber is present, the peripheral axonal process may not be present. When it is absent, the target element for electrical stimulation consists only of the cell body and its centrally projecting axon. For fibers in this condition, the activating function calculations have little relevance. The present model addresses field patterns and neuronal responsiveness only in the region of the peripheral axonal process.

The significance of activating functions for predicting neuronal responsiveness is now considered for the pure radial electrode configuration with a positive monophasic stimulus (cathode lateral). In Figure 5.12*a* the largest activating function value occurs at the most peripheral node (n_2) of the fiber closest to the electrode pair (f_4). Actually node position n_2 is the only position that would be stimulated for any given fiber in the target field for this polarity stimulus since the activating function is positive only at this position. It is important to note that in this cathode lateral condition, more centrally positioned nodes (n_3 through n_5) are hyperpolarized, raising the possibility of anodal blockage. In Figure 5.12*b* the magnitude of the activating function for node n_2 position diminishes rapidly (−40 dB/mm between f_4 and f_5) as a function of longitudinal fiber location. Assuming that a high activating function value correlates with a low fiber threshold, very high thresholds would be expected at all locations within the cochlea except near the radial-pair location. Here a sharp decrease in threshold would occur, forming a sharp, symmetrical threshold dip centered at the electrode-pair location. This exact single-unit threshold behavior has been observed by van den Honert and Stypulkowski (1987a, Fig. 6) in the cat using radial bipolar pair electrical stimulation in an acoustically intact ear. They monitored fiber electrical threshold and measured acoustic characteristic frequency to establish each fiber's location along the basilar membrane. The variability in their data is most likely due to uncertainties in scala tympani electrode placement.

For a negative stimulus polarity (cathode medial) applied to the same electrode configuration, the model predicts stimulation of a completely different set of nodes. In this case, the most strongly depolarizing node (signified now by the maximum negative activating function value) again lies along fiber f_4 but is now the most centrally positioned node n_5. This central node (n_5) is driven only about half as much under cathode medial conditions as the most peripheral node (n_2) on the same fiber with the cathode lateral. The two adjacent, but more peripherally positioned, nodes (n_2 and n_4) are also activated but to a lesser degree. Looking across the ensemble of fibers, we see again a diminishing depolarization drive for fibers more distant from the electrode pair (-27 dB/mm between f_4 and f_5). In both polarity conditions, the widths of the target fields of depolarized fibers along the basilar membrane are the same. Predictions of unit thresholds versus fiber location for the cathode medial condition would provide a similar picture of a sharp threshold dip centered at the electrode location, with two qualifications: (1) with the cathode lateral, the depth of the threshold dip should be less pronounced, and (2) the maximum width of the dip should be the same in both conditions. This again is consistent with observed unit data (van den Honert and Stypulkowski, 1987a, Fig. 6).

The neural response patterns for the pure longitudinal bipolar configuration are quite different. For a positive monophasic stimulus (cathode basal), Figure 5.13*a* shows the largest positive activating function (hence depolarizing) values located at the central node positions (n_5). Figure 5.13*b* indicates that these nodes lie along fibers (f_2 and f_3) nearest the more basal electrode. In contrast, fibers located near the more apical, anodic electrode (f_5 and f_6) are only moderately stimulated at the most peripheral nodes (n_2) but are strongly hyperpolarized at the most central nodes (n_5). A plot of predicted fiber thresholds versus basilar membrane location would show high thresholds everywhere across the cochlea except in the vicinity of the electrode pair. Near the electrode pair, two threshold dips would be expected. One dip, near the basal cathode and including fibers f_2 and f_3, would be relatively deep, but not as deep as the dip seen with the pure radial, medial cathode configuration. The width of this dip should be approximately half that for the pure radial configuration. Midway between the electrodes the thresholds should rise to high values. Near the apical anode, including fiber locations f_5 and f_6, another dip is expected that would be even shallower in depth. For fibers in this region, anodal blockage is a possibility since more centrally positioned nodes are hyperpolarized. A negative monophasic (cathode apical) stimulus would produce a similar distribution, with the anodic and cathodic threshold dips reversed in position.

Van den Honert and Stypulkowski (1987) observed this pattern in experiments with longitudinal bipolar electrodes. In their report the cathode basal condition demonstrates a modest threshold dip near the anode, whereas a very narrow, deeper threshold dip occurs near the cathode for the anode basal condition (van den Honert and Stypulkowski, 1987a, Fig. 5). Insufficient unit data from the basal cochlea prevented a full demonstration of the bimodal threshold distribution. Our present model fails to predict the small, but broadly distributed, decrease in thresholds they observed when the cathode was most apical. We interpret that decline as due to the influence of the apically positioned cathode on fibers from apical regions of the cochlea passing through the modiolus. Because van den Honert and Stypulkowski's electrode was inserted only about 5 mm into the first turn, the more basal electrode of the longitudinal pair was substantially further away and somewhat shielded by the apical electrode from the core of the modiolus. Only when the cathode is apically located could it influence the modiolus. This geometry is not described by the present field model.

The neural response patterns for the offset radial configuration are similar to the pure radial configuration for node site selection but more closely resemble the pure longitudinal configuration in fiber distribution. For a positive monophasic stimulus (cathode more basally and peripherally located), the depolarized nodes are those only at the most peripheral node position n_2, as shown in Figure 5.14*a*. This pattern is very similar to that computed for the pure radial configuration (Figure 5.12*a*). Figure 5.14*b* indicates that the most strongly depolarized node sites are on fibers f_2 and f_3 near the cathodic electrode. Fibers near the central plane (f_4) and near the anodic electrode (f_5 and f_6) are also depolarized at the n_2 node position. These fibers are, however, hyperpolarized at more central node positions, raising the possibility of anodal blockage. In contrast, for a negative monophasic stimulus (cathode more apical and central), the depolarized nodes will be those closer to the ganglion at position n_5 and lie on fibers f_5 and f_6 near the cathode. In this case, the field of excitation is substantially smaller in extent along the basilar membrane than with a positive monophasic stimulus.

There are no VIII nerve single-unit studies of fiber thresholds using an offset radial electrode pair for stimulation. Merzenich and White (1977) recorded unit thresholds in the central nucleus of the inferior colliculus of the cat while electrically stimulating with pure radial, pure longitudinal, and offset radial electrode configurations. They acoustically stimulated the contralateral ear to determine characteristic frequencies, taking advantage of the binaural organization of the central nucleus. Although limited in the number of animals, their results suggest an ordering of unit thresholds based on electrode configuration. All three configurations stimulated a narrow region of the cochlea, with pure radial being most selective. The authors found that collicular unit thresholds were either low, intermediate, or high, depending on whether the electrode configuration was offset radial, pure longitudinal, or pure radial, respectively. This ordering is exactly opposite the order expected from the model threshold predictions for these configurations. This ordering, however, is consistent with the ordering of the expected ensemble widths, and hence the number of fibers, for each stimulus configuration. Interpretation of these results is problematic. The relationship between central nucleus thresholds and cochlear fiber activity is not well understood, particularly with regard to how intermediate neuronal pathways process temporally and spatially complex activity, occurring across an ensemble of peripheral fibers. Also, this study recorded thresholds using continuous sine-wave stimuli instead of the single monophasic pulses discussed here. While the binaural, collicular recording method may provide useful estimates of fiber place, especially in deafened ears, interpretation of collicular unit threshold levels in terms of peripheral stimulation mechanisms should be questioned until their validity is confirmed experimentally.

The neural activation pattern for the banded longitudinal configuration (Figure 5.15) deviates from the patterns previously described. Here the activating functions for positive monophasic stimulation predict very small depolarization at the most peripheral node positions (n_2 and n_3) of fibers f_5 and f_6 lying near the cathodic electrode band. Note n_3 on fiber f_7 is slightly depolarized also. Near the anodic electrode band the field is symmetrical, but opposite in effect, where the most peripheral nodes (n_2 and n_3) are hyperpolarized along fibers f_1, f_2, and f_3. With negative monophasic stimulation a similar pattern of nodal stimulation occurs, however now with the cathodic and anodic band positions reversed. Taken to their logical extension, these activating function patterns suggest that stimulation with the banded longitudinal electrode pair would produce a very high threshold for a neural response. In addition, in the case of pathological loss of the peripheral process, the threshold would jump to exceedingly high values. These predictions are clearly not the case based on the extensive clinical experience using the Melbourne implant system. It is possible that the primary nodes of neural stimulation lie in a more central position, perhaps near the cell body or along the centrally projecting axons. Indeed, this possibility cannot be ruled out with regard to the use of the other configurations discussed as well. As described in the discussion on the field patterns, expansions of the model are planned to better describe field patterns in the modiolus. It can be stated, however, that the banded longitudinal configuration, as described here, produces a broadly spreading field that stimulates a wider distribution of fibers than would be expected with the pure radial, pure longitudinal, or offset radial configurations. The full extent of this influence is not yet appreciated.

Limitations of the Present Neural Model

Analysis of neuronal responsiveness using activating functions is at best simplistic. There are numerous aspects of neuronal anatomy and physiology that are not addressed by this analysis. In the present analysis, only initial sites of excitation, along uniform myelinated fibers, are predicted. No insight into behavior involving temporal integration of membrane currents or multiple spike firing is provided. Additionally, anatomical variability, due to pathological loss of peripheral processes, and the presence of the cell body, are not accounted for. To address these limitations, an expanded, anatomically and physiologically based neural model of electrical stimulation has been developed.

The expanded model extends the work of the previous neural models (Colombo and Parkins, 1987; McNeal, 1976; Rattay, 1987; Reilly, Freeman, and Larkin, 1985) by providing for impedance characterization of myelin, by incorporating mammalian node characteristics, and by allowing for geometrical scaling to account for varying anatomical dimensions. A portion of this model is presented in Figure 5.16. The neuron model

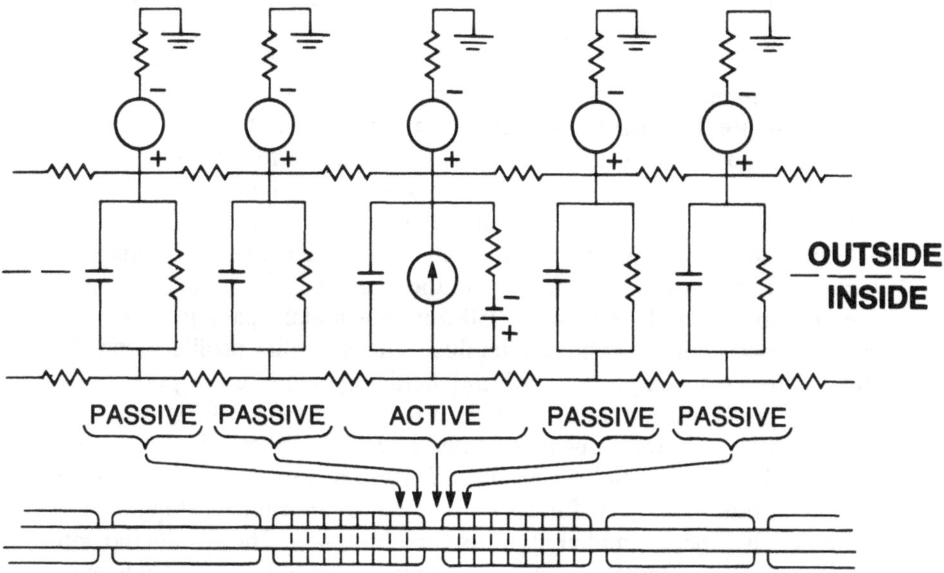

FIGURE 5.16. Lumped-element model of a myelinated neuron stimulated by an extracellular electrical field. See text for full description.

comprises a section of a myelinated axon containing 19 active nodes of Ranvier. Each node is isolated from adjacent nodes by 9 myelinated segments. The ends of the neuron consist of 9 myelinated segments terminating in a sealed membrane. In all, 199 computational segments are included in the model. Nodes of Ranvier are located at segments 10, 20, . . . , 180, 190. The myelin segments are assumed to be passive and comprise simply a parallel combination of the transmembrane capacity and resistivity. Each myelinated segment is specified by the geometrical dimensions of the segment (i.e., radius, length, myelin thickness). The lumped-element electrical properties are then computed assuming a cylindrical model of the segment and using specific tissue characteristics (i.e., axoplasm and myelin resistivities and myelin dielectric constant). Each node is described electrically by a transmembrane capacity in parallel with both a voltage-controlled current source and a series combination of a leakage resistance and a battery source. The behavior of the current source is described by Frankenhaeuser-Huxley–type equations in the present configuration. Future versions will use Hodgkin-Huxley–type equations adjusted for mammalian node characteristics (Sweeney, Mortimer, and Durand, 1987). Transmembrane capacity and leakage resistances are calculated in a manner similar to the passive properties of the myelinated segments. The battery sources are adjusted to provide the normal resting membrane potential for the cell at each of the active nodes. External to the axon at each segment is a voltage source, which drives through the impedance of the extracellular medium. These external voltage sources are set to define the extracellular potential along the cell. Cell body characteristics are incorporated by varying the length and diameter of the myelinated segments between two nodes so as to approximate the longitudinal cross-sectional profile of the cell body in a stepwise manner. At present the model is solved iteratively using Euler approximations for the differential equations and fixed time steps (1.0 μs).

Work with this model is preliminary; however, we present one result that illustrates the significance of the cell body in neural responsiveness to electrical stimulation. We computed the response of a single 1.0-μm-diameter myelinated fiber with 250-μm internodal spacing to a step-function extracellular voltage stimulus. The stimulus profile along the fiber is an idealized version of the field expected for a pure radial electrode configuration and is shown in the upper panel of Figure 5.17*a*. This field profile spans a distance of two internodal lengths between peak anodic and cathodic levels. The lower portion of Figure 5.17*a* shows the transmembrane potentials for each computational segment along a short section of the fiber, sampled at 40-μs time intervals. The results indicate that the maximal depolarization of the fiber occurs at the node (9) nearest the peak cathodic region of the stimulus field. This also is the site that activating function analysis would predict for initial depolarization. Hyperpolarization occurs maximally at the node (11) nearest the peak

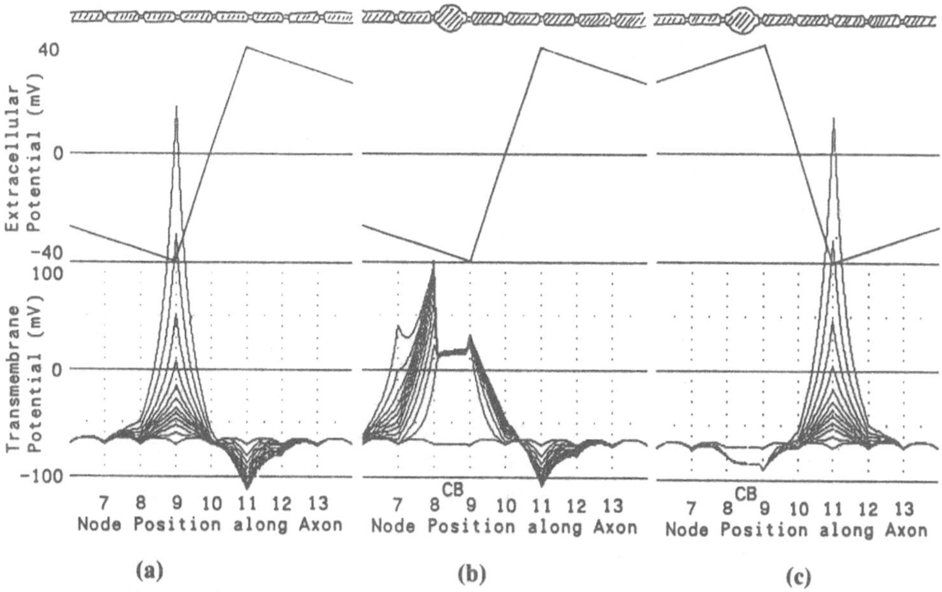

FIGURE 5.17. Neural model transmembrane potentials as a function of position along the axon in response to extracellular stimulation. Potentials are plotted at rest condition and at every 40 μs after application of a step-function extracellular field. The field profile along the fiber is shown in the central portion of each panel. The upper portion of each panel describes the anatomical configuration of the modeled neural element. Panel (*a*) shows the response of a constant-diameter fiber to a field profile that is maximally cathodic at node position 9 and maximally anodic at node position 11. Panel (*b*) shows the response of the same fiber with a cell body included between node positions 8 and 9 to the same electrical field. Panel (*c*) shows the response to the same neural element of panel (*b*) but with the polarity of the extracellular field reversed.

anodic region. The response in Figure 5.17*b* is computed with an identical stimulus condition, except a myelinated, egg-shaped cell body (20 μm in diameter and 30 μm in length) has been introduced between node positions 8 and 9. This cell body position relative to the potential profile peaks was chosen to re-create the potential profile distribution computed for the pure radial bipolar electrode configuration (Figure 5.8). The modeled neuron's response is dramatically affected by the cell body presence. Node 9 is no longer the principal node of activation. Now node 8, on the opposite side of the cell body, is depolarized the most. Note also that node 7 is depolarizing rapidly as well, giving rise to an action potential propagating centrally along the axon. In the vicinity of node 11, the hyperpolarization pattern is very similar to the pattern generated without the cell body present (Figure 5.17*a*). The model conditions for

Figure 5.17*c* are similar to the conditions for Figure 5.17*b*, only now the stimulus polarity is reversed. Node 11 is now nearest the peak cathodic region and is depolarized the most. Nodes 7 and 8 are hyperpolarized along with the cell body region of the fiber. The depolarization pattern at node 11 is similar to what would be expected for the uniform fiber of Figure 5.17*a* without the cell body, but with the stimulus polarity reversed. These results indicate that the presence of the cell body significantly alters the distribution of sites of excitation along the fiber. The effect is clearly dependent on stimulus polarity and probably on the magnitude and shape of the extracellular potential profile. These findings may have bearing on the explanation of the bimodal latency distributions of single units to biphasic pulsatile stimuli (Javel et al., 1987; van den Honert and Stypulkowski, 1987b; and see Javel, Chapter 18, this volume) and the compound action potential to monophasic stimuli (Stypulkowski and van den Honert, 1984). Both of these phenomena are under active investigation using the integrated field-neuron model. In any case, realistic models of neuronal responsiveness to electrical stimulation must account for these mechanisms.

An additional component of neural behavior that must be incorporated into these models is the stochastic behavior of the neuron. Verveen (1968) has shown that neuronal responsiveness to electrical stimulation fluctuates over time in a manner that is consistent with the presence of noise sources at the nodal membrane. Threshold fluctuations are observed routinely in recordings of electrically stimulated VIII nerve fibers (Javel et al., 1987). We have shown that a model based on simple anatomical measurements of nodal membrane area can predict the shape of these fibers' probability-of-firing input-output functions (White, Finley and Wilson, 1987). When combined with the anatomical variability that exists between fibers (Liberman and Oliver, 1984), we feel that stochastic neuronal behavior may have a large influence on the characterization of the responsiveness of the general population of fibers comprising an ensemble. Such a stochastic model of neuronal responsiveness to electrical stimulation is proving useful in predicting psychometric, intensity discrimination, and dynamic range functions.

Summary

Although simple in principle, the mechanisms involved in electrical stimulation of the cochlea are very complex in practice. We have presented an integrated field-neuron model that describes electrical field patterns for a variety of electrode systems and the responsiveness of neurons lying in those electrical fields. The electrical fields are very much a function of the configuration and placement of the electrode array, and the neuronal responsiveness is dependent on the location and detailed anatomy and physiology of the fiber itself. In addition, the population response of an ensemble of simultaneously stimulated fibers must be considered as well.

When considered en masse, the electrically stimulated cochlea appears as a highly nonlinear, uncontrollable interface that limits the ultimate performance goals of cochlear prostheses. However, when considered separately, electrical stimulation of the cochlea appears as an ordered set of biophysically based mechanisms. Knowledge of these mechanisms will allow us to identify the fundamental limitations of the peripheral electrical interface and will provide many opportunities for optimization of electrode systems and stimulation protocols, ultimately leading to improved cochlear prostheses and greater insight into basic hearing mechanisms.

Acknowledgments. This work was supported by NIH Contracts NO1-NS-3-2356 and NO1-NS-5-2396 from the Neural Prosthesis Program of NINCDS and a Professional Development Award from Research Triangle Institute to CCF. The authors are indebted to F. Terry Hambrecht for continued encouragement and support and to Dewey T. Lawson for editorial review.

References

Békésy, G. von (1951). The course pattern of the electrical resistance in the cochlea of the guinea pig (electro-anatomy of the cochlea). *J. Acoust. Soc. Am.* 23:18–28. Reprinted in *Experiments in Hearing,* by G. von Békésy (McGraw-Hill, New York), 1960, pp. 684–703.

Black, R.C., and Clark, G.M. (1980). Differential electrical excitation of the auditory nerve. *J. Acoust. Soc. Am.* 67:868–874.

Cannon, M.W., Jr. (1976). Electrical impedances, current pathways and voltage sources in the guinea pig cochlea. Institute for Sensory Research Report ISR-S-14, Syracuse University, Syracuse, N.Y.

Coburn, B. (1980). Electrical stimulation of the spinal cord: Two-dimensional finite element analysis with particular reference to epidural electrodes. *Med. Biol. Eng. Comp.* 18:573–584.

Colombo, J., and Parkins, C.W. (1987). A model of electrical excitation of the mammalian auditory-nerve neuron. *Hearing Res.* 31:287–312.

Finley, C.C., and Wilson, B.S. (1985). An integrated field-neuron model of electrical stimulation by intracochlear scala tympani electrodes. *Abstracts of the 8th Midwinter Research Meeting of the Association for Research in Otolaryngology,* pp. 105–106.

Finley, C.C., Wilson, B.S., and White, M.W. (1987). A finite-element model of bipolar field patterns in the electrically stimulated cochlea—A two-dimensional approximation. *Proceedings of the Ninth Annual Conference of the IEEE Engineering in Medicine and Biology Society,* Boston, pp. 1901–1903.

Frankenhaeuser, B., and Huxley, A.F. (1964). The action potential in the myelinated nerve fiber of *Xenopus laevis* as computed on the basis of voltage clamp data. *J. Physiol.* (*London*) 171:302–315.

Grizon, G. (1987). Investigation of current flow in the inner ear during electrical stimulation of intracochlear electrodes. MS thesis in EE&CS, MIT, Cambridge, Mass.

Hinojosa, R., and Marion, M. (1983). Histopathology of profound sensorineural deafness. *Ann. N.Y. Acad. Sci.* 405:459–484.

Honrubia, V., Strelioff, D., and Sitko, S. (1974). Electroanatomy of the cochlea: Its role in cochlear potential measurements. *Proceedings of the International Congress in Electrocochleography,* Bronx, N.Y.

Javel, E., Tong, Y.C., Shepherd, R.K., and Clark, G.M. (1987). Responses of cat auditory nerve fibers to biphasic electrical current pulses. *Ann. Otol. Rhinol. Laryngol.* 96, Suppl. 128:26–30.

Johnstone, B.M., Johnstone, J.R., and Pugsley, I.D. (1966). Membrane resistance in endolymphatic walls of the first turn of the guinea-pig cochlea. *J. Acoust. Soc. Am.* 40:1398–1404.

Laurence, M. (1980). Factors in the continuing development of auditory prostheses. In *Controversies in Otolaryngology,* edited by J.B. Snow (Saunders, Philadelphia), pp. 433–442.

Leake-Jones, P.A., and Rebscher, S.J. (1983). Cochlear pathology with chronically implanted scala tympani electrodes. *Ann. N.Y. Acad. Sci.* 405: 203–223.

Liberman, M.C., and Oliver, M.E. (1984). Morphometry of intracellularly labeled neurons of the auditory nerve: Correlations with functional properties. *J. Comp. Neurol.* 223:163–176.

Loeb, G.E., Byers, C.L., Rebscher, S.J., Casey, D.E., Fong, M.M., Schindler, R.A., Gray, R.F., and Merzenich, M.M. (1983). Design and fabrication of an experimental cochlear prosthesis. *Med. Biol. Eng. Compt.* 21:241–254.

McNeal, D.R. (1976). Analysis of a model for excitation of myelinated nerve. *IEEE BME* 23(4):329–337.

Merzenich, M.M., and White, M.W. (1977). Cochlear implant. The interface problem. *Biomed. Eng. Instrum. Funct. Electr. Stimul.* 3:321–340.

Miller, C.E., and Henriquez, C.S. (1988). Three-dimensional finite element solution for biopotentials: Erythrocyte in an applied field. *IEEE BME* 35(9): 712–718.

Misrahy, G.A., Hildreth, K.M., Shinabarger, E.W., and Gannon, W.J. (1958). Electrical properties of the wall of the endolymphatic space of the cochlea (guinea pig). *Am. J. Physiol.* 194:396–402.

Patrick, J.F., Crosby, P.A., Hirshorn, M.S., Kuzma, J.A., Money, D.K., Ridler, J., and Seligman, P.M. (1985). Australian multi-channel implantable hearing prosthesis. In *Cochlear Implants,* edited by R.A. Schindler and M.M. Merzenich (Raven Press, New York), pp. 93–100.

Pernkopf, E. (1960). *Topographische Anatomie des Menschen* IV. Band: Topographische and stratigraphische Anatomie des Kopfes. Zweite Halfte, Urban and Schwarzenberg, Berlin, p 599. (Note: 3rd English edition published in 1989 by Urban and Schwarzenberg, Baltimore-Munich).

Ranck, J.B. (1975). Which elements are excited in electrical stimulation of mammalian central nervous system: A review. *Brain Res.* 98:417–440.

Rattay, F. (1986). Analysis of models for external stimulation of axons. *IEEE BME* 33(10):974–977.

Rattay, F. (1987). Ways to approximate current-distance relations for electrically stimulated fibers. *J. Theor. Biol.* 125:339–349.

Reilly, J.P., Freeman, V.T., and Larkin, W.D. (1985). Sensory effects of transient electrical stimulation—Evaluation with a neuroelectric model. *IEEE BME* 32(12):1001–1011.

Reilly, J.P., and Bauer, R.H. (1987). Application of a neuroelectric model to electrocutaneous sensory sensitivity: Parameter variation study. *IEEE BME* 34(9):752–754.

Rubinstein, J.T., Soma, M., and Spelman, F.A. (1985). Mixed boundary value problem in the implanted cochlea: An analytical model of a cylindrical banded electrode array. *IEEE/7th Conf. EMBS,* 1120–1123.

Shepherd, R.K., Clary, G.M., Pyman, B.C., and Webb, R.L. (1985). The banded intracochlear electrode array: An evaluation of insertion trauma. *Ann. Otol. Rhinol. Laryngol.* 94:55–59.

Sitko, S. (1976). Electrical network properties of the guinea pig cochlea. Doctoral dissertation, University of California, San Diego, Calif.

Soma, M., Spelman, F.A., and Rubinstein, J.T. (1984). Fields produced by the cochlear prosthesis: The ear as a multilayered medium. *IEEE Frontiers of Engineering & Computing in Health Care,* pp. 401–405.

Spelman, F.A., Clopton, B.M., and Pfingst, B.E. (1982). Tissue impedance and current flow in the implanted ear. Implications for the cochlear prosthesis. *Ann. Otol. Rhinol. Laryngol.* Suppl. 98, 91:3–8.

Spelman, F.A., and Clopton, B.M. (1987). Measurement of the specific impedance of bony tissues in the guinea pig cochlea. *Abstracts of the 10th Midwinter Research Meeting of the Association for Research in Otolaryngology, #41.*

Strelioff, D. (1973). A computer simulation of the generation and distribution of cochlear potentials. *J. Acoust. Soc. Am.* 54:620–629.

Stypulkowski, P.H., and van den Honert, C. (1984). Physiological properties of the electrically stimulated auditory nerve. I. Compound action potential recordings. *Hearing Res.* 14:205–223.

Sweeney, J.D., Mortimer, J.J., and Durand, D. (1987). Modeling of mammalian myelinated nerve for functional neuromuscular stimulation. *Proceedings of the Ninth Annual Conference of the IEEE Engineering in Medicine and Biology Society,* Boston, p. 1577.

van den Honert, C., and Stypulkowski, P.H. (1987a). Single fiber mapping of spatial excitation patterns in the electrically stimulated auditory nerve. *Hearing Res.* 29:195–206.

van den Honert, C., and Stypulkowski, P.H. (1987b). Temporal response patterns of single auditory nerve fibers elicited by periodic electrical stimuli. *Hearing Res.* 29:207–222.

Verveen, A.A., and Derksen, H.E. (1968). Fluctuation phenomena in nerve membrane. *Proc. IEEE* 56:906–916.

White, M.W., Finley, C.C., and Wilson, B.S. (1987). Electrical stimulation model of the auditory nerve: Stochastic response characteristics. *Proceedings of the Ninth Annual Conference of the IEEE Engineering in Medicine and Biology Society,* Boston, pp. 1906–1907.

Wilson, B.S., and Finley, C.C. (1984). Speech processors for auditory prostheses. 2nd–4th Quarter Progress Reports. Contract NO1-NS-3-2356, NINCDS, NIH.

Charles Finley: Discussion

Question: At this point, do we know the actual position of the UCSF electrode? Is it really close to the modiolar wall? And if so, how useful is it to provide highly restricted stimulation if degeneration may be extensive or variable?

Dr. Finley: The understanding I have from UCSF is that with insertions of the electrode and followed by dissections, they find it adjacent to the modiolar wall. Mike, would you like to comment?

Dr. Merzenich: Insertion trials were done in cadavers in simulated surgeries and that's where it ended up with high reliability.

Dr. Finley: I think the question related to the location of surviving fibers also. This clearly is an important agenda in this type of work and one that will be pursued very quickly. You note that I have specified tissue characteristics as separated as dendrites versus ganglion cells, as opposed to one continuous structure. That was to allow us to assess such conditions as the loss of dendrites, where we still have ganglion cells present. We can change the resistivity of the dendrites at that point to perilymphatic resistivities and see what impact it has upon the potential calculations.

Dr. van den Honert: Have you done that?

Dr. Finley: No. I have not.

Dr. van den Honert: We found that we had difficulty exciting ganglion cells with a strictly radial orientation in the cat. These cells, however, in the cats are not anatomically identical to humans.

Dr. Johnstone: You raise a major problem I have with this whole discussion. You have a lot of animal data and yet it is my understanding, Mr. Hawkins will correct me, that in man the ganglion cells are not myelinated or only marginally myelinated. This is a very different situation from that of cats. Can we apply these models to man? I think one has to be very concerned with the anatomical differences.

Dr. Finley: I agree fully. My comment here is that the problem exceeds the technique. We need to refine the techniques further. We have tried to develop a simulation model of the nerve fiber that includes the ganglion cell and tried to incorporate varying myelinization. One of the things that perhaps I can show you later in the course of the meeting is some unusual phenomenon that we see in terms of the response of the fiber with regard to the presence or absence of the myelinated ganglion cells. For the same potential profile outside of the neuron, we can find some very interesting characteristics in which particular nodes of the fiber are selectively favored for initial stimulation over other nodes of fiber. Some of these differences might explain some of the B-to-A response characteristics that we see in the single-unit data.

Dr. van den Honert: First, I would like to congratulate you on the very clear presentation of a great deal of complex data. Given that your profiles change without lateral displacement, would it be appropriate to normalize the functions, say relative to the highest slope in each case?

Dr. Finley: Using the maximal gradient along the fiber won't work in all cases. For instance, with the Nucleus electrode condition, we really don't have substantial gradients. Basically we are dealing with a local field with very gradual gradients. This suggests to me that we may be dealing with multiple stimulation mechanisms, which differ in the case of the neural membrane in a field with steep gradients from the field that is essentially an isocontour.

Dr. van den Honert: Still that gradient has to exist because the current is indeed going to flow out of the cell somewhere. Your model has to go farther out.

Dr. Finley: Exactly! And the model must be expanded to include more of the modiolar structure. We just have not had time to do that yet.

Dr. Spelman: I agree with Chris; that was a very clear presentation. I'm wondering if you can suggest any experiments which could be done to determine whether your model represents the actual situation.

Dr. Finley: One approach that we are trying to pursue is to extend our neural model to include a description of the entire interface from field to electrode response. We will then attempt to predict single-unit responses. That is the most direct approach that we can take at this point. Sandy will be the first, I think, to comment that as soon as you interrupt these bony structures to go in and measure potentials, you have disrupted the field considerably and cannot make accurate invasive measures of the potentials. Sandy, would you have any ideas as to how more direct monitoring of these potential profiles could be done short of trying to model it through a single-fiber response?

Dr. Spelman: Well, I think you could use Don Eddington's techniques with the Nucleus electrode, at least to look at the potentials that would obtain at each of the 22 electrodes along the scala tympani. The other possibility is to go into scala media with micropipettes to measure potentials. One might try to get some data within the scala media with reference to the internal auditory meatus. You could look at potentials along the scala media, scan the source of current along the array, and see whether the profiles change in the way you predict as you move from electrode to electrode.

6 Observations on Current Pathways in the Cochlea and Their Computer Modeling

BRIAN M. JOHNSTONE

Despite at least 10 years of passing current through electrodes into the cochlea, we still are not at all sure of the paths taken by the current.

This is best illustrated by taking a common, and what on the surface appears to be the simplest, case, e.g., passing current between the round window and the body.

In 1984, van den Honert and Stypulkowski used pulsatile current from round window to neck and concluded that the current flow was initially all along scala tympani and then back to the body. This conclusion was derived from their experimental results of an almost identical threshold for nerve fibers independent of their characteristic frequencies (CFs). Other observations about the latencies reinforced their conclusion. This may be contrasted with the findings from Schreiner, Synder, and Johnstone (1986) and Cousillas, Patuzzi, and Johnstone (1988), who passed direct current between round window and neck and found a variety of effects, all confined to the basal coil unless very high currents (in excess of 400 μA) were used.

It would appear that there are at least two explanations for these divergent views.

1. The data of van den Honert and Stypulkowski are certainly valid, but their interpretation—that the nerves are stimulated near their site of origin—may not be valid; instead the nerves may be stimulated within the internal auditory meatus.
2. The spread of current and current pathways may be heavily frequency-dependent; i.e., the pathway for DC and current pulse may be quite different. If this is the case, then the implications for a cochlear prothesis are profound.

This illustrates the problem with some of the models of the cochlea that have been discussed in this volume. The measurements of the impedance of various parts of the cochlea have not been performed, so only the crudest modeling is possible no matter how highly sophisticated the modeling and computing techniques.

The technique proposed by Dr. Spelman (Chapter 4, this volume) is certainly interesting and will make a valuable contribution. However, it is only one very small part; and as someone who has spent considerable time poking around in the living cochlea, I am impressed with the variability and inhomogeniety of the spiral lamina and its changes with age.

There is no doubt in my mind that more direct measurements of current flow are needed. Possibly microprobes (tungsten carbide microelectrodes?) pushed into the various turns, the spiral lamina, and the modiolus can be used and measurements can be made with varying frequencies or pulse widths.

Then there is the problem of choosing the right candidates. In whom should we be trying to stimulate the nerve? It seems to be generally assumed that a good cochlea implant patient is one with good nerve survival—a reasonable supposition—and a bad patient is one with poor nerve survival—not a reasonable supposition. We now know that the auditory system exhibits plasticity at the cortex at least, so some of the poorer patients may well have a substantially modified CNS, changed because of their deafness.

It is also possible that the site of stimulation is not well chosen. If the bipolar electrodes are near the basilar membrane, then even crude modeling suggests that most of the current flow is near the distal process of the ganglion cell. All experimental evidence suggests that this process is the first part of the nerve to degenerate in the deaf cochlea. Hence it would seem best to try to concentrate the current so as to stimulate the proximal process.

It may well be that the Nucleus electrode, composed of rings, does just this and may well be a factor in the success of that system. Discovering what sort and disposition of electrodes are best to stimulate the proximal process constitutes a formidable task for the modeling; however, given appropriate physical and physiological data, it would seem that the techniques of Dr. Finley (Chapter 5, this volume) would be adequate for the task.

References

Cousillas, H.C., Patuzzi, R.B., and Johnstone, B.M. (1988). Post-stimulatory effects of direct current stimulation of the cochlea on auditory nerve activity. *Hearing Res.* 36:21–40.

Schreiner, C.E., Synder, R.L., and Johnstone, B.M. (1986). Effects of extracochlear direct current stimulation on the ensemble auditory nerve activity of the cat. *Hearing Res.* 21:213–226.

van den Honert, C., and Stypulkowski, P.H. (1984). Physiological properties of the electrically stimulated auditory nerve: II. Single fibre recordings. *Hearing Res.* 14:225–243.

7
Session I: General Discussion

Dr. Johnstone: I would like to start the discussion by proposing that all excitation takes place in the modiolus. I believe that the data are consistent with this notion, even if the models are not.

Dr. van den Honert: The thresholds and the latencies we saw were not consistent with what we would expect with excitation within the modiolus. The latencies were consistently long whether we were exciting a low- or high-CF fiber. The chronaxes were appropriate for excitation of the dendritic process, and they were certainly not different in the base than in the apex, that is, for low- or high-frequency fibers.

Dr. Johnstone: So the current that goes through the round window goes through the modiolus.

Dr. van den Honert: Ultimately, it has to. But I'm just saying where it enters the modiolus is still an issue. Whether it enters through the avenue of the apex or the base is unclear.

Dr. Geisler: Your data would not be inconsistent with current going through the stria and then going through the bony spiral lamina into the modiolus. So the current paths are still very much up in the air.

Dr. Johnstone: This is one of the points I was trying to make. Measurement of where current flows must be made. These measurements should start with the simple model of an electrode on the round window. The multiple electrode in the cochlea is more complex.

Dr. Spelman: I disagree with that heartily. The geometry and the distribution of the tissues and their electrical properties remain the same no matter where you place the electrode. The stimulation scheme may be simple, but the interpretation of the data based on the construction of the system which underlies it is very complex. This is true whether you are using one or many electrodes. I don't see it as being any simpler in the first case than the second.

Dr. Johnstone: Oh, to model it and understand it, I agree. I'm simply pointing out that experimentally, what could be simpler? And one can make very simple measurements on such preparations. However, the measurements haven't been done yet, and what looks simple on the surface may not be. That doesn't eliminate the need for such data. I wonder if, in fact, anybody has any ideas of what happens to current passed through the round window.

Dr. Hartmann: We measured unit activity the same way as Chris van den Honert. We stimulated at the round window, and we could find no threshold differences in our single-fiber recordings. Then we stimulated with the Nucleus electrode inside the scala tympani, referred to an indifferent electrode outside. We can see a little dependency on place. It's calculated as a slope of 2.3 dB/mm. So the dependency that exists is weak. To interpret this, I think we should compare it to the data from Charlie Finley's model. We have to look where the electrode rings are inside the scala tympani. We can't implant the electrode ring beyond the first half turn of the cat cochlea because the duct is so narrow after the first half turn. It should be possible to determine the distances between the electrodes at different locations and the basilar membrane, and make predictions of response characteristics from the Finley model.

Dr. Finley: It's interesting that there is a set of data that we could compare the model to. We look forward to doing that. I would like to comment on the issue of modeling of the round-window stimulation configuration. From a modeling viewpoint, in terms of handling the field interpretations, that is the most complex configuration that we can have with regard to stimulation of the cochlea and is one that we would like to build toward. Since we were talking about such complex currents, we have to account for all the fine anatomical detail in terms of vascular pathways and have a much more accurate model of the system than currently exists. I have started with a bipolar electrode pair, which provides a very focused stimulation site. It is well placed close to the target fibers we are trying to stimulate. For modeling purposes this is much simpler than a round-window electrode.

Part II Neural/ Behavioral Models

Guido F. Smoorenburg, Moderator
Josef M. Miller, Discussion Leader

8
Physical versus Perceptual Dimensions in Cochlear Implants

GUIDO F. SMOORENBURG

The Intimate Relation between the Physical and the Perceptual World

Man lives in interaction with his physical environment. Actually, he lives in his perception of this environment. Our contacts with the outside physical world are primarily established by way of our senses. As a consequence, the definitions of some physical quantities are based on our perception of these quantities. Light is the visible part of electromagnetic radiation; sound the audible part of vibrating matter. As a second consequence, occasionally physical and perceptual quantities are not well distinguished from one another. "Sound" is a term used for both the physical and the perceptual quantity, and so is the term "tone." Moreover, units are sometimes confused. The percept "pitch" is occasionally expressed in the physical unit "Hertz" rather than the perceptual unit "Mel" without any clarification of the improper use of the physical unit. In studying perception, however, it is mandatory to make a clear distinction between physical dimensions on the one hand and perceptual dimensions on the other. Only then will it be possible to present a precise description of perception, a description in terms of transformations from the physical world into the perceptual world (Smoorenburg, 1970).

The confusion between physical and perceptual dimensions may also be fostered by the close relation between some physical and perceptual dimensions. Pitch may be expressed in Hertz because the percept pitch and the physical quantity frequency are closely related. Likewise, there is a close relation between the percept loudness and the physical quantity intensity. These close relations may seem trivial, but they are, in fact, properties of the ear. This is illustrated by the imperfection of these properties. Loudness depends, to some extent, on stimulus frequency, and pitch may depend on stimulus intensity (the Broca phenomenon). Yet these imperfections are not of an essential nature. When we study the just-noticeable differences in frequency and intensity and the just-noticeable differences in combined changes in frequency and intensity, we find that frequency and intensity are represented independently in the perceptual space (Coninx, 1978).

The Perceptual World in Electrostimulation

Turning to electrostimulation, we may now wonder whether its perceptual space still resembles the familiar normal one. Are physical quantities and units that are based on normal perception still useful? Do we again find basic psychoacoustic phenomena like masking? Do the close relations between physical and perceptual dimensions found in normal hearing still hold?

Some quantities based on normal perception may loose significance. A simple example is the quantity "sound." It represents vibrations between, say, 20 Hz and 16 kHz. Electrostimulation of the ear at higher frequencies than 16 kHz, however, does produce a sound sensation. The acoustically and the electrically evoked sensations are not identical.

A more interesting example is the intensity scale. In view of loudness perception in normal hearing and the just-noticeable difference in intensity, we have decided to express intensity in decibels—equal steps in decibels corresponding to equal steps in loudness. In electrostimulation, however, the just-noticeable difference in intensity decreases markedly with stimulus level (Shannon, 1983). The logarithmic scale is clearly not an appropriate metric.

The phenomenon of simultaneous masking appears to be completely absent in electrostimulation. The absolute threshold remains unaffected, or may even show some decrease, when the level of a masker is increased from below threshold up to about the uncomfortable loudness level. Figure 8.1 presents a typical example. It shows no difference among the absolute threshold and the thresholds for masker levels at one-fourth, two-fourths, and three-fourths of the dynamic range. The thresholds were measured as a function of probe duration. Absence of simultaneous masking and even unmasking was reported previously (Müller, 1981). Yet it received little attention, probably because it means that masking cannot be used as a technique to scan the representation of a sound in the ear. It is, however, an important finding in itself. The constant threshold in our results implies a constant increment on a linear intensity scale; and thus, in line with the conclusion in the previous paragraph, it implies that the logarithmic decibel scale is inappropriate.

The experiments on masking revealed another interesting phenomenon. The probe tones were presented at constant time intervals, omitting every fourth probe. This gives a rhythmic stimulus which is easily recognized. When the probe was added to an intense masker, near uncomfortable loudness level, some subjects reported that the sensation of the previously almost painful masker disappeared; only the triads of probes were

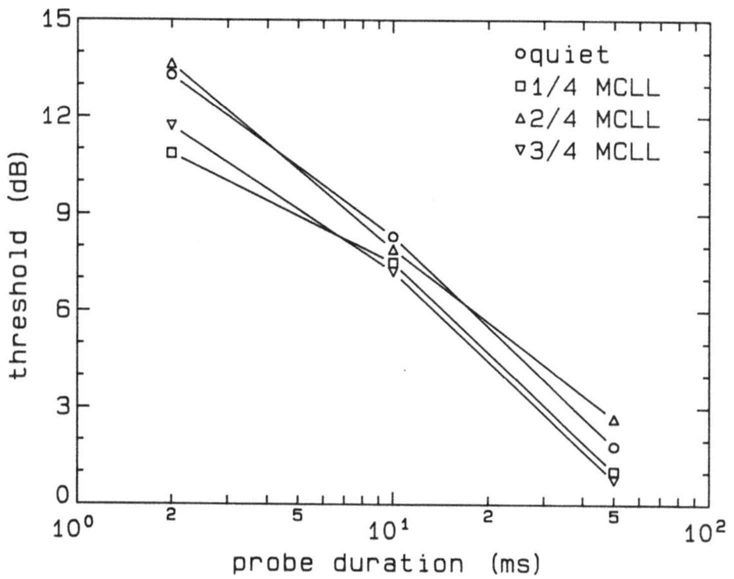

FIGURE 8.1. Detection threshold as a function of probe duration in quiet (without masker) and for maskers at levels one-fourth, two-fourths, and three-fourths of the distance from absolute threshold to maximum comfortable loudness level (MCLL). The masker was presented continuously. Masker frequency was 16 kHz; probe frequency, 15 kHz.

perceived. This is certainly not found in normal hearing. It suggests that changes in the stimulus may be more important for perception in electrostimulation than continuously present tones.

An example of imperfect correspondence between physical and perceptual dimensions is the following. When we were measuring the just-noticeable difference in duration using a two-alternative forced-choice paradigm, one subject demonstrated a much smaller just-noticeable difference than three others (Figure 8.2). When we mentioned this to her, she remarked that she had used not only duration as the cue but also a difference in sharpness of the signals. Thus, the duration of the physical quantity affects the perceptual quantity sharpness, while sharpness may also be affected by stimulus frequency and intensity. The result for this one subject may be misleading when it is used as an estimate of temporal resolution in predicting speech discrimination capabilities. The sharpness cue becomes useless in the discrimination of duration when, as in speech signals, frequency and intensity change continuously.

Another example is found in the frequency-pitch relation. When we are stimulating via one electrode, there is no place coding of frequency. This unique representation of frequency has disappeared, and consequently the close relation between frequency and pitch may have disappeared too.

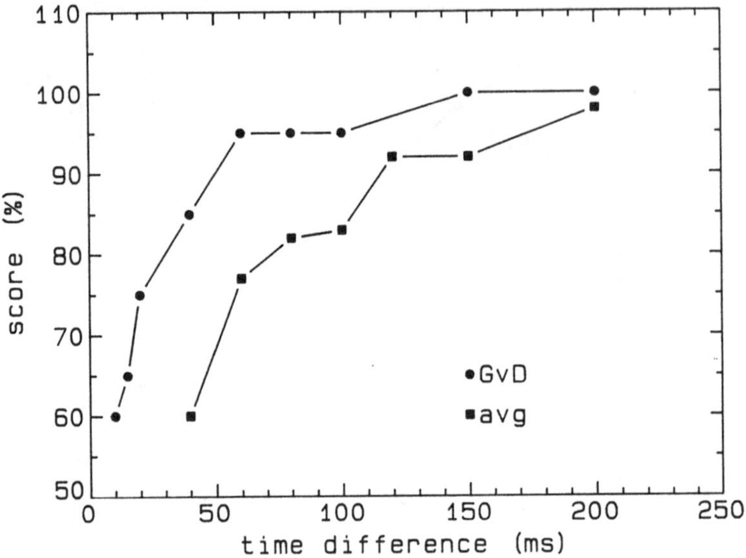

FIGURE 8.2. Percentage of correct identification of a difference in duration, T, of two tone bursts (300 ms and 300+T ms, 16 kHz). Subject GvD used an unexpected cue: a difference in sharpness.

The question of whether frequency is still related to a basic factor in the perceptual space of electrostimulation has not yet been studied systematically. When stimulus intensity is changed at constant stimulus frequency, our implanted subjects report, when asked for higher, lower, or same pitch, that the pitch changes clearly. However, at the same time they mention that a description in terms of higher or lower pitch is not adequate; sharper would be a better description. We are not at all sure whether the two perceptual dimensions known from normal hearing, the timbre scale from dull to sharp and the pitch scale from low to high, coexist in electrostimulation. In fact, we don't know what perceptual dimensions are present, and this simple example shows that we should not ask for certain percepts by means of a verbal description. The implanted subjects frequently indicate that it is almost impossible to describe a sensation in terms of the sensations they experienced when they still had normal or near-normal hearing, and the investigator may, perhaps unwittingly, depart from his knowledge of normal hearing and ask the wrong question. A reasonable approach would be to map out the perceptual space of electrostimulation using nonverbal techniques, for example, triadic comparisons, where the subject is asked to choose that pair of stimuli out of a set of three that is most similar and that pair that is most dissimilar. The perceptual dimensions may subsequently be found using scaling techniques. In this way we may gain insight into the basic dimensions of the perceptual space and their relation to the physical dimensions.

The Open Relation between the Physical World and the Perceptual World in Electrostimulation

Once we have found the basic dimensions of the perceptual space in electrostimulation, we know what sensations can be produced and how they should be produced. It is very interesting to note that we then have the freedom to relate certain aspects of sounds (the physical quantity) to certain sensations. We do not have to hold on to the intimate relation between the physical and perceptual world in normal hearing, described above.

The freedom to relate aspects of sounds to sensations may be questionable in the moderately hearing impaired who use hearing aids. The moderately hearing impaired, still hearing without hearing aid, should, when using their hearing aid, be presented with stimuli that are compatible with the acoustic signals. Signal processing, such as translation of the frequencies in the acoustic signal to lower stimulus frequencies that would better fit into the restricted audible range, may be very confusing.

In the severely hearing impaired, those subjects who hear virtually nothing without a hearing aid, and in deaf implanted subjects, however, we do not have to reckon with unaided perception. This is certainly true for those who became deaf at an early age before hearing became a significant part of their learning and memory. One may argue, though, that we should reckon with previous acoustic perception in those who became deaf at a later stage of life. It is likely, however, that this will turn out to be an indecisive factor. First of all, there is doubt about whether the present implant systems designed to evoke sensations corresponding to those in normal hearing indeed do so. We noticed already that there are differences with respect to normal hearing. Moreover, the distribution of the neural activity evoked by these systems is abnormal, even if they are designed on a physiological basis. Second, present systems have transformation errors which seem to go unnoticed by postlingually deafened subjects. For example, the Cochlear/Nucleus device projects the first formant, which does not exceed 1000 Hz, into a region of the first cochlear turn normally tuned to frequencies above 1000 Hz. The upward shift of the formants is not reported. It would correspond to "Donald Duck" or divers' speech. Third, implanted subjects seem to adopt cues in their perception that are not related to previous normal hearing. Often, they find it very difficult to explain to the therapist what exactly they do use. This, in turn, makes it very difficult for the therapist to provide adequate guidance. Fourth, the brain demonstrates an amazing plasticity. Within 2 weeks, subjects adapt to spectacles that invert the retinal image. We may expect that subjects will also be able to build a new auditory perceptual space. In fact, speech performance measurements in postlingually deafened subjects show continuous learning, even after periods exceeding a year. The intriguing question here is, What do they learn? Are they recovering their former speech perception, or are they building a new perceptual space?

In summary, it seems to me that the percepts in electrostimulation of the auditory nerve are quite different from normal hearing. It is therefore questionable whether we should strive for sensations that correspond to those in normal hearing. In view of the plasticity of the brain it may be more beneficial to consider different signal coding schemes, making optimal use of the basic dimensions and resolution in the perceptual space.

An Information Transfer Approach for Hearing by Electrostimulation

Having accepted the idea of freedom of coding, it becomes very important to assess the information handling capacity of the impaired ear. This capacity will determine which aspects of the acoustic signal will be eligible for coding into the stimulus. The bandwidth of acoustic signals is high, but there is considerable redundancy in the signals, and thus there is a possibility of reducing the bandwidth without loss of information. Consider speech signals (although environmental sounds are just as important). The signal is adequately sampled at a rate of 20 kHz and a resolution of 10 bits—thus at a rate of 200 kbits/s. There is not much loss in quality (evaluated perceptually) when the signal is represented in linear predictive coding using 14 points at 64 bits and a sample time of 22.5 ms. This implies a rate of about 3 kbits/s. The information rate, however, is very low when we consider the sequence of phonemes: at most 50 phonemes (5 to 6 bits) at a rate of at most 20 Hz. Including some prosodic information, the rate is not higher than 120 bits/s. Thus if we would have a good speech recognizer at the phonemic level, the information handling capacity of the impaired ear need not be greater than 120 bits/s. Coding the individual phonemes in different sounds is, in my view, not such a far-fetched idea. The blind learn to read with their fingertips.

At present, there are no techniques to assess the information handling capacity of the impaired ear. However, for normal hearing some schemes have been developed to predict speech intelligibility. The best known, the articulation index (AI), has also been applied to hearing impairment. Although the predictions are not perfect, the procedure has proved its merits. An important aspect of the AI procedure is that information in different frequency bands can be added in a linear fashion. To a first approximation this is also true for applications in the hearing impaired.

This suggests that something similar may successfully be developed for multichannel implants.

The AI approach was successfully extended by Houtgast and Steeneken (1985) to the temporal aspects of information transfer per channel. They interpreted speech as intensity modulations in contiguous frequency bands. In their notion, perfect speech intelligibility would require that the slow and fast modulations relevant to the speech signal be fully transferred. Loss of speech intelligibility in communication systems could be predicted quite accurately from a decrease in the amplitude of the modulations (from the so-called modulation transfer function, MTF).

Figure 8.3 shows the intensity of the modulations as a function of frequency (the spectrum of the envelope). The speech signal contains modulations from about 0.1 to 20 Hz. The frequency range considered important for speech perception is indicated by the bar (0.6 to 12.5 Hz). The envelope spectrum does not depend on the frequency band. Figure 8.4 shows a first experimental result following the above line of thought. The modulation transfer function was measured in a subject provided with the House/3M single-channel implant. The House/3M signal processor was not used. A 16-kHz carrier, modulated with a sine wave at the indicated frequency, was directly transmitted to the internal coil. The figure shows a typical result. It reveals a cutoff frequency of about 5 Hz, a value about one order of magnitude lower than the cutoff frequency found

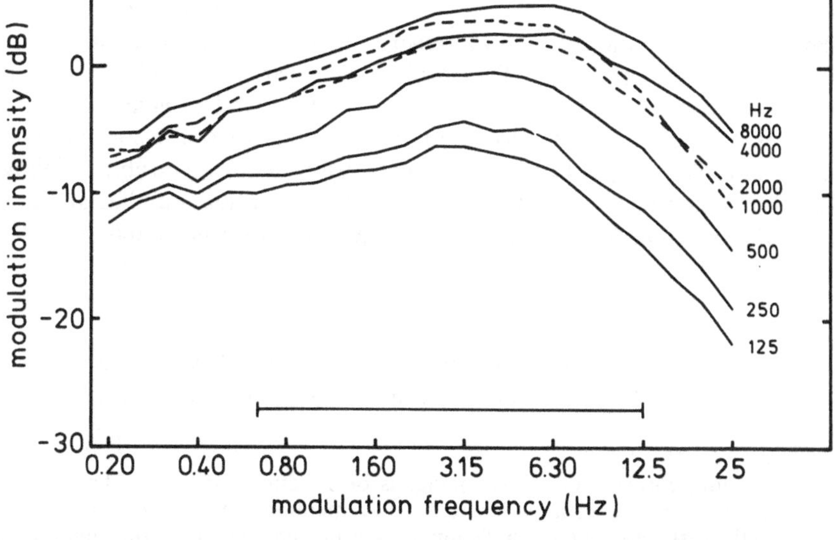

FIGURE 8.3. Spectral distribution of the envelopes of the speech signal filtered in octave bands from 125 Hz to 8 kHz.

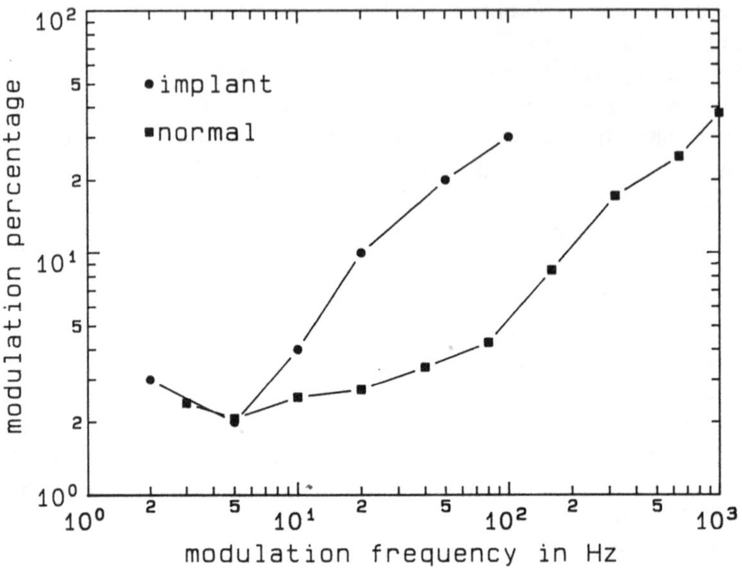

FIGURE 8.4. Modulation depth in percent as a function of modulation frequency required to just detect the modulation. A typical result for the House/3M implant and for normal hearing.

by Rodenburg (1972) in normal hearing using a comparable paradigm. The cutoff frequency is lower than the highest modulation frequencies in speech, and thus this finding indicates that the auditory system is not capable of following the rapid intensity fluctuations in speech using this type of electrostimulation. The result suggests that the auditory system reverberates with a reverberation time of about 1 s.* As suggested above, this result can now be used to determine what feature of the speech signal can usefully be coded. For example, the system seems to be able to follow the slow variations in prosodic features (like intonation, emphasis), but it is probably too slow to follow spectral changes associated with the sequence of phonemes.

Acknowledgments. The author gratefully acknowledges the cooperation of Arjan Bosman and Martin Stollman in the research reported above.

---

* This finding corresponds to spontaneous observations of our implanted subjects. In frequency-discrimination tasks they mentioned that it was difficult to perform the task when the second stimulus was presented within a time interval of abut 0.5 s from the first stimulus. The after-sensation of the first stimulus affected the second stimulus.

This research was supported by the Fonds ter Bevordering van de Gezondheidszorg (Fund for the Advancement of Health Care).

References

Coninx, F. (1978). The detection of combined differences in frequency and intensity. *Acustica* 39:137–150.

Houtgast, T., and Steeneken, H.J.M. (1985). A review of the MTF concept in room acoustics and its use for estimating speech intelligibility in auditoria. *J. Acoust. Soc. Am.* 77:1069–1077.

Müller, C. (1981). Survey of cochlear implant work, 102nd Meeting of the Acoustical Society of America.

Rodenburg, M. (1972). Sensitivity of the auditory system to differences in intensity. Dissertation, Erasmus University, Rotterdam, The Netherlands.

Shannon, R.V. (1983). Multichannel electrical stimulation of the auditory nerve in man. I. Basic psychophysics. *Hearing Res.* 11:157–189.

Smoorenburg, G.F. (1970). Pitch perception of two-frequency stimuli. *J. Acoust. Soc. Am.* 48:924–942.

9 Reproducing Auditory Nerve Temporal Patterns with Sharply Resonant Filters

CHRIS VAN DEN HONERT

Introduction

Despite the variety of electrode configurations and signal processing strategies which have been employed for multielectrode cochlear prostheses, all such devices share one underlying intent. That intent is to determine from the incoming sound spectrum which cochlear nerve fibers should be excited at any given moment. The presence of high-frequency components causes excitation of basal fibers, while low-frequency components cause excitation of apical fibers. In some cases as many as 10 separate fiber populations may be stimulated simultaneously, each with a different intensity. This spectral-to-spatial mapping is motivated by the compelling spatial organization of the cochlea itself.

Considerable effort has been devoted to the development of electrode arrays which can independently excite small groups of tonotopically related nerve fibers. Physiological measures have indicated that in cases of good radial axon survival, 10 or more nonoverlapping excitation regions may be achieved with existing intrascalar electrodes (van den Honert and Stypulkowski, 1987a).

Nevertheless, stimulation of a single (presumably narrow) cochlear region does not produce a single tonal sensation. This cannot be attributed entirely to inadequate spatial selectivity, because a moderately loud acoustic tone would normally activate a region of similar size. This suggests that we must look beyond the spectrum-to-place mapping of existing devices in order to generate more natural sensations, and presumably to improve intelligibility. In particular, the temporal aspects of neural firing patterns have been largely neglected in the design of strategies to convey spectral information. In cases where temporal patterning has been explicitly incorporated into signal processing, it has generally been used to convey voicing information (Clark, Tong, and Dowell, 1984; Wilson et al., 1987).

This paper will explore an approach to spectral representation through temporal patterning which is based upon the sharply tuned resonances of the normally functioning basilar membrane and auditory nerves.

The Missing Transformation

It is well established that nerve spike patterns generated by electrical current waveforms differ markedly from those produced by identical acoustic pressure waveforms. Those differences include smaller dynamic range, higher driven rates, higher synchrony, and a broad frequency response which is independent of cochlear place (Hartmann, Topp, and Klinke, 1984; Javel et al., 1987; Moxon, 1971; van den Honert and Stypulkowski, 1987b). In considering these apparently dramatic differences, it is helpful to bear in mind that even in the normally functioning cochlea, the afferent neuron is excited by electrical current: that current is the ionic membrane current which flows as a result of neurotransmitter arrival at the postsynaptic membrane beneath the inner hair cell. But that current waveform is not equivalent to the original acoustic pressure waveform. Several significant transformations of the signal occur between the vibrations of cochlear fluid and the flow of postsynaptic membrane current. These transformations include (at least):

- Sharp bandpass filtering of the mechanical vibrations by the locally tuned basilar membrane
- Compression of the inner hair cell generator potential
- Rectification, quantification, and introduction of noise at the excitatory synapse

The function of every cochlear implant is to substitute for those missing transformations, sometimes with the specific intent of duplicating them as closely as possible. All implants provide some form of amplitude compression. Multiple electrode implants also reproduce to some extent the frequency-to-place mapping of the cochlear bandpass filtering. But it will be argued below that the bandpass filtering also serves an important temporal encoding function which is not reproduced by existing processing methods.

Spectral Encoding in the Auditory Nerve

Young and Sachs (1979) and others since (Carney and Geisler, 1985; Horst, Javel, and Farley, 1986; Palmer, Winter, and Darwin, 1986; Sachs and Young, 1980; Sachs, Voigt, and Young, 1983; Sinex and Geisler, 1983; Voigt, Sachs, and Young, 1982) have demonstrated that the acoustic spectrum is well represented by a combination of spatial and temporal codes in the discharge of auditory nerve fibers. The magnitude of a particular frequency component can be determined by analyzing the activity among neurons whose characteristic frequencies (CFs) are near the frequency of interest. If the analysis involves only a measure of mean discharge rate, contrasts between strong and weak components are lost at moderate and high sound intensities (Sachs and Young, 1979). If, on the other hand, spike timing is examined for activity synchronized to the frequency of interest, the spectrum remains well represented over a larger intensity range. For purposes of this discussion it will be assumed that the central nervous system (CNS) exploits this spatial-temporal encoding, although there is no direct evidence that it does.

In the absence of external timing references, any synchrony analysis performed by the CNS must be based upon intervals between spikes (on the same or different fibers). Sachs and Young (1980) measured such interval synchrony for each fiber by computing the Fourier transform of its interspike-interval histogram, and examining the transform component at the frequency of interest. However, one need not postulate that the CNS performs Fourier transforms in order to extract such a measure. Very simple neural circuits can be hypothesized which would respond preferentially to incoming spikes with a particular periodicity.

Perhaps the simplest such circuit consists of a delay equal to the preferred interval and a secondary neuron which requires simultaneous arrival of a direct spike and a delayed spike in order to fire (Figure 9.1*a*). With additional cascaded delays (Figure 9.1*b*) the secondary neuron might respond to multiples of the preferred interval, or might respond only when several multiples are present.* More elaborate circuits are also possible which would respond to synchrony among several fibers with the same CF. This is by no means a new concept, as is apparent from Licklider's proposal in 1959 of a neural autocorrelator for periodicity detection.

In summary, we will assume here that the CNS uses some form of interval detection matched to fiber CF in order to exploit both place and

---

*It is possible that multiples of the base period *must* be present in order to generate a response from the interval detector. This is implicit in the Fourier analysis of interval histograms by Sachs and Young (1980). That analysis assumes an underlying Poisson process, (Johnson, 1974) giving rise to many multiples of the base interval. A tone therefore generates a periodic interval histogram with peaks at multiples of the base interval, and a corresponding component in its Fourier transform.

If, on the other hand, a fiber responds to a tone with a single spike at the same point during *every* cycle, *only* the base interval is present. The interval histogram is then nonperiodic (an impulse) and has equal energy at all frequencies. Such rigid synchronization is in fact possible with some electrical stimuli (Hartmann, Topp, and Klinke, 1984. Javel et al., 1987; van den Honert and Stypulkowski, 1987b), CNS interval detectors might be adapted to reject spike trains without multiples in order to minimize spurious responses to subharmonics of CF.

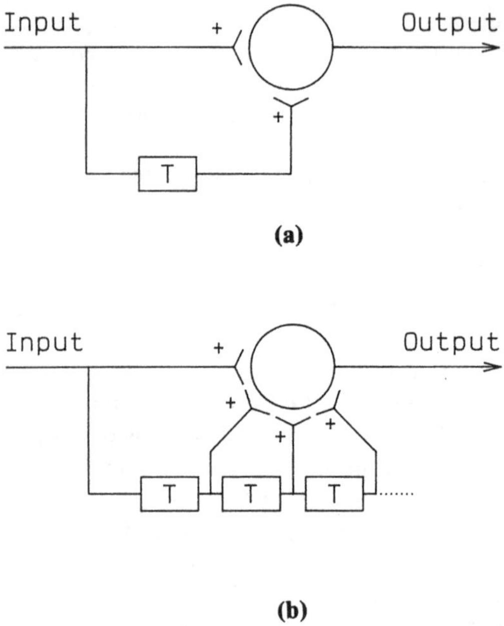

FIGURE 9.1. Neural interval detectors. In each case the output neuron requires simultaneous arrival of two or more synaptic inputs to generate a spike. Boxes labeled "T" represent a delay equal to one base interval. The circuit of (*a*) is sensitive only to the base interval, while that of (*b*) responds to multiples of the base interval as well.

periodicity cues in evaluating the magnitude of a particular frequency component. For example, to determine whether a sound contains a component at 500 Hz, the CNS would examine the 500-Hz CF fibers for intervals of 2 ms (or multiples of 2 ms) between spikes. A 400-Hz tone could entrain those fibers, but the resulting 2.5-ms intervals would be ignored by the 2-ms interval detectors. This hypothesized ability to ignore off-CF intervals has important implications for prosthesis design, as we shall see later.

Before proceeding, we must acknowledge that periodicity cannot convey information about spectral components above 4–6 kHz, where neural phase locking disappears (Johnson, 1978). No dichotomy of central circuitry is necessary to accommodate this, however. Most interval detection circuits (and those of Figure 9.1 in particular) become simple integrators when the incorporated delays become small compared with spike duration. As such, the same circuit can function as a simple rate detector for fibers from basal regions of the cochlea where only rate-place coding is available.

The Function of Cochlear Filters

Figure 9.2*a* shows several typical isorate tuning curves from auditory nerve fibers of a cat. Tuning is sharpest for high-CF fibers, which may have Q_{10dB} factors up to 20 (Kiang et al., 1965). Even the lowest-CF fibers

FIGURE 9.2. (*a*) Isorate tuning curves from auditory nerve fibers of cats (10 Hz above spontaneous rate). Sharpness of tuning increases with CF. (*b*) Composite poststimulus-time histogram from a fiber with CF = 1.25 kHz. Stimuli were 80-dB peak-SPL 100- μs clicks presented 1000 times (each polarity) at 17/s.

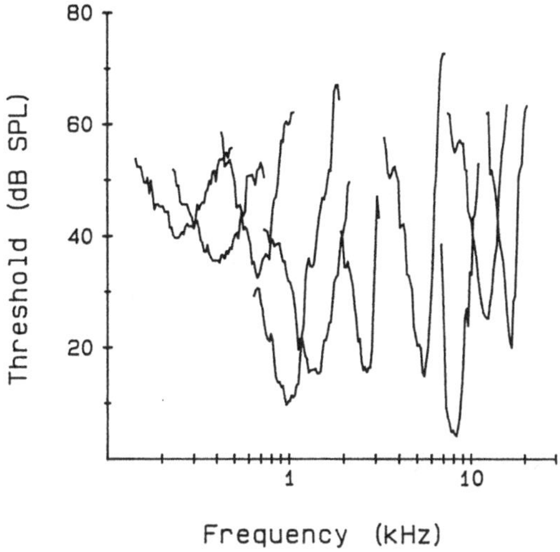

(a)

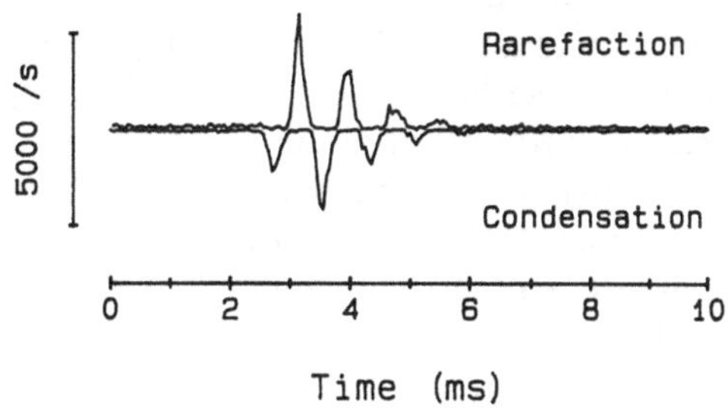

(b)

have Q_{10dB} factors of approximately 2, which is representative of a resonant, underdamped filter.

This sharp tuning is clearly essential to the spatial aspect of spectral coding described above, but it has important implications in the time domain as well. The click-evoked poststimulus-time (PST) histogram provides a measure of the rectified impulse response for the corresponding cochlear filter. By combining histograms for rarefaction and condensation clicks, a composite impulse response can be constructed as in Figure 9.2*b*. Such a strongly oscillatory impulse response is the time domain counterpart of sharp frequency domain tuning.

The convolution of such an oscillatory impulse response with the acoustic input signal tends to produce a highly periodic output whose periodicity is close to the filter's resonant frequency (the fiber's CF). The temporal patterns of neuronal spikes are directly determined by this driving signal from the basilar membrane filter.

The time domain behavior of the cochlear filters becomes particularly important in the context of the discussion of temporal coding above. If spike timing is an important element in conveying spectral information (as we have assumed), this implies that each cochlear filter performs the dual functions of frequency selection and temporal encoding, each of which is place-specific.

Comparison of Broadband and Narrowband Filters

Digital implementations of two filter sets were designed to illustrate the temporal ramifications of filter bandwidth. Figure 9.3 shows frequency and impulse responses for the four bandpass filters of the first set. These filters were designed to approximate the bandpass characteristics described by Eddington (1983). Details of the filter specifications appear in the figure caption. They are intended to be representative of the relatively flat-topped bandpass filters generally used for frequency band extraction. The second filter set, shown in Figure 9.4, also comprises four bandpass filters. These filters were designed to approximate the sharp resonances and steep roll-off of auditory nerve tuning curves of the cat.

Comparison of impulse responses of the two filter sets underscores their time domain differences. Like the click PST histograms, the impulse responses of the sharp filter set (Figure 9.4*b*) are strongly oscillatory and weakly damped. In contrast, impulse responses of the broader filters (Figure 9.3*b*) are brief and more heavily damped. It should be noted that time domain properties were not explicit design criteria. The filters were designed solely on the basis of *frequency domain* criteria (corner or center frequencies, *Q* factors, skirt slopes) using Laplace plane techniques. The corresponding time domain properties follow as a natural consequence of minimum-phase implementations of those frequency responses. [The steep roll-off above 10 kHz apparent in the broad filter responses is due to bilinear transformation (Rabiner and Gold, 1975) of analog filter designs for the digital simulation.]

Figure 9.5 shows the response of each of the filters to a synthetic vowel "eh." This vowel is perfectly periodic with a fundamental of 128 Hz, and first and second formants at 512 Hz and 1792 Hz, respectively. It is identical to that described by Sachs and Young (1979). The sharp filters centered at 500 Hz and 2 kHz respond with highly periodic waveforms to the energy from nearby formant peaks. These regular oscillations would be appropriate electrical waveforms for generation of the appropriate

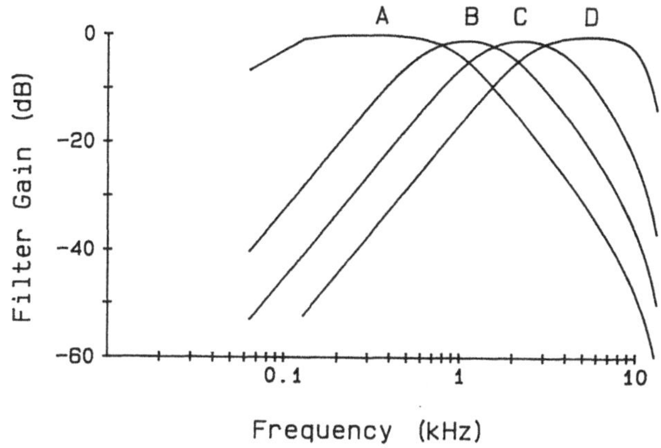

(a)

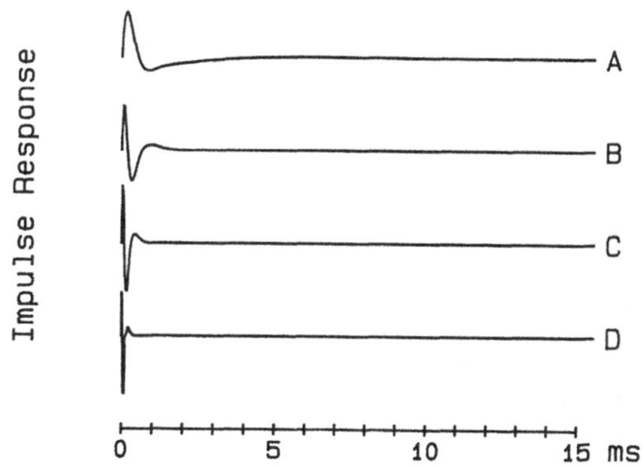

(b)

FIGURE 9.3. (*a*) Frequency response curves for four broad bandpass filters. Each was designed by cascading second-order Butterworth high-pass and low-pass sections: A: 88 to 917 Hz; B: 648 to 1792 Hz; C: 1345 to 3691 Hz; D: 2537 to 9941 Hz. IIR Digital implementation by bilinear transform with 32,786-Hz sampling rate. (*b*) Impulse responses of the same four filters.

interspike intervals on neurons at the corresponding tonotopic locations. They would presumably be inappropriate stimuli for neurons located elsewhere.

In comparison, the waveforms from the broader filters are relatively complex. Periodicity of the first formant appears in both of the lower band-filter outputs, although with less regularity than shown by the the

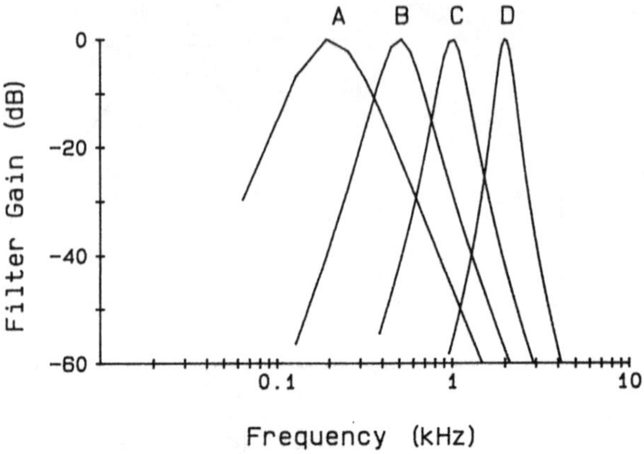

(a)

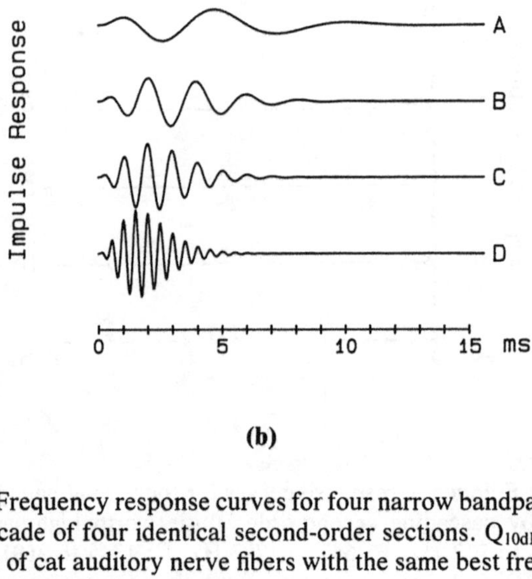

(b)

FIGURE 9.4. (*a*) Frequency response curves for four narrow bandpass filters. Each represents a cascade of four identical second-order sections. Q_{10dB} for each filter is representative of cat auditory nerve fibers with the same best frequency (Kiang et al., 1965), computed from:

$$Q = 2.82(\mathrm{CF}/1000)^{.638}$$

Digital implementation as above. (*b*) Impulse responses of the same four filters.

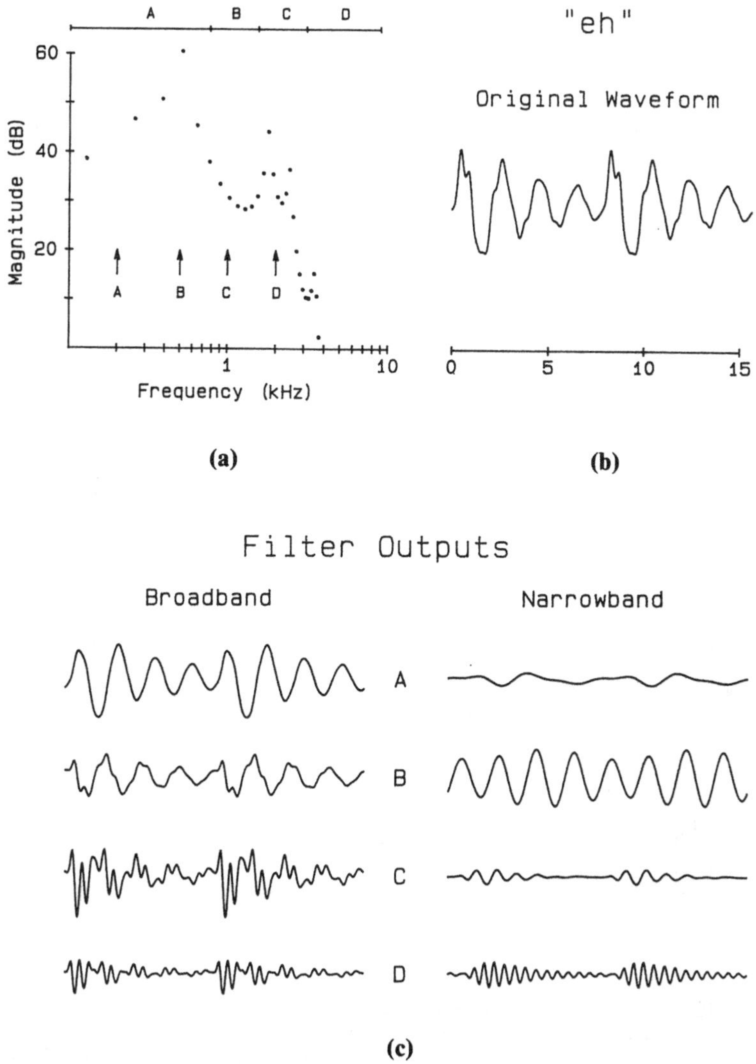

FIGURE 9.5. Responses of bandpass filters to synthetic vowel "eh," $F_0 = 128$ Hz, $F_1 = 512$ Hz, $F_2 = 1792$ Hz, sample rate = 32,786 Hz. (*a*) Vowel magnitude spectrum—vertical arrows indicate center frequencies of narrowband filters; horizontal bar indicates crossover frequencies of broadband filters. (*b*) Two periods of the unfiltered waveform. (*c*) Output signals from each of the filters.

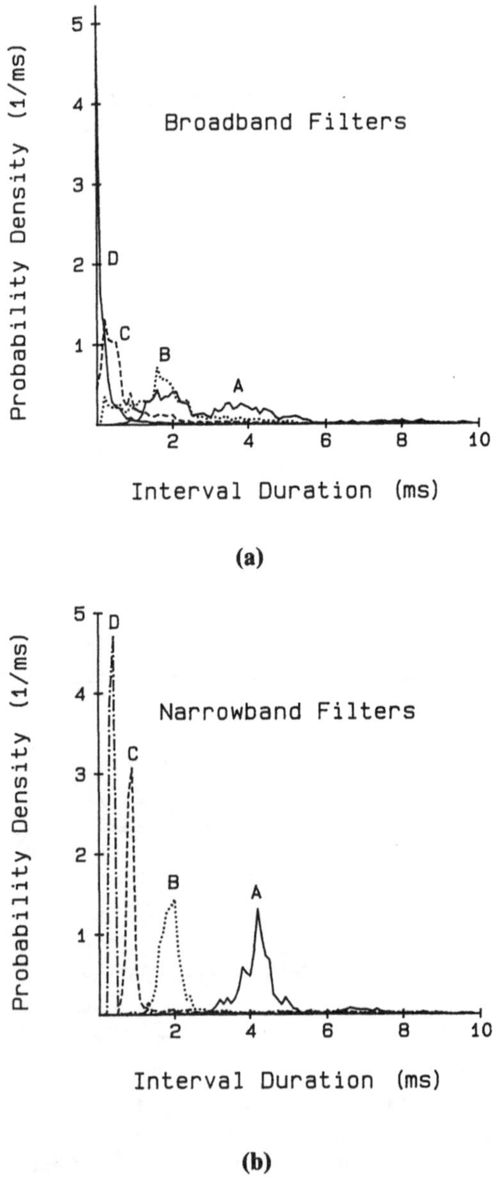

FIGURE 9.6. Distribution of intervals between positive-going zero crossings in filter output signals. The input signal was a set of 10 CID Everyday Sentences (list 1A) spoken by a male talker. Total duration = 20 s, sampling rate = 32.786 kHz. Hysteresis in zero crossing detection was adjusted individually for each filter to ignore noise. (*a*) Distributions from broadband filters of Figure 9.3; (*b*) distributions from narrowband filters of Figure 9.4.

500-Hz resonator. There is no regular periodicity corresponding to higher formants, even in the two higher band filters whose complex outputs would tend to generate irregular interspike intervals.

Response patterns to a more comprehensive speech sample were computed by passing a set of 10 CID sentences spoken by a male talker through each of the filters. Figure 9.6 shows distributions of intervals between positive-going zero crossings in each of the filter output signals. The tendency toward regular periodic behavior is apparent in the narrow interval distributions of the sharp filters. In contrast, intervals in the broad filter outputs are widely distributed. It should be noted that these are not equivalent to interspike interval histograms, because a spike would not necessarily be elicited by every peak of the stimulus signal. Interspike intervals would tend to reflect combinations of stimulus intervals. In the case of the sharp filters, this would imply multiples of the base interval.

Implications for Design of Signal Processing Filters

Mimicking the sharp resonances of basilar membrane tuning provides a simple method of implementing what otherwise appears to be a relatively complex temporal code. Appropriate temporal responses to transient and dynamic signals (e.g., diphthongs, plosives, consonant-vowel transitions) are much less obvious than those of the steady-state vowel shown above, but may nevertheless be important to their perception. Duplication of those complex patterns can be simply achieved by reproducing the resonant structure which gives rise to them in the normal cochlea.

Given their narrow bandwidth, more than four such resonances are needed to encompass the speech spectrum. From 10 to 15 resonances can be constructed between 100 Hz and 5 kHz without excessive passband overlap (Figure 9.7). Each electrode (or pair) in a multielectrode array should stimulate a correspondingly narrow tonotopic region. It is a convenient coincidence that at least 10 nonoverlapping stimulation regions should be available with the most selective electrode geometries (van den Honert and Stypulkowski, 1987a).

When only a few large stimulation regions are available (because of electrode number or sparse neural survival), it might still be useful to utilize a larger number of resonances, but to apply only one output at a time to any one electrode. This would require real-time selection of one signal for each electrode from among those resonances whose center frequencies fell within its tonotopic region. The strongest of those would become the signal for that electrode, thus preserving appropriate temporal coding for at least some fibers within its stimulation region. This approach depends upon the prior assumption that other fibers, though stimulated, would be largely ignored by the CNS interval detectors because the stimulated spike intervals would not match their CFs.

The Traveling Wave

In addition to the within-fiber temporal patterning discussed above, simulation of cochlear resonances also duplicates one aspect of across-fiber spatial temporal patterning: the cochlear traveling wave. This is

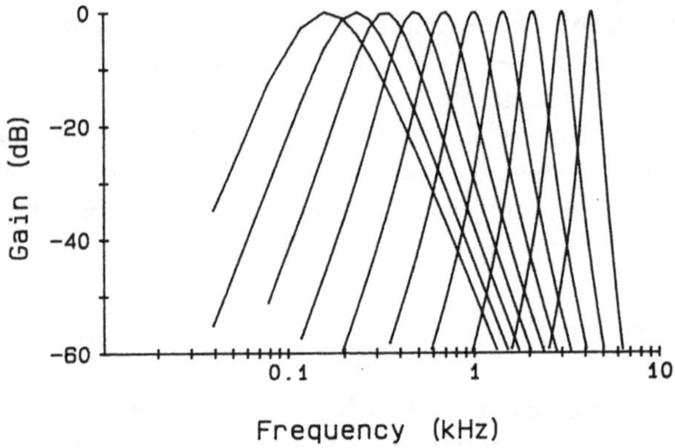

(a)

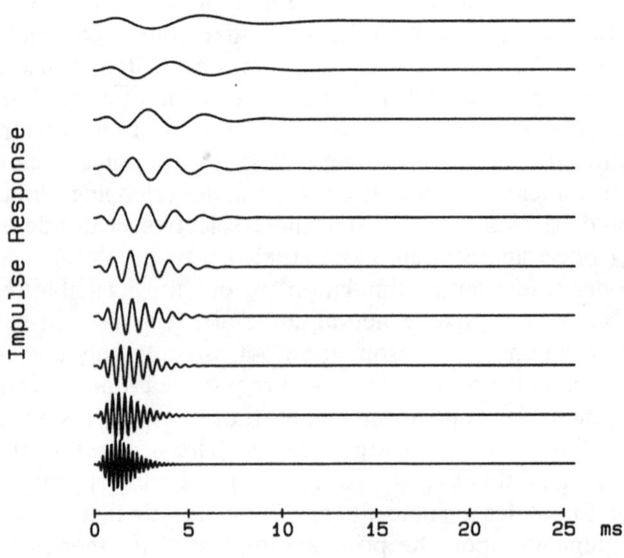

(b)

FIGURE 9.7. (*a*) Frequency response curves for 10 narrowband filters designed as in Figure 9.4. Center frequencies at equal logarithmic intervals between 160.25 and 4326 Hz. (*b*) Impulse responses of the same filters.

suggested by the impulse responses of Figure 9.4 which mimic the increasing latency of the propagated click response as CF decreases (Kiang et al., 1965). Goldstein, Baer, and Kiang (1971) have demonstrated that group delays of cochlear neurons are well modeled by linear filters whose slopes match those of the neural tuning curves.

Figure 9.8 shows traveling waves explicitly computed from simulated cochlear resonances with sinusoidal inputs of 300 Hz, 1 kHz, and 3 kHz. Each solid curve represents one of five instants in time, equally spaced within a single period of the stimulus. Each horizontal location represents the output of a different cochlear resonance. Thus the curves plot stimulating current versus cochlear place. Place has been determined from CF according to Liberman's (1982) frequency map for the cat cochlea. For clarity the continuous lines were generated with an unrealistically dense set of several hundred very closely spaced resonances. The discrete circles represent a more realistic set of 10 resonances spaced within the speech frequency range.

Figure 9.9 similarly shows the spatial-temporal response to a click (impulse). Each curve represents stimulating current versus cochlear place for a different instant in time, progressing from time 0 at the bottom. The solid curves were computed with 100 closely spaced resonances. The circles represent a smaller set of 9 resonances distributed across the speech frequencies.

The point of these illustrations is that simulation of cochlear resonances preserves normal macroscopic-phase relationships among different cochlear places. Signals "propagate" from high-CF to low-CF electrodes due to the dynamic properties of the filters, just as in the normal cochlea. This may or may not be important perceptually, but is a natural consequence of the processing.

Implications for Electrode Design

It was assumed above that the CNS uses detection of place-specific intervals to make spectral judgments, and that central interval detectors are unresponsive to spike trains whose periodicity does not match the tonotopic place of the fiber. If follows from this that for normal spectral encoding, *periodicity must match place*. If this is true, then the resonance which drives a particular electrode must be tuned to match its actual site of stimulation. The potential benefits of simulating cochlear resonances may be lost entirely if the resulting signals do not activate the appropriate auditory nerve fibers.

This raises the issue of electrode insertion depth. The speech frequency range of 200 Hz to 4 kHz occupies approximately the region between 29 and 11 mm from the stapes in the human cochlea (Schuknecht, 1974). Current electrodes generally achieve maximum insertion depths of 23 to

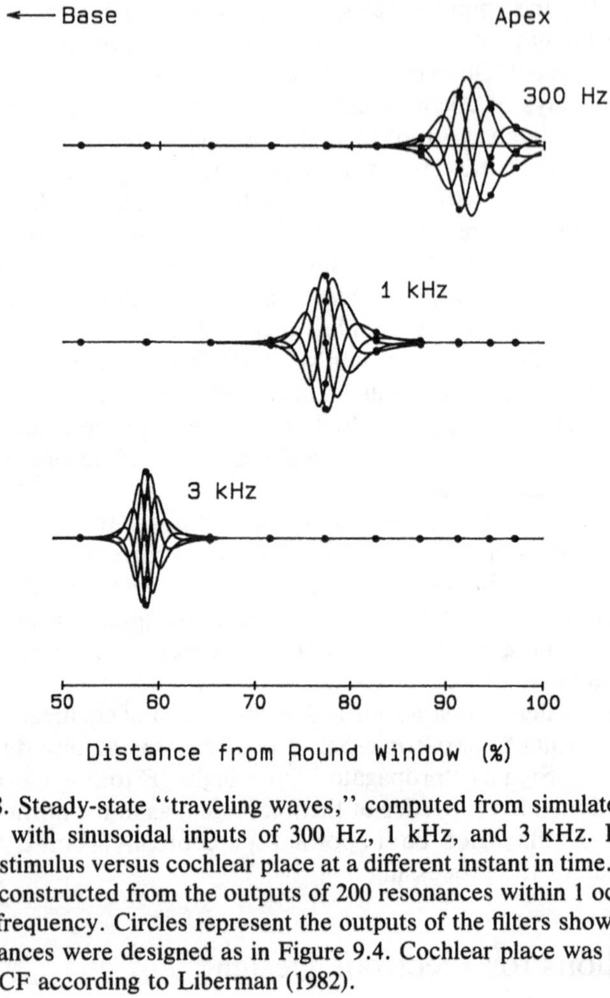

FIGURE 9.8. Steady-state "traveling waves," computed from simulated cochlear resonances with sinusoidal inputs of 300 Hz, 1 kHz, and 3 kHz. Each curve represents stimulus versus cochlear place at a different instant in time. Each solid curve was constructed from the outputs of 200 resonances within 1 octave of the excitation frequency. Circles represent the outputs of the filters shown in Figure 9.7. Resonances were designed as in Figure 9.4. Cochlear place was determined from filter CF according to Liberman (1982).

25 mm. Therefore tonotopic locations below 500–700 Hz are probably not accessible with selective bipolar geometries. Indeed, contact placement may actually be limited to tonotopic regions even higher than 500 Hz for two reasons: (1) human frequency maps based upon postmortem experiments probably underestimate CFs which are higher in the intact cochlea (Rhode, 1986); and (2) electrodes sometimes cannot be inserted to intended design depths due to ossification or other obstructions.

If adequate electrode insertion depths can be achieved, the problem remains of determining, for a given subject, the actual tonotopic locations

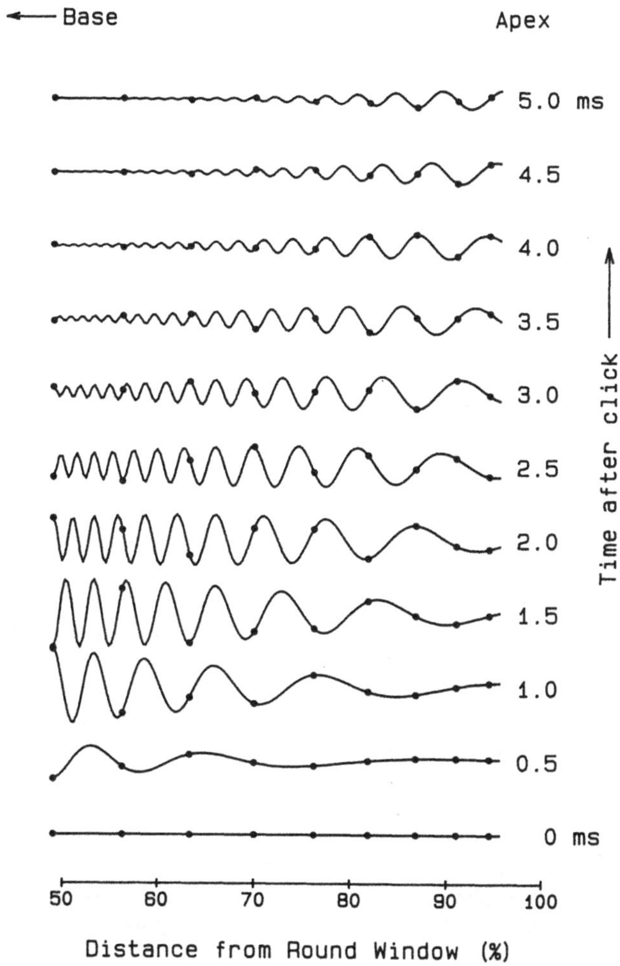

FIGURE 9.9. Transient "traveling wave" produced by an impulse (click) stimulus. Each curve represents stimulus versus cochlear place at a different instant in time. Solid curves were constructed from the outputs of 100 resonances between 231 Hz and 5 kHz. Circles represent the outputs of 9 resonances from Figure 9.7 (160.25-Hz resonance not shown).

of his or her electrode contacts. Processing resonances must be adjusted to match the actual regions of stimulation, which vary from one subject to another. Imaging technology (e.g., X-ray, CAT, NMR) may be adequate for this purpose, but it is likely that some psychophysical measure will be necessary.

Conclusion

The success of multielectrode cochlear implants has demonstrated the benefit provided by spatial encoding of sound spectrum. The addition of site-specific temporal encoding is a logical next step in duplicating the missing functions of the basilar membrane and hair cells. Although the necessary temporal patterns may be complex, they can be readily reconstructed by simulation of the natural cochlear resonances which ordinarily generate them.

References

Carney, L.H., and Geisler, C.D. (1985). A temporal analysis of auditory-nerve fiber responses to spoken stop consonant-vowel syllables. *J. Acoust. Soc. Am.* 79:1896–1914.

Clark, G.M., Tong, Y.C., and Dowell, R.C. (1984). Comparison of two cochlear implant speech processing strategies. *Ann. Otol. Rhinol. Laryngol.* 93:127–131.

Eddington, D.K. (1983). Speech recognition in deaf subjects with multichannel intracochlear electrodes. *Annals N.Y. Acad. Sci.* 405:241–258.

Goldstein, J.L., Baer, T., and Kiang, N.Y.S. (1971). A theoretical treatment of latency, group delay, and tuning characteristics for auditory-nerve responses to clicks and tones. In *Physiology of the Auditory System,* edited by Murray B. Sachs (National Educational Consultants, Inc., Baltimore, Md).

Hartmann, R., Topp., G., and Klinke, R. (1984). Discharge patterns of cat primary auditory fibers with electrical stimulation of the cochlea. *Hearing Res.* 13:47–62.

Horst, J.W., Javel, E., and Farley, G.R. (1986). Coding of spectral fine structure in the auditory nerve I. Fourier analysis of period and interspike interval histograms. *J. Acoust. Soc. Am.* 79:398–416.

Javel, E., Tong, Y.C., Shepherd, R.K., and Clark, G.M. (1987). Responses of cat auditory nerve fibers to biphasic electrical current pulses. *Ann. Otol. Rhinol. Laryngol.* Suppl. 128:26–30.

Johnson, D.H. (1974). The response of single auditory nerve fibers in the cat to single tones: Synchrony and average discharge rate. Ph.D. thesis, MIT, Cambridge, Mass.

Johnson, D.H. (1978). The relationship of post-stimulus time and interval histograms to the timing characteristics of spike trains. *J. Biophys. Soc.* 22:413–430.

Kiang, N.Y.S., Watanabe, T., Thomas, E.C., and Clark, L.F. (1965). *Discharge Patterns of single fibers in the cat's auditory nerve.* MIT Research Monograph No. 35. MIT Press, Cambridge, Mass.

Liberman, M.C. (1982). The cochlear frequency map for the cat: Labeling auditory-nerve fibers of known characteristic frequency. *J. Acoust. Soc. Am.* 72:1441–1449.

Licklider, J.C.R. (1959). Three auditory theories. In *Psychology: A Study of Science,* edited by Sigmund Koch (McGraw-Hill, New York), vol. 1.

Moxon, E.C. (1971). Neural and mechanical responses to electric stimulation of the cat's inner ear. Doctoral dissertation, MIT, Cambridge, Mass.

Palmer, A.R., Winter, I.M., and Darwin, C.J. (1986). The representation of steady-state vowel sounds in the temporal discharge patterns of the guinea pig cochlear nerve and primarylike cochlear nucleus neurons. *J. Acoust. Soc. Am.* 79:100–113.

Rabiner, L.R., and Gold, B. (1975). *Theory and Application of Digital Signal Processing* (Prentice-Hall, Englewood Cliffs, N.J.).

Rhode, W.S. (1986). Basilar membrane motion: Results of Mossbauer measurements. *Scand. Audiol.* Suppl. 25:7–15.

Sachs, M.B., Voigt, H.F., and Young, E.D. (1983). Auditory nerve representation of vowels in background noise. *J. Neurophysiol.* 50:27–45.

Sachs, M.B., and Young, E.D. (1979). Encoding of steady-state vowels in the auditory nerve: Representation in terms of discharge rate. *J. Acoust. Soc. Am.* 66:470–479.

Sachs, M.B., and Young, E.D. (1980). Effects of nonlinearities on speech encoding in the auditory nerve. *J. Acoust. Soc. Am.* 68:858–875.

Schuknecht, H.E. (1974). *Pathology of the Ear* (Harvard University Press, Cambridge, Mass.), pp. 114–116.

Sinex, D.G., and Geisler, C.D. (1983). Responses of auditory nerve fibers to consonant-vowel syllables. *J. Acoust. Soc. Am.* 73:602–615.

van den Honert, C., and Stypulkowski, P.H. (1987a). Single fiber mapping of spatial excitation patterns in the electrically stimulated auditory nerve. *Hearing Res.* 29:195–206.

van den Honert, C., and Stypulkowski, P.H. (1987b). Temporal response patterns of single auditory nerve fibers elicited by periodic electrical stimuli. *Hearing Res.* 29:207–222.

Voigt, H.F., Sachs, M.B., and Young, E.D. (1982). Representation of whispered vowels in discharge patterns of auditory-nerve fibers. *Hearing Res.* 8:49–58.

Wilson, B.S., Finley, C.C., White, M.W., and Lawson, D.T. (1987). Comparisons of processing strategies for multi-channel auditory prostheses. *Proceedings of the 9th Annual Conference of the IEEE Engineering in Medicine and Biology Society,* pp. 1908–1910.

Young, E.D., and Sachs, M.B. (1979). Representation of steady state vowels in the temporal aspects of discharge patterns of populations of auditory nerve fibers. *J. Acoust. Soc. Am.* 66, 1381–1402.

Chris van den Honert: Discussion

Dr. Pfingst: In your model you have a very large number of filters. If it is not possible to achieve a corresponding number of independent channels with electrical stimulation, would you combine the outputs of adjacent filters, or use only the outputs of selected filters?

Dr. van den Honert: Bryan's question is "Well what if we don't have that many channels, should we pick and choose amongst these signals?" My answer is decidedly yes. The 10-channel case was chosen because I think it represents a number of discrete stimulation sites that are achievable with existing technology. But I would be inclined to try to do this, even if we had fewer channels available. I wouldn't reduce the number of resonances necessarily. One approach might be to take all of the resonances whose center frequencies fall within the stimulus range of electrode A, even though it may be very broad, examine those in real time, and try to select one at a time so that the temporal pattern is at least appropriate for some of the neurons under the influence of that electrode. We've done experiments with trying to mix them together and have found a hopeless mixture of artifactual periods, as well as those of the resonances themselves. My approach would be to try in real time to select from among them.

Dr. Shannon: I don't know if there are any hard data on this, but I suggest an approach to introduce the delays and successive filters needed to reproduce traveling-wave phenomenon in the analog devices that are available. At least that may satisfy the broad filter requirements of the auditory nerve. However, I believe that has been tried and patients couldn't even tell the difference when appropriate delays were added.

Dr. van den Honert: That could be. My principle objective certainly is not re-creation of the traveling wave. I threw it in because it is available at no cost. Introduction of delay, incidentally, is by no means the same as creating a large group delay on account of having a narrowband filter. The time domain implications are very different for those two and that is really my primary motive, to try to get that periodic behavior from the filter.

Question: In answer to Bryan's question: It could still be advantageous to have many filters to choose from. To be able to select the set that could generate the most information.

Dr. van den Honert: To elaborate on my answer to Bryan's question, if you have an electrode and you are going to drive it from several channels, you must pick one at a time. How do you do that? If you divide it up into many narrow filters, you have more outputs than you have electrodes. Do you think it is better to divide it up into many narrow channels at the input level if you have only a small number at the output? It might be better. We've done some work on our four-channel patients, the results of which were not very compelling, but there were a number of problems associated with those studies. We were unable to test this hypothesis very effectively in those subjects. Principally, the electrodes weren't in the right place and they weren't at the right orientation to produce the narrow stimulation that we needed.

Dr. Smoorenburg: Is there any compelling evidence that the CNS detects intervals?

Dr. van den Honert: No, but with electrical stimuli and the ability to separate place and periodicity, we have an ideal opportunity to test that.

10
Response Characteristics of Nerve Fibers to Patterned Electrical Stimulation

RAINER HARTMANN AND RAINER KLINKE

Introduction

The main interest of our group is the establishment of optimal coding strategies for cochlear implant patients, based on data gained in animal experiments. Obviously two features of normal auditory nerve performance have to be offered to the patient's brain: an adequate time structure of the discharge pattern in the nerve fibers and a sufficient place-frequency coding. Correct time structure will be most important for single-channel devices, as it is the only means of information transfer in this type of prosthesis. Multichannel implants are capable of a certain place-frequency coding. Yet it may be difficult to obtain good place coding because of channel interaction and resrictions in the correct placement of the electrodes. Therefore, preserving the signal time structure in the impulse pattern will also be important for multichannel devices. In addition, there are even more difficulties, as the performance of any device will depend on the particular status of the patient, e.g., survival of nerve fibers, preservation of central synapses, competence of language (prelingually or postlingually deafened), and so on. Thus there may be patients in whom a perfect imitation of peripheral mechanisms will still not lead to sufficient speech comprehension. Entirely different approaches, such as preprocessing of speech and feature extraction, may have to be used in such cases.

Methods

Normally hearing and deafened cats were used as experimental animals. Single-fiber recordings from primary auditory nerve fibers were made with glass micropipetes (for details see Hartmann, Topp, and Klinke, 1984). Extracochlear electrical stimulation was performed with 0.8-mm-diameter Ag-AgCl ball electrodes placed at the round-window membrane. The same type of electrode was placed as an indifferent lead at the ipsilateral bulla wall. For intracochlear stimulation, cat-adapted electrode arrays (University of California at San Francisco, 4 Pt-Ir mushroom-shaped contacts: Merzenich and White, 1977) or human-type electrode arrays (University of Vienna, 8 Pt-Ir ball electrodes: Hochmair-Desoyer, Hochmair, and Burian, 1983; and Nucleus-Cochlear, 22 Pt-Ir electrode rings: Clark et al., 1983) were inserted into the scala tympani.

One or two optically isolated current sources were used for sinusoidal, gated sinusoidal, and monophasic or biphasic pulsatile electrical stimulation. For parallel bipolar stimulation with two sources, a phase shifter in one pathway could shift the current phase between 0 and 360°.

Special care was taken to minimize the electrical artifiact in the single-fiber recordings by electronic bridge circuits and by a running cross-correlation between the recorded action potentials (APs) and a stored example of an uncontaminated AP.

Acute deafening of the cats was performed by instillation of neomycin sulfate (Upjohn) into the scala tympani through the opened round window. To achieve a high degree of hearing loss, cats were chronically treated with kanamycin (200 mg/day, IM, over three 16-day periods) or neomycin (Leake-Jones et al., 1982).

Before and after implantation of electrode arrays, the acoustically evoked compound action potentials (ACAPs) were recorded via an additional small monitor electrode in the round-window niche.

The recordings were stored with a PDP-11 computer, and period and interval histograms were calculated. Pulse rate and synchronization index (Goldberg and Brown, 1969) were also calculated.

Results

Extracochlear Stimulation at the Round Window

Cats with Normal Hearing

In the low-stimulus frequency range (50 to 300 Hz) the auditory fibers showed the lowest thresholds for sinusoidal stimulation. The threshold increase of impluse rate (threshold criterion, 20 impulses above spontaneous activity) was 40.1±SD 19.5-μA rms (n = 35 fibers). To achieve a synchronization index of 0.1 calculated from period histograms (Figure 10.1) 4 dB of lower current levels (26.3±SD 11.8-μA rms, n = 65) were sufficient (Hartmann, Topp, and Klinke, 1984). These thresholds were independent of spontaneous activity and characteristic frequencies (CFs) of the fibers determined by acoustic stimulation. This means that with this monopolar electrical stimulation the apical and basal fibers showed the same sensitivity. The impulse rate increased with current levels over a range of 10 to 15 dB at low frequencies. The sychronization index reached values up to 0.95 at 100-μA rms depending on spontaneous activity

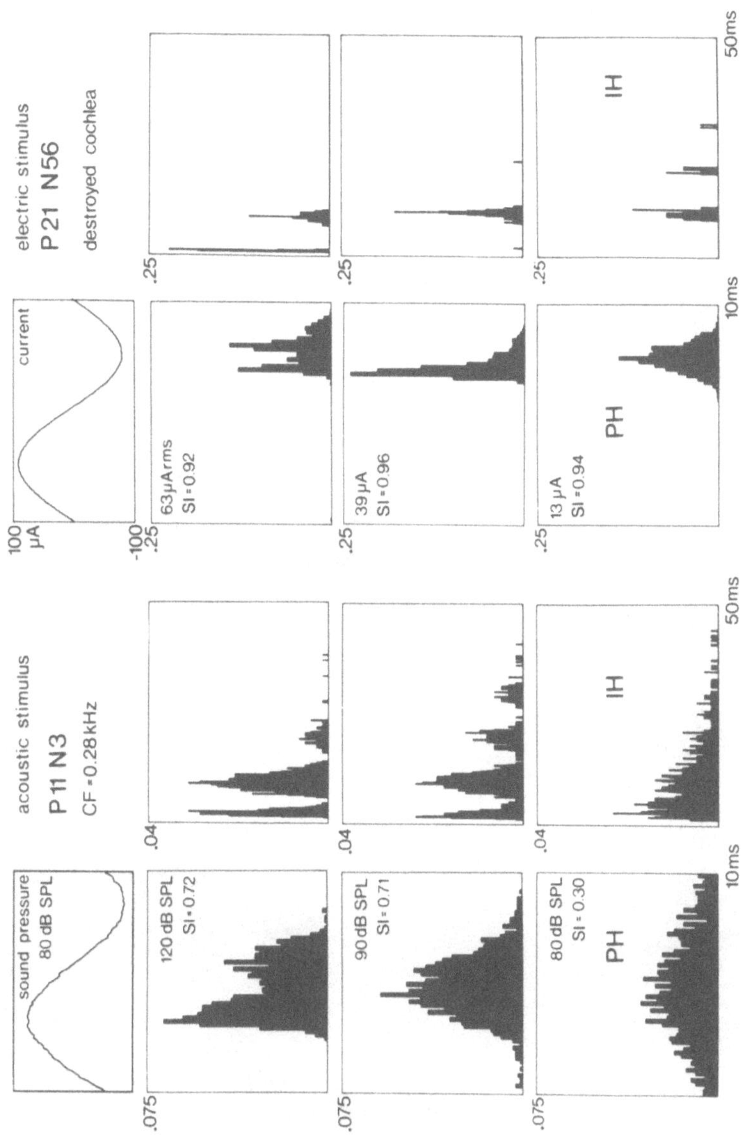

FIGURE 10.1. *Left*: 100-Hz acoustic stimulation; period histograms (PHs) and interval histograms (IHs) from one auditory fiber at different sound pressure levels. *Right*: 100-Hz electrical stimulation at the round window of a deaf cat with increasing current. PHs: 64 bins; IHs 320 bins; ordinate scaling: counts per bin/total number of counts.

(Figure 10.2). The thresholds for sinusoidal stimulation increased with frequency and in the intact cochlea can show sharp minima at the CF of the fiber (Figure 10.4*a*) due to the so-called electromechanical effect (Moxon, 1971). This effect was also present with pulsatile electrical stimulation and could evoke phase locking of action potentials not only immediately after the pulse onset (< 0.7 ms) but also at delay times

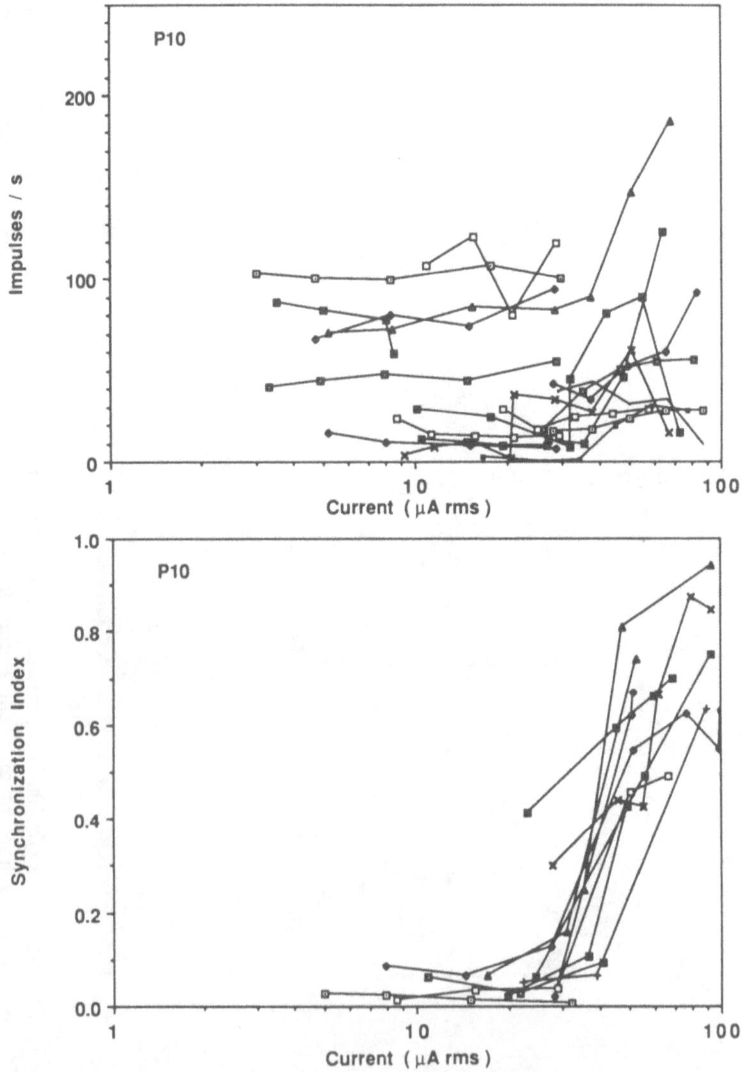

FIGURE 10.2. 19 rate-level (*top*) and 12 SI-level functions (*bottom*) from fibers of a cat with normal hearing. 100-Hz sinusoidal electrical stimulation at the round window.

similar to the N1 component (> 1.2 ms) of the acoustically evoked compound action potential (Figure 10.8*b*). It is supposed that the late response is elicited by a mechanical vibration of the basilar membrane brought about by the electrical stimulus.

Deafened Cats

After instillation of neomycin sulfate into the scala tympani through the opened round window, the ACAP decreased to zero in approximately 5 min. The spontaneous activity of the auditory fibers decreased also, and after half an hour these fibers had spontaneous rate < 2 imp/s or were silent. The thresholds for low-frequency sinusoidal electrical stimulation were in the same current range as in cats with normal hearing. As a consequence of missing spontaneous activity, the rate-current level and the SI-current level functions (Figure 10.3) showed less variability and high synchronization values. This can already be seen at threshold. With increasing current levels, 1 to 3 APs could be locked to the cathodal phase of the sinusoidal current (Figure 10.1). The current thresholds increased with higher frequencies with ≤ 6 dB/octave. The interindividual threshold differences in one animal were 17.2 dB (n = 30) at 100 Hz. The dynamic range measured with isorate contours (Figure 10.4) decreased with higher frequencies. In this example it was 4.2 dB at 100 Hz and only 1.7 dB at 6.4 kHz between the activation threshold and the 100-imp/s contour.

Cats chronically treated with antibiotics (kanamycin, neomycin) showed severe hearing losses or total deafness as monitored by the acoustically evoked brain-stem responses. In a cat chronically treated with neomycin and tested 36 months after total deafness, with a severe degeneration pattern of the organ of Corti, afferent nerve endings, and ganglion cells (Leake and Hradek, 1988), 65 single-fiber recordings could be recorded under electrical stimulation. Forty-seven of them showed spontaneous activity with low rates (< 2/s) and an irregular firing pattern. High spontaneous rates (up to 126/s) with regular intervals or double and triple spiking were also found. Despite the severity of the cochlea damage, 5 fibers responded to acoustic stimulation in the 1–3-kHz region with sound pressure levels above 100-dB SPL. Figure 10.5 shows the current thresholds of all investigated neurons. Because it was impossible to activate most of the fibers with sound stimuli, some vestibular fibers could be present in this sample. As previously has been shown (Hartmann, Topp, and Klinke, 1984), vestibular fibers have electrical thresholds that are similar to those of auditory fibers; and in this particular cat, the structure of the auditory nerve was degenerated to such an extent that histological controls of the recording tracks were inconclusive.

The synchronization of action potentials of auditory fibers from acutely deafened cats was measured with the running cross-correlation technique from 50 Hz to 12.8 kHz. The synchronization indices were calculated

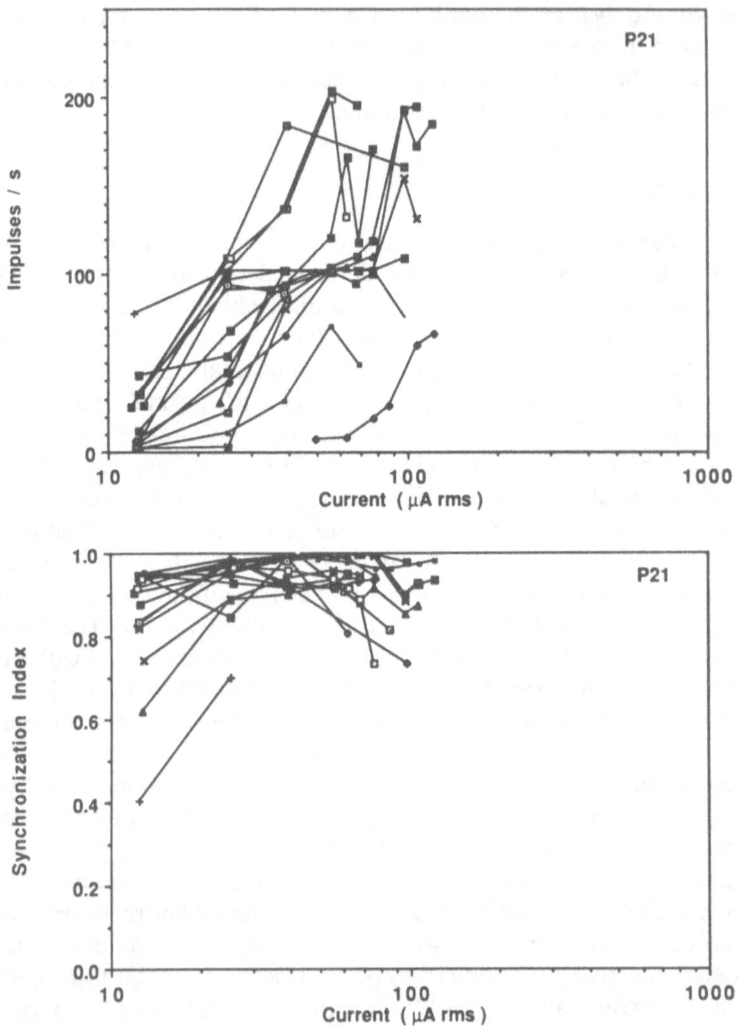

FIGURE 10.3. 21 rate-level (*top*) and 23 SI-level functions (*bottom*) from an acutely deafened cat. 100-Hz sinusoidal electrical stimulation at the round window.

from the period histograms at current levels 3 dB above threshold. Figure 10.6 shows the electrical sychronization versus frequency in comparison to the maximum values of acoustically achieved phase locking in a cat with normal hearing. The maximum electrically evoked synchronization is higher than the acoustically evoked one, expecially in the high-frequency range. Figure 10.7 shows the synchronization of APs to gated sinusoidal currents (3 dB above threshold) at different frequencies.

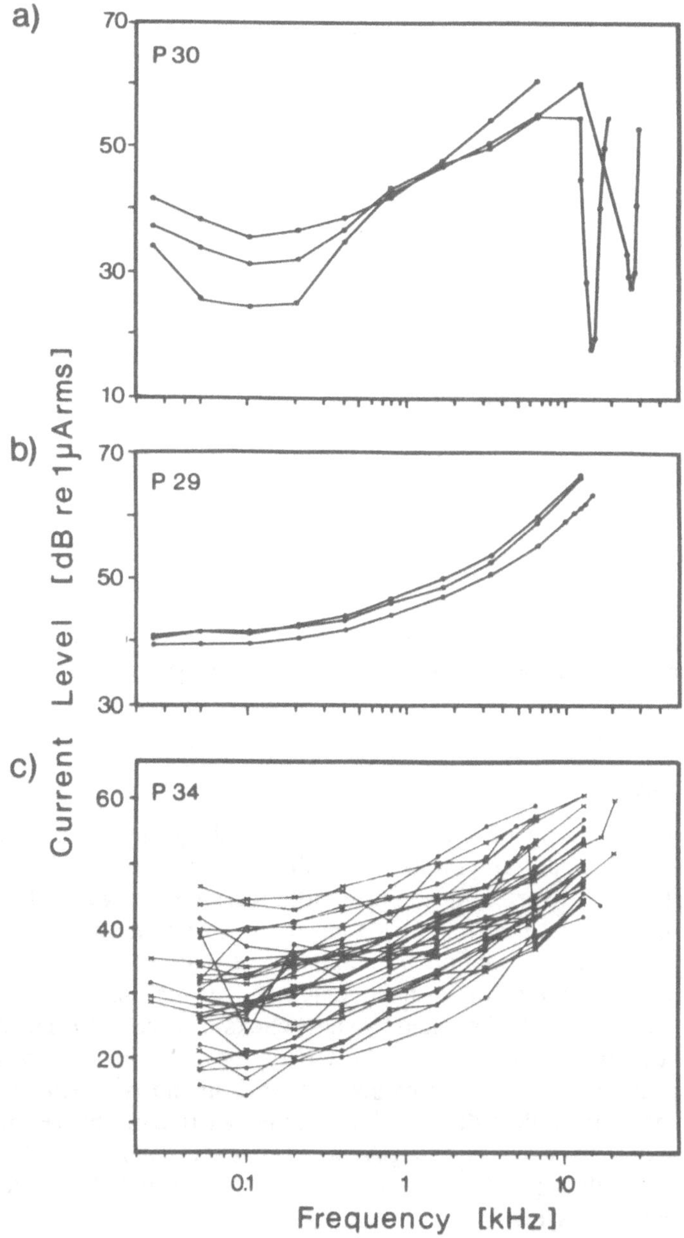

FIGURE 10.4. (*a*) Three single-fiber threshold current levels obtained with sinusoidal electrical round-window stimulation of a cat with normal hearing thresholds. (*b*) Three single-fiber threshold current levels from an acutely deafened cat. (*c*) Thirty-one single-fiber threshold current levels recorded from the VIIIth nerve of a deaf cat (chronically treated with neomycin sulfate 50 mg/kg daily, IM) 36 months after ABR; threshold > 100-dB SPL. Sixteen threshold functions from spontaneous active fibers (×——×); fifteen from nonspontaneously firing fibers (○——○).

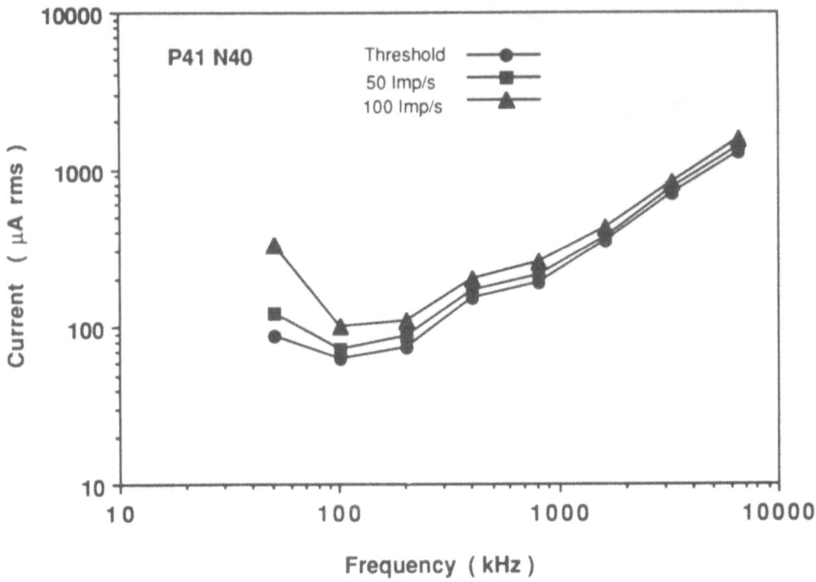

FIGURE 10.5. Isorate contours from one auditory fiber of an acutely deafened cat. Sinusoidal electrical stimulation at the round window. Threshold = 20 imp/s.

Pulse Stimuli

The synchronization of action potentials by short electrical pulses depends on the current amplitude, pulse duration, polarity, and interpulse delay. Thresholds for biphasic pulses (0.2 ms/phase, negative first, 10/s repetition rate) were 60 to 350 μA pp in cats with normal hearing. As already stated above, action potentials were elicited either with short latencies (0.3–0.6 ms) or with latencies (> 1.0 ms) similar to the N1 component of the ACAP evoked by short clicks (Figure 10.8). The latency of this later peak depended on the CF of the fiber. In deafened cats, however, only short latency peaks appeared in the post stimulus-time histograms. Threshold values for biphasic pulses (0.2 ms/phase, negative first) reached from 67 to 600 μA pp. The synchronization of APs to pulsatile stimuli depended on the current strength and the presence of spontaneous activity. In the case of an acutely deafened cat without spontaneous activity, every superthreshold current pulse was followed by an AP if the pulse interval between two pulses was longer than 2 ms. Double-pulse stimulation (repetition rate 33/s) in this case led to a 100% synchronization of the APs to both leading and second pulse if the pulse delay was not shorter than 1.5 ms (Figure 10.9). With a 1.3-ms delay, only 76% of the second pulses were followed by an AP; and with a 1-ms delay, no second APs were evoked.

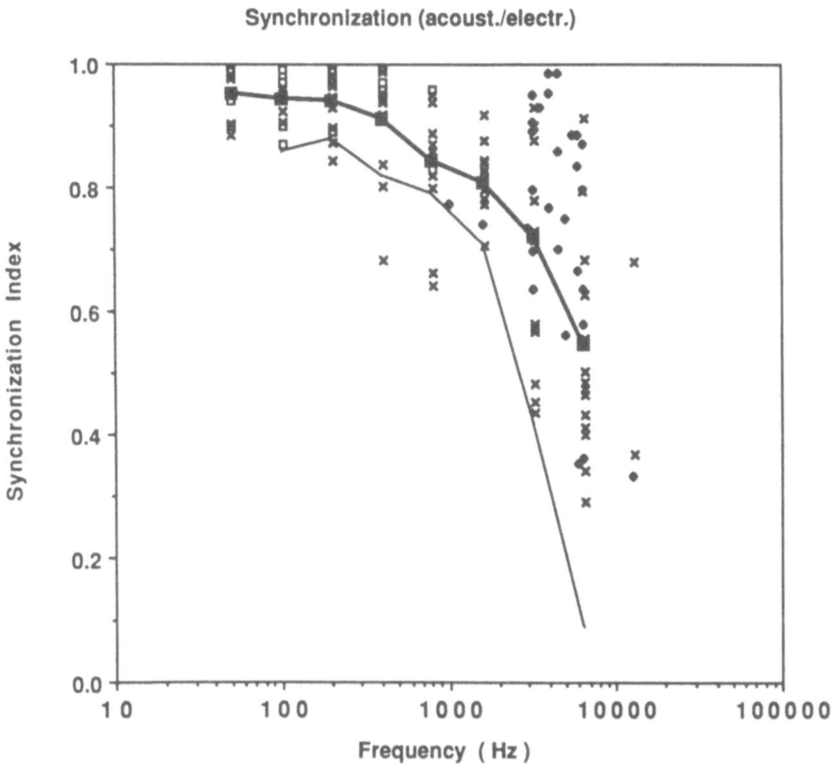

FIGURE 10.6. Synchronization indices (scatter) calculated from PHs from 54 single-fiber registrations from 3 acutely deafened cats with sinusoidal electrical stimulation (3 dB > threshold) at the round window. *Heavy line:* SI mean value of the scatter. *Thin line:* Maximum SI—values obtained with acoustical sinusoidal stimulation in the CF region of fibers from a cat with normal hearing thresholds.

Intracochlear Stimulation

Single-Channel Stimulation

The opening of the round window in a cat with normal hearing thresholds does not normally cause a decrease in the ACAP. The insertion of an electrode array in the first half of the basal turn of the cochlea, however, led to a threshold elevation of 40 dB. The remaining frequency responses of the fibers to 50-ms sinusoidal tone bursts were no longer sharply tuned. There was always a low-frequency response, but tuning curve tips at frequencies over 5 kHz were never found.

Rate-current level functions were measured with 100-Hz sinusoidal stimulation using different electrode combinations. An electrode array with four mushroom-shaped contacts (Merzenich and White, 1977) em-

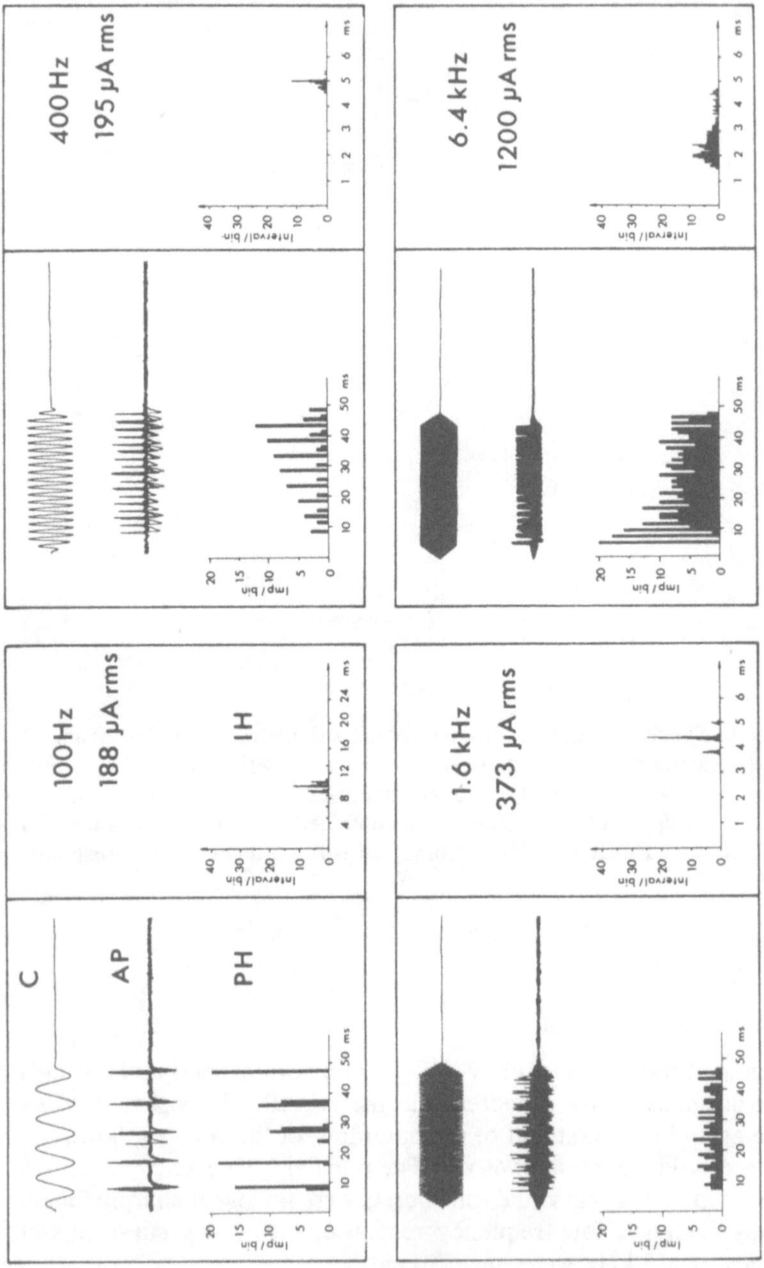

FIGURE 10.7. Current (C), 10 superimposed original recordings of action potentials (APs), period histograms (PHs), and interval histograms (IHs) during sinusoidal electrical burst stimulation at the round window of an acutely deafened cat 3 dB above threshold. Current bursts: Duration 50 ms, ramp 5 ms, repetition rate 10/s.

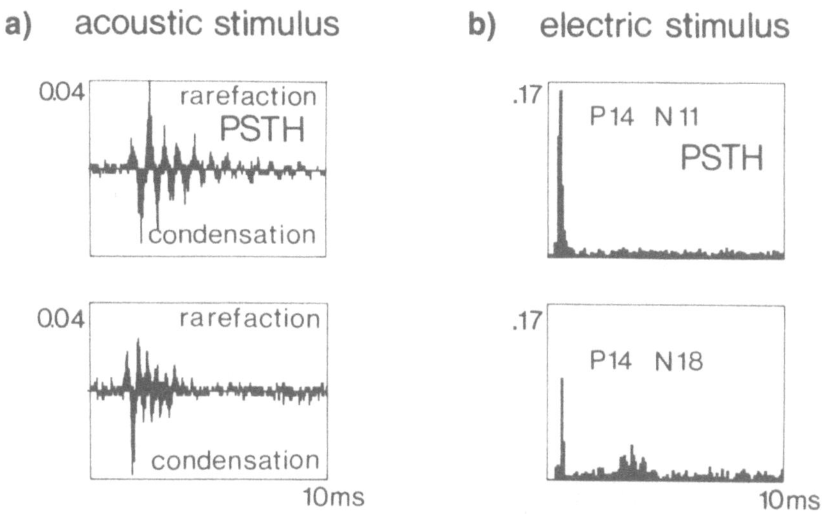

FIGURE 10.8. (*a*) Normalized compound poststimulus-time histograms (PSTHs) to acoustic click stimulation (1.3 N/m^2pp, 100 μs) from two fibers with different CF of cat P14 with normal hearing threshold. (*b*) Normalized PSTHs evoked by pulsatile electrical stimulation at the round window of the same cat. Current 150 μApp, 100 μs, monophasic AC-coupled, repetition rate 33/s.

bedded in silastic carrier was inserted in the first half turn of a cat cochlea. The shape of the rate functions was similar for monopolar and bipolar stimulation. The thresholds for bipolar stimulation were about 14 dB higher than for the monopolar configuration (Figure 10.10). Similar results were obtained with human-type electrode arays Vienna, 8 Pt-Ir ball electrodes; Melbourne, 22 Pt-Ir ring electrodes in silastic carrier. The necessary current level to activate a fiber depends on the electrode configuration (shape, silastic embedding, monopolar/bipolar, longitudinal/radial, distance between the electrodes), the place inside the scala tympani, and the origin of the auditory fiber in the cochlea duct. To measure the effect of electrode position in the cochlea on the threshold current, the current level which evoked an impulse rate of 20/s above spontaneous rate was used. Figure 10.11 shows that with increasing distance between the electrodes, the thresholds for bipolar 100-Hz stimulation decreased. The thresholds for monpolar stimulation (indifferent electrode outside the cochlea) were lower for the most apical electrodes and increased slightly to the basal electrodes. The mean slope of these functions was 1.7 dB/mm, or 5.8 dB/octave as calculated from Liberman's (1982) map of the cat cochlea. The thresholds for bipolar stimulation of electrode pairs were in this case about 20 dB higher, and

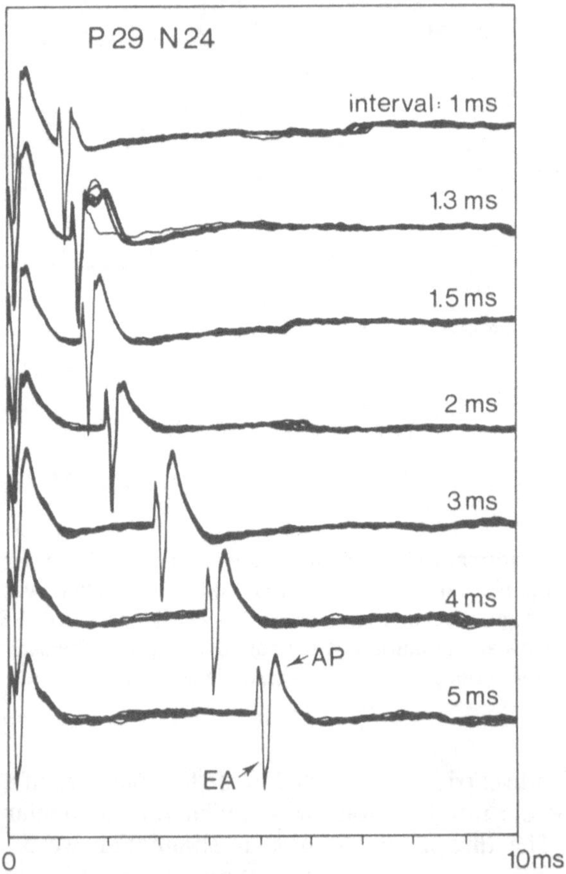

FIGURE 10.9. Original recordings (each row shows 10 superimposed sweeps) with action potentials (APs) and electrical artifact (EA) from electrical double-pulse stimulation at the round window of an acutely deafened cat. Pulses: Biphasic (negative first) 2000 mA_{pp}, 100 μs/phase, repetition rate 10/s.

FIGURE 10.10. Impulse rate-current functions from four single fibers from four different cats during single-channel electrical stimulation inside the scala tympani at different locations. 100-Hz monopolar sinusoidal stimulation with electrode 1,2,..., 6 (electrode 1 most apical) against the extracochlear indifferent electrode and bipolar stimulation with electrode pairs 1/2, 3/4, and 5/6. P35: Cat electrode (San Francisco type). Interelectrode distance: 1.2 mm; distance from electrode 1 to round window: 5 mm. P44: Human electrode (Vienna type). Interelectrode distance 1-2: 1.5 mm, 2-3: 2.5 mm, 3–4: 1.5 mm; distance from electrode 1 to round window: 6 mm. P37: Human electrode (Melbourne type). Interelectrode distance: 0.75 mm; distance from electrode 1 to round window: 5.3 mm. P48: Human electrode (Melbourne type). Distance from electrode 1 to round window: 7.5 mm.

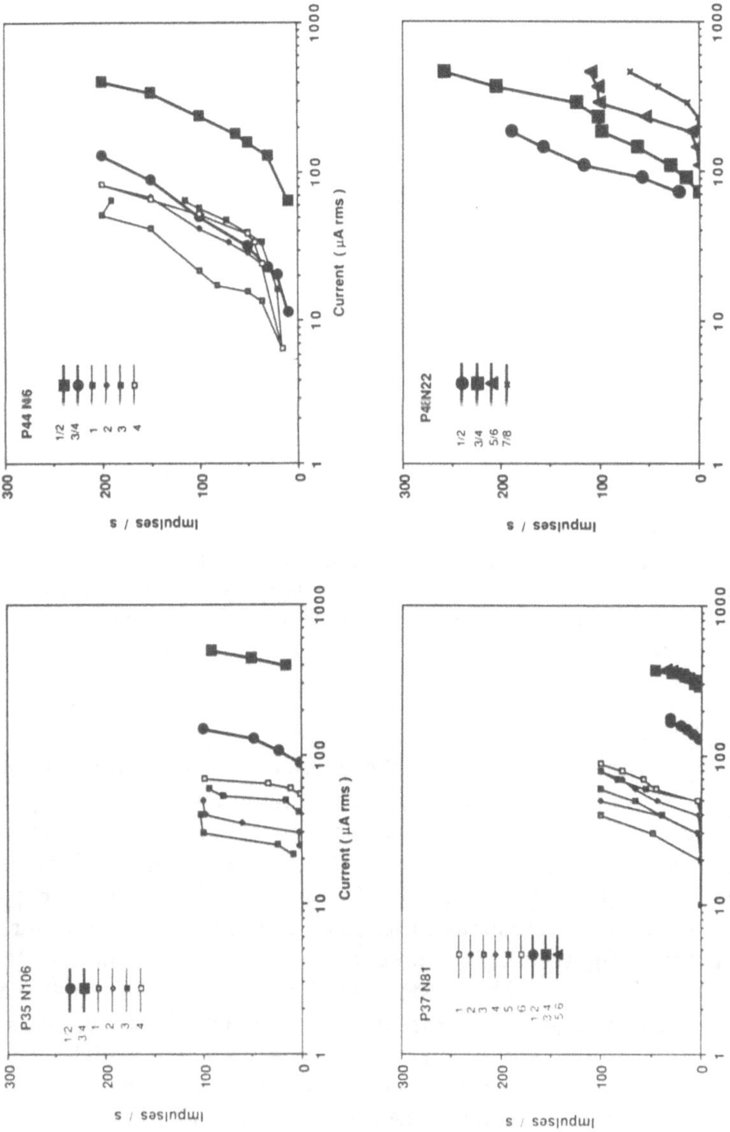
P44 N6
P35 N106
P37 N81
Impulses / s
Current (μA rms)

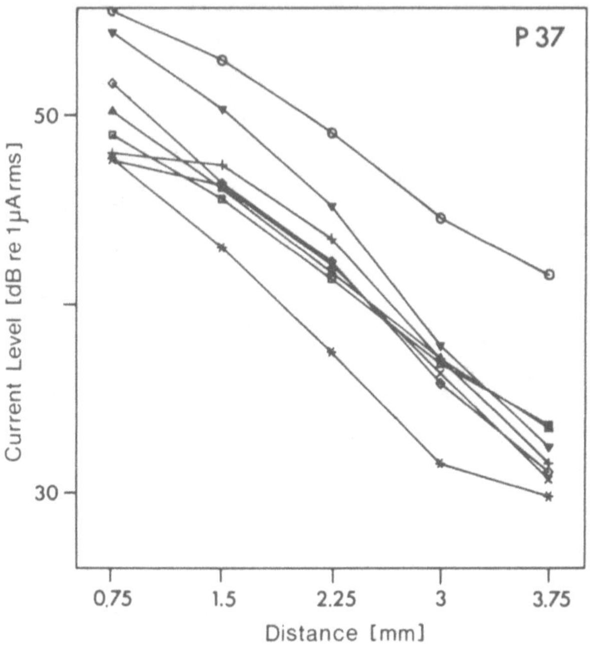

FIGURE 10.11. Eight single-fiber threshold current levels (re 1-μA rms) and mean value (symbols) for 100-Hz sinusoidal bipolar stimulation with different electrode spacing using a Melbourne electrode array inserted in the first turn of a cat scala tympani (see Figure 10.10).

the mean slope of the steepest part of these functions was 3.3 dB/mm, or 11.1 dB/octave (Figure 10.12). These functions showed no V-shaped threshold minimum at a distinct stimulation place, because the electrode array could not be inserted deeply enough to reach the optimum place for these fibers. Such an optimal place could be obtained in another experiment, and the bipolar threshold functions from these two cats were plotted together (Figure 10.13). Three of these functions showed V-shaped threshold curves, with the steepest slopes of 12.8 dB/mm at the high- and 4.3 dB/mm at the low-frequency side. On the other hand, threshold variance within the fibers from one cochlea is high. The maximum threshold differences found in one cat between different fibers stimulated at the optimal place was 19 dB (see Figure 10.13).

Multichannel Stimulation

To measure the channel interaction between adjacent electrode pairs, two channels were stimulated parallel via two independent optically isolated current sources. The inputs were connected to the same signal generator,

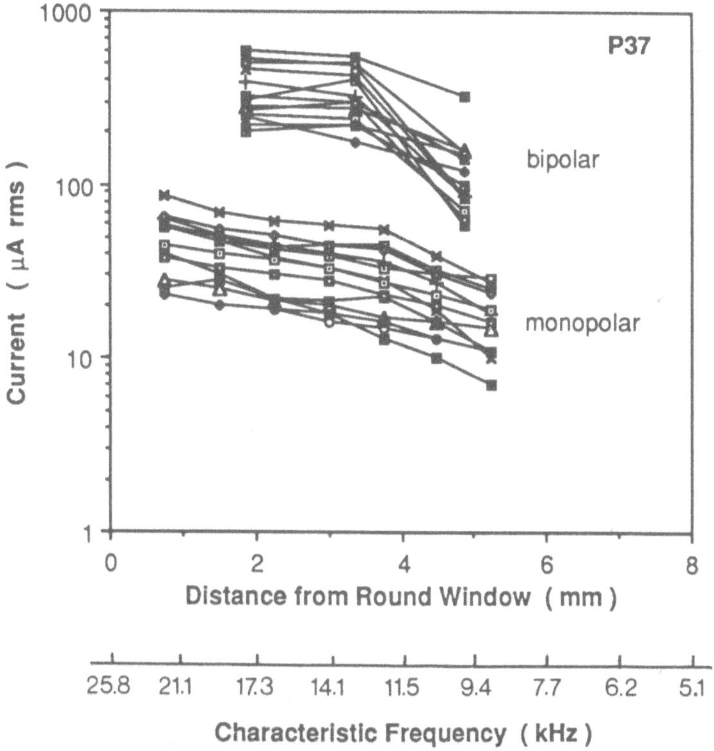

FIGURE 10.12. Single-fiber threshold currents with 100-Hz sinusoidal bipolar and monopolar stimulation (Melbourne electrode; for configuration see P37 Figure 10.10) at different locations inside the first turn of the cat cochlea. Frequency-distance scale calculated from Liberman's formula (Liberman, 1982).

but with a phase shifter in one pathway. In the first step the rate-current level functions of the same neuron were determined with stimulation at the different channels (Figure 10.14). Subsequently, for the two-channel parallel stimulation a current level, which gave sufficient activation of the fiber, was chosen for each channel. Depending on the location of the two channels and the phase between the currents, the impulse rate increased or decreased because of the interaction (Figure 10.15). In the neurons illustrated in Figure 10.15, the more sensitive apical channel 1/2 together with 3/4 showed higher modulations of the rate-phase functions than channel 3/4 together with the insensitive basal channel 5/6.

This channel interaction can be explained by the hypothesis that the current densities of both sources interact at the excitable membrane of this neuron. Assuming a linear superposition of the current density vectors at this place, a simple model with complex transfer functions a_{mn} for the

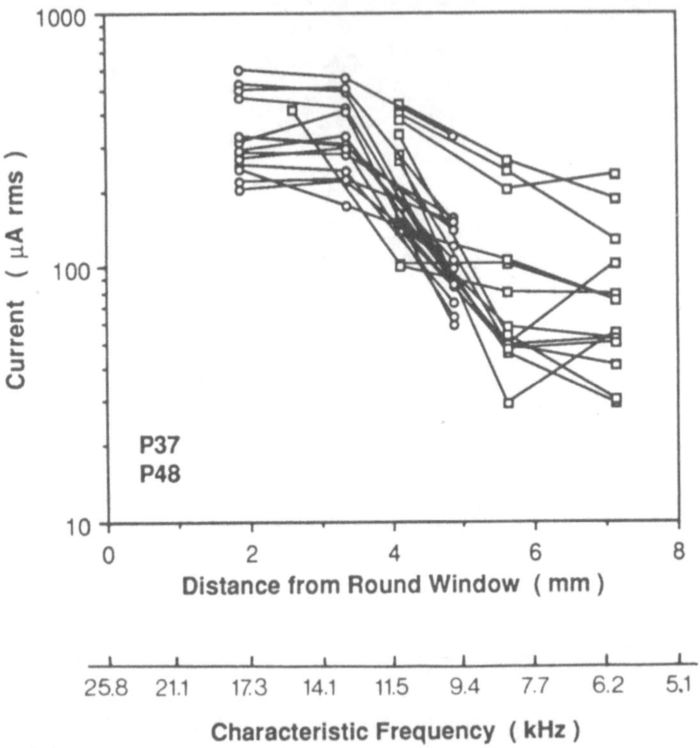

FIGURE 10.13. Single-fiber threshold currents from two cats (P37 ○——○, P48 □——□) obtained with bipolar 100-Hz sinusoidal stimulation of adjacent electrode pairs (Melbourne electrode, see Figure 10.10) at different locations inside the scala tympani.

different current pathways and a neuronal membrane model with a saturation function for the rate-current density relation explain the measured data sufficiently (Figure 10.16). The gain of the transfer functions could be determined from the difference of the individual rate-current level functions from each channel and the phase from the rate-phase relations from the two-channel parallel stimulation experiments. Figure 10.17 shows a comparison of a measured modulation function and the model's rate fuction for the two channels 1/2 and 3/4.

These data show that in cochlear implants with true bipolar stimulation inside the cochlea, a place-dependent stimulation of auditory nerve fibers is possible. On the other hand, there is also a strong channel interaction during parallel stimulation if the distance of the channels is of the same order as the distance between the stimulated electrode pairs.

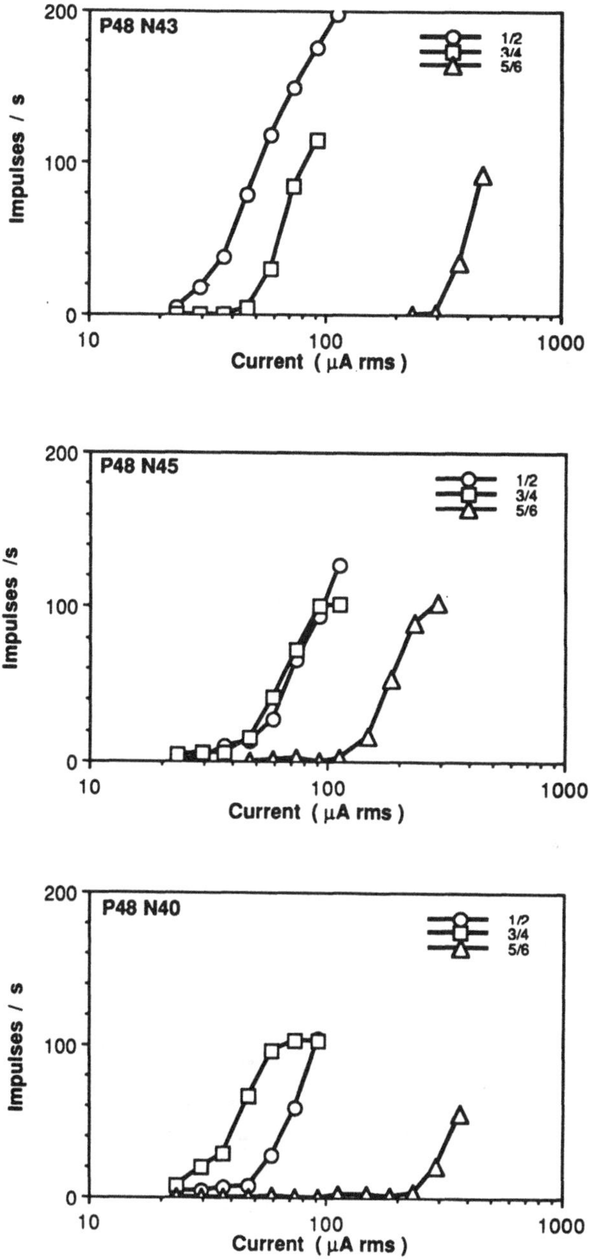

FIGURE 10.14. Channel sensitivity of single-fiber impulse rate functions to 100-Hz single-channel bipolar stimulation with different electrode pairs (Melbourne electrode, see Figures 10.10 and 10.15).

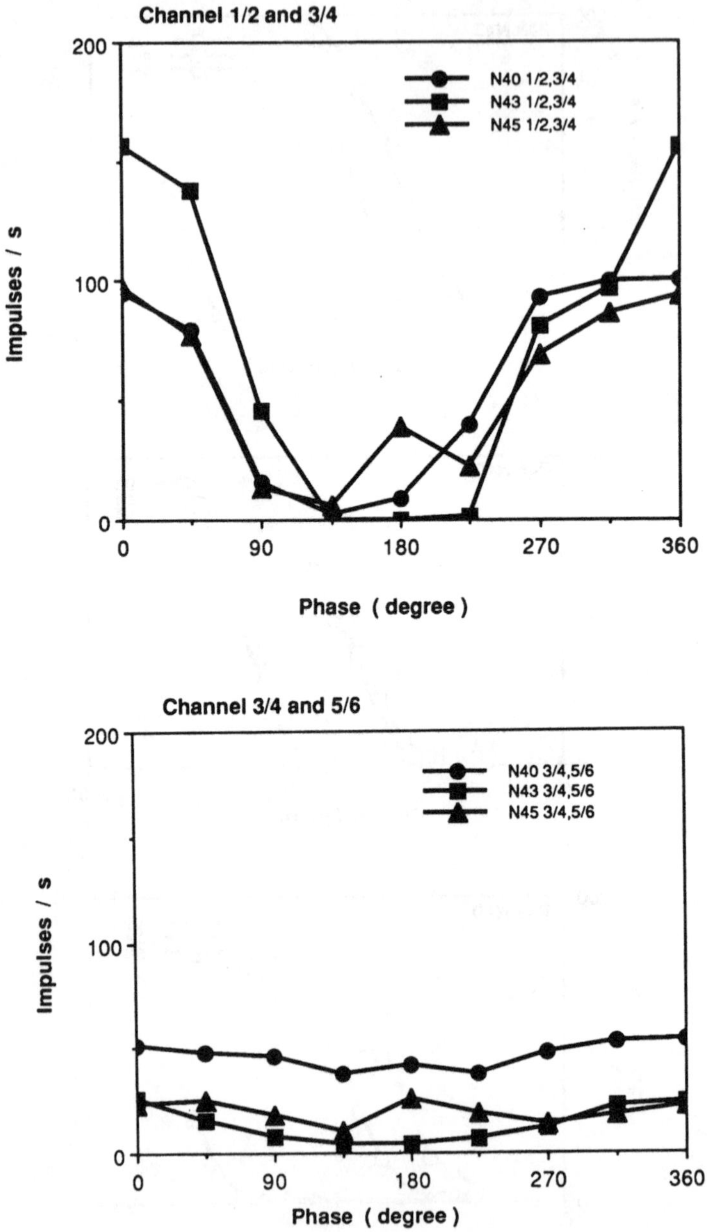

FIGURE 10.15. *Top:*Impulse rate functions from three fibers from Figure 10.14 during 100-Hz sinusoidal electrical stimulation (Melbourne electrode, see Figures 10.10 and 10.14). Parallel stimulation with two current sources of electrode pairs $\frac{1}{2}$ (apical) and $\frac{3}{4}$ at different phase shifts between the currents. *Bottom:* Rate functions of the same fibers with parallel stimulation of electrode pairs $\frac{3}{4}$ and $\frac{5}{6}$ (basal).

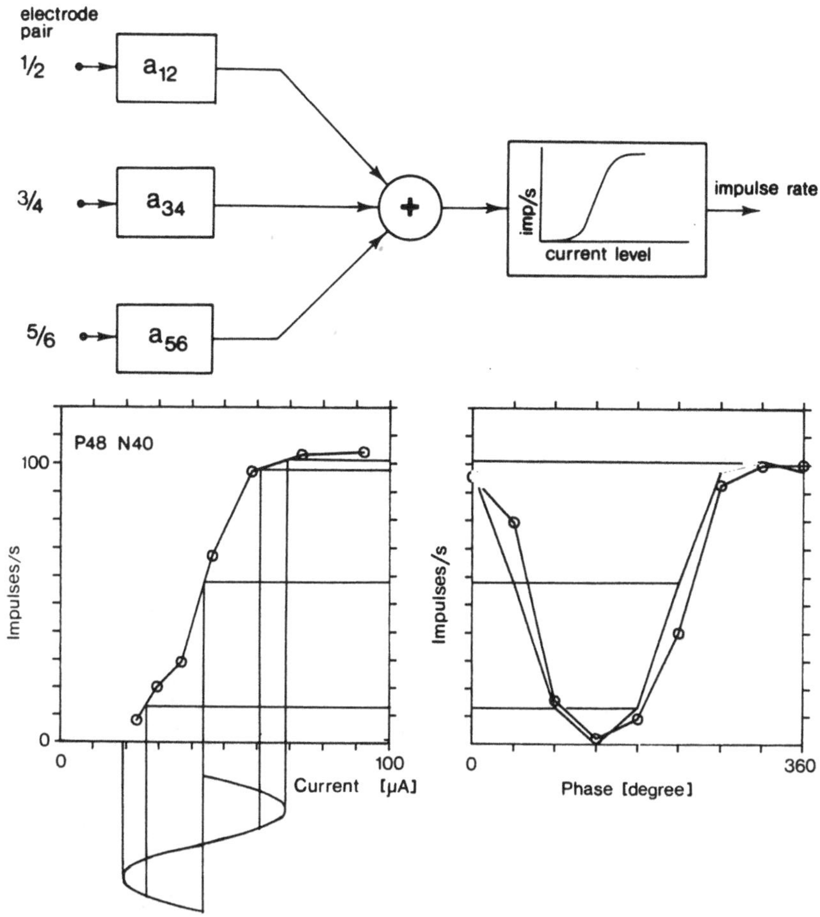

FIGURE 10.16. *Top:* Model of channel interaction by current spread. a_{nm}: linear transfer functions from electrode pair to neuronal membrane input. Membrane model with a saturation rate level function. *Bottom:* Mirror image of the calculated superimposed current values from the two-channel parallel stimulation (electrode pairs $\frac{1}{2}$ and $\frac{3}{4}$, 100 Hz) at the rate function of fiber N40 (pair $\frac{1}{2}$) and the measured impulse rate of the fiber (○——○) in comparison with the model output function (———) during two-channel parallel stimulation with different phases.

If the main effect of the channel interaction is due to the linear superposition of the current densities in the tissue, then one can generate a "lateral inhibition" effect. During the stimulation of a given channel the current sources of the neighboring channels get an inverted fraction of the input signal of the activated channel to minimize the cross talk. Such an inhibition network (Figure 10.17) can be calculated for our fiber sample using the deconvolution technique.

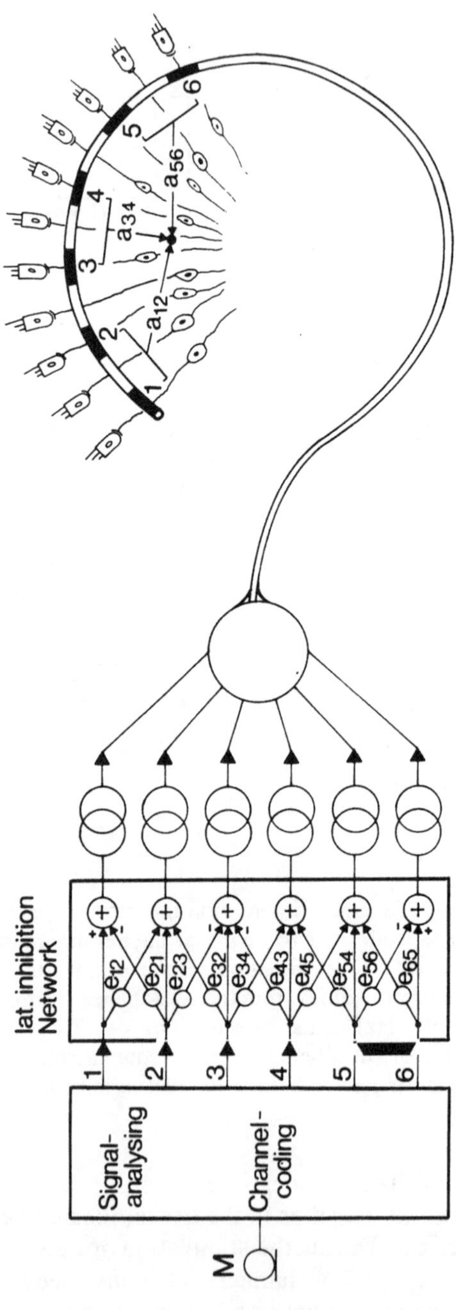

FIGURE 10.17. Multichannel stimulation system with a lateral inhibition network with the inhibition coefficients e_{nm} to improve the channel separation for intrascalar bipolar stimulation with the transfer functions a_{nm} of the current pathway from the electrode array to the excited neuronal membranes along the cochlea duct.

Discussion

The impulse pattern in auditory nerve fibers evoked by single-channel extracochlear stimulation depends of the conditon of the cochlea and the nerve fibers. In cats with normal auditory functions one has the advantage of normal responses to acoustic stimulation. No degeneration pattern has to be taken into account in this case, and the spontaneous activity, the rate-sound level functions, and the CFs of the recorded fibers are known before the electrical stimulation. The only problem with this method is the presence of the so-called electrophonic effect (Moxon, 1971). This is a mechanical vibration of the cochlea by forces caused by the electrical stimulation. It can be observed as a tip at the CF in the electrical threshold function of fibers with a high CF (Figure 10.4). The low-frequency parts of the threshold current fucntions versus frequency look similar to those of fibers from deafened cats. A contamination of these threshold functions by the "electrophonic" effect at low frequencies is therefore unlikely. With the single-channel round-window stimulation, no significant correlation was found between the electrical low-frequency threshold and the CF of the fibers (Hartmann, Topp, and Klinke, 1984). This was confirmed by studies from van den Honert and Stypulkowski (1987). This means that with a single extracochlear electrode the current spread inside the cochlea is so large that no place-dependent thresholds can be obtained. There is also no correlation between the spontaneous activity and the threshold for low-frequency current stimulation (Hartmann, Topp, and Klinke, 1984). The reason for interfiber threshold differences measured in the same cat has to be different fiber diameters and membrane properties and the location of the nodes of Ranvier in relation to the electrical field rather than the cochleotopic organization of the fibers.

For a comparative interpretation of the impulse pattern in the auditory nerve of cochlear implant patients, one has to consider the status of the hair cells, afferent nerve endings, myelinization, and ganglion cells of these subjects. As a model for human deafness, acutely deafened cats were used. Mechanical destruction of the basilar membrane or instillation of antibiotics (neomycin) in the scala tympani induced severe damage to the inner hair cells and a pathological alteration of the afferent nerve endings (Leake-Jones et al., 1982). The threshold values for low-frequency (50–300 Hz) sinusoidal current stimulation were in the same range as before deafening. They are also comparable to sensation thresholds obtained from cochlear implant patients with direct stimulation at the round window (Fourcin et al., 1979) but higher than the thresholds measured in behavioral studies in monkeys (Pfingst, 1988).

Deafening of the cats caused the spontaneous activity of the fibers to disappear. Therefore only electrically evoked APs, which are strongly synchronized with the current signal, occur. Thus, with suprathreshold electrical activation, a large population of auditory fibers carries the identical impulse pattern. Parkins and Colombo (1987) showed with intrascalar electrical stimulation in monkeys that the thresholds for sinusoidal and biphasic pulse stimulation are the same if the same rms current level is used. The strength of the synchronization depends on the current level and waveform (see Figures 10.1 and 10.3). Phase locking of APs to sinusoidal currents occurs at low frequencies during the cathodal stimulation phase (round-window electrode negative re indifferent electrode). At higher frequencies, when the stimulus period is of the same order as or less than the refractory period, phase locking occurs during both the negative and the positive phases, with intervals between the APs of multiples of the signal period. This is also the case with sinusoidal burst stimulation. In this case the first AP is triggered by the ramp of the envelope, and the synchronization of the next APs is determined by both the relative refractory period and the stimulus cycles (Figure 10.7). Intervals shorter than 1.25 ms were rarely observed. This holds also for pulse stimulation (Figure 10.9). This means that a direct representation of the stimulus period in the firing pattern of a single fiber is only possible up to 800 Hz. Shorter interval detection may be possible assuming parallel processing networks in the central auditory system (a review of relevant hearing theories is given by Javel and Mott, 1988).

These neurophysiological data fit nicely with our measurements of the ability of cochlear implant patients with a single-channel extracochlear and intracochlear Vienna/3M device. They show a clear periodicity pitch sensation with sinusoidal or pulsatile stimulation up to 1 kHz. One of the better patients can distinguish between octave band-filtered noise with center frequencies from 125 to 4000 Hz presented at the most comfortable loudness level. This observation and the speech test results by Hochmair and Hochmair-Desoyer (1983) with low-pass-filtered analog-coded speech show that for a single-channel prostheses it is absolutely necessary to achieve an optimal image of the signal time structure in the auditory fibers. This does not say that the firing pattern should be identical in all fibers. The "hypersynchronization" of the electrically stimulated fibers may be quite unnatural to the brain. In particular, the problem of the transmission of short intervals leads to difficulties in discriminating vowels with similar F1 and F2 formants in these implant subjects (White, 1983).

Our attempt to individually stimulate subgroubs of auditory fibers with intrascalar electrode arrays in the cat cochlea shows that, with single-channel stimulation, the timing of the impulse pattern is not substanially different from that obtained with extracochlear round-window stimulation. The restriction of the stimulation to a distinct place inside the cochlea is possible but depends on many parameters. One major problem is the exact location of the electrodes with respect to the nearest excitable membrane of the fibers, e.g., the beginning of the myelin sheath at the habenula perforata. However, the electrical stimulus does not necessarily become effective at the first node of Ranvier. In our own experiments instillation of glutaraldehyde into the scala tympani, which certainly fixates the peripheral dendrites, did not abolish electrical excitability of the auditory afferents. Even the thresholds remained the same as before the glutaraldehyde fixation. Thus it has to be considered that the ganglion cell membranes possess lower thresholds than the peripheral dendrites and may be the normal site of excitation. With the monopolar electrode configuration the electrical threshold–stimulation place functions show only weak slopes of 1–3 dB/mm caused by the large current spread inside the cochlea. Better results were obtained with the true bipolar stimulation. Here the single-fiber threshold functions showed maximum slopes of up to 13 dB/mm, if there is threshold minimum at a distinct stimulation position. This is the case when the origin of the fiber inside the cochlea is close to the stimulating electrode pair. Van den Honert and Stypulkowski (1987) used optimally placed radially oriented electrodes to measure spatial tuning curves, with a result of $Q10$ dB = 4. Our measurements with the Melbourne human-type array with electrode rings showed only $Q10$ dB values <1.2, because of the longitudinal orientation of the electrodes and the fluid space between the silastic carrier and the scala tympani wall, which is relatively large near the round window. Merzenich et al. (1973) and Black and Clark (1980) showed also CF-dependent thresholds of inferior-colliculus neurons with bipolar electrical stimulation with a fixed electrode pair in the scala tympani. The computed $Q10$ dB values obtained with this indirect method are also < 1.

Up to now, no implant with radially oriented electrode arrays has been tested in a cochlear implant because of the difficulties of the proper orientation inside the cochlea. The Vienna and the San Francisco array have a small radial component additional to the longitudinal orientation, but the measured spatial tuning curves looked similar to those with the pure longitudinal Melbourne array. The slopes of the electrically measured spatial tuning curves (6–13 dB/mm) are much shallower than the high-frequency slopes of auditory frequency tuning curves (> 50 dB/mm) in the 8-kHz CF region.

The poor electrical place tuning leads to heavy interference between neighboring channels during parallel stimulation and restricts the number of independent channels. Some of our patients with a Nucleus device are able to rank the electrode number tested with the same stimulus at the comfortable loudness levels; others are not. This is obviously a question of nerve survival. A patchy degeneration pattern along the cochlea duct would cause a problem for pure place-coding strategies.

Beside the possibility of using more sophisticated electrode arrays, channel separation could be improved by sharpening the electrical field inside the cochlea with a lateral inhibition effect (Figure 10.17). This requires a network inside the speech processor modifying the input to the individual stimulation channel. This method may be an improvement for patients if their excitable membranes are close to the habenula or ganglion cells (Ifukube and White, 1987). But this is obviously not always the case. Therefore one has to demand that for further improvements of cochlear prostheses, time- and place-coding strategies should be combined. The proper time structure of the signals should be preserved as far as possible for each frequency channel. It may be that the limiting factor then is the status of the patients. For patients with no place pitch sensation and poor time resolution of the signal time structure, a speech processor with feature extraction and simplified stimulation pattern may be more helpful.

Acknowledgments. The authors are grateful to Professor P. Leake, San Francisco, for her collaboration, and in particular for the gift of a long-term chronically deafened cat. We thank also Professor G. Clark, Melbourne; Dr. I. Hochmair-Desoyer, Innsbruck; Professor M. Merzenich, San Francisco; and the Nucleus-Cochlear Company for the electrode arrays; and we thank Dr. D. Caird for critically reviewing the English manuscript. This work was supported by the Deutsche Forschungsgemeinschaft SFB-45 B13 and Schilling-Stiftung.

References

Black, R.C., and Clark, G.M. (1980). Differential electrical excitation of the auditory nerve. *J. Acoust. Soc. Am.* 67:868–874.

Clark, G.M., Shepherd, R.K., Patrick, J.F., Black, R.C., and Tong, Y.C. (1983). Design and fabrication of the banded electrode array. In *Cochlear Prostheses: An International Symposium,* edited by Ch.W. Parkins and S.W. Anderson (New York: New York Academy of Sciences), *Ann. N.Y. Acad. Sci.* 405:191–201.

Fourcin, A.J., Rosen, S.M., Moore, B.C.J., Douek, E.E., Clarke, E.G.P., Dodson, H., and Bannister, L.H. (1979). External electrical stimulation of the cochlea: Clinical, psychophysical, speech-perceptual and histological findings. *Br. J. Audiol.* 13:85–107.

Goldberg, J.M., and Brown, P.B. (1969). Response of binaural neurones of dog superior olivary complex to dichotic tonal stimulation; some physiological mechanisms of sound localization. *J. Neurophysiol.* 32:613–636.

Hartmann, R., Topp, G., and Klinke, R. (1984). Discharge patterns of cat primary auditory fibers with electrical stimulation of the cochlea. *Hearing Res.* 13: 47–62.

Hochmair, E.S., and Hochmair-Desoyer, I.J. (1983). Percepts elicited by different speech coding strategies. In *Cochlear Prostheses: An International Symposium,* edited by Ch.W. Parkins and S.W. Anderson (New York: New York Academy of Sciences), *Ann. N.Y. Acad. Sci.* 405:268–279.

Hochmair-Desoyer, I.S., Hochmair, E.S., and Burian, K. (1983). Design and fabrication of multiwire scala tympani electrodes. In *Cochlear Prostheses: An International Symposium,* edited by Ch.W. Parkins and S.W. Anderson (New York: New York Academy of Sciences), *Ann. N.Y. Acad. Sci.* 405:173–182.

Ifukube, T., and White, R.L. (1987). A speech professor with lateral inhibition for an 8 channel cochlear implant and its evaluation. *IEEE Trans. Biomed. Eng.* 34:876–882.

Javel, E., and Mott, J.B. (1988). Physiological and psychophysical correlates of temporal processes in hearing. *Hearing Res.* 34:275–294.

Leake, P.A., and Hradek, G.T. (1988). Cochlear pathology of long term neomycin induced deafness in cats. *Hearing Res.* 33:11–34.

Leake-Jones, P.A., Vivion, M.C., O'Reilly, B.F., and Merzenich, M.M. (1982). Deaf animal models for studies of a multichannel cochlear prosthesis. *Hearing Res.* 8:225–246.

Liberman, M.C. (1982). The cochlear frequency map for the cat: Labeling auditory-nerve fibers of known characteristic frequency. *J. Acoust. Soc. Am.* 72:1441–1449.

Merzenich, M.M., Michelson, R.P., Pettit, C.R., Schindler, R.A. and Reid, M. (1973). Neural encoding of sound sensation evoked by electrical stimulation of the acoustic nerve. *Ann. Otol. Rhinol. Laryngol.* 82:486–503.

Merzenich, M.M., and White, M.W. (1977). Cochlear implant. The interface problem. In *Biomedical Engineering and Instrumentation: Functional Electrical Stimulation*, F.T. Hambrecht, and J.B. Reswick (New York: Dekker), pp. 321–340.

Moxon, E.C. (1971). Neural and mechanical responses to electric stimulation of the cat's inner ear. Thesis, MIT, Cambridge, Mass.

Parkins, C.W., and Colombo, J. (1987). Auditory-nerve single-neuron thresholds to electrical stimulation from scala tympani electrodes. *Hearing Res.* 31: 267–286.

Pfingst, B.E. (1988). Comparison of psychophysical and neurophysiological studies of cochlear implants. *Hearing Res.* 34:243–252.

van den Honert, C., and Stypulkowski, P.H. (1987). Single fiber mapping of spatial excitation patterns in the electrically stimulated auditory nerve. *Hearing Res.* 29:195–206.

White, M.W. (1983). Formant frequency discrimination and recoginition in subjects implanted with intracochlear stimulating electrodes. In *Cochlear Prostheses, Ann. N.Y. Acad. Sci.* 405:348–359.

Rainer Hartmann: Discussion

Dr. Pfingst: In the experiments where you looked at current spread, i.e., threshold versus electrode position, was there any effect of frequency on these functions?

Dr. Hartmann: At the moment we have these functions only in the low-frequency range. As in these experiments we want to show that we are recording from auditory fibers we must be able to drive the fibers acoustically. The problem is that when we deafen the cat, we cannot say whether it is an auditory fiber or whether it is a vestibular fiber. There is an initial high-frequency hearing loss of about 40 dB, but to avoid electrophonic effects we must be on the low-frequency side. It is a problem with this type of experiement.

Dr. Johnstone: Yes, well you still have to know where your recording electrode is, or your system doesn't work anyway; you've got to know what part you're looking at.

Dr. Hartmann: In the acutely deafened cat I have recorded a track before deafening, that is, in the normal hearing situation. So I know the position of the electrode and I know where the track is, and so I'm sure that I am recording from auditory fibers.

Dr. Johnstone: If you could go a bit higher, in the higher frequency the electrophonic effect would be less of a problem. If you are getting a fiber that may be at the 6- or 7-kHz place, you could perhaps then use a 10- or 12-kHz signal, and your electrophonics should not affect that fiber.

Dr. Hartmann: Yes, we can do this. Or the other way around is to stimulate with short pauses as Chris van den Honert did and look to see whether there is an electrophonic long latency response, and then you look only for the short latencies.

Dr. Josef Miller: With the Nucleus electrode and monopolar stimulation you were seeing a slope change of about 3.3 dB/mm. I'm under the impression that Chris van den Honert's data don't show that much of a change, nor Delgutete's, for monopolar stimulation. Your stimulation was monopolar, right?

Dr. Hartmann: It was monopolar with one ring inside the scala tympani, and the indifferent electrode was at the bulla wall on the ipsilateral side. You can also see the effects with the special cat-adapted San Franciso–type electrode.

Dr. Sachs: In your measurements of phase locking to sinusoidal stimuli, how did you rule out possible artifacts?

Dr. Hartmann: I mentioned that we used a special cross-correlation technique to avoid additional phase locking to the signal artifact. We have an artifact reduction system that you saw in the first slide, and then we feed these signals through a cross-correlator. In the cross-correlator an original action potential was stored, and then we looked for the maximum of the output of the running cross-correlation and took this time event as the occurrence of a spike. So this gives an additional reduction. I did some checks that, even down to synchronization values of 0.1, it was detectable, so that you get no additional artifacts.

11 Psychophysical Constraints on Biophysical/Neural Models of Threshold

BRYAN E. PFINGST

Introduction

Models of cochlear prosthesis function serve the purpose of specifying, preferably in a mathematically tractable fashion, the relationship between the physical parameters of electrical stimulation and the psychophysical behavior of the subject. Given a perfect model, we should be able to assign values to all relevant parameters of electrical stimulation and accurately predict the resulting psychophysical behavior. Two classes of models may be considered: phenomenological "black-box" models which make no assumptions about the intervening variables but simply try to characterize the relationship between the physical variables and the psychophysical behavior, and biophysical/neural models which attempt to specify the mechanisms that link the physical stimus to the behavior. In both classes of models, psychophysics plays the role of specifying values that the model must predict. In the case of biophysical/neural models, it may play the additional role of helping estimate to what extent the possible intervening variables influence the behavior. Table 11.1 lists some of the variables that may be considered in formulating a biophysical/neural model of electrical stimulation of the cochlea.

Regrettably, few stimulus parameters can be expected to cleanly affect one and only one of the possible physiological responses underpinning an observed behavior. By studying, one at a time, the psychophysical responses to multiple variables, each of which may be expected to influence a diffferent subset of neural responses, we hope to identify the mechanisms that most significantly influence the behavior. Data from other disciplines such as anatomy, biophysics, and neurophysiology are also important, if not essential, in this effort.

A key issue in the development of a model of electrical stimulation of the cochlea is to understand the pattern of activity in the auditory nerve array at the level of psychophysical detection thresholds. This issue is fundamental because most, if not all, psychophysical performance is dependent on the level of the stimulus above threshold. Frequency

TABLE 11.1. Formulating a biophysical/neural model.

Independent variables (physical)	Intervening variables (biophysical and neural)	Dependent variables (psychophysical)
Stimulus parameters	Number of fibers activated	Detection thresholds
Frequency	Current spread	Frequency difference limens
Level	Fiber thresholds	Level difference limens
Phase	Discharge rate	Electrode-place difference limens
Periodicity	Discharge synchrony to stimulus	Etc.
Pulse shape	Across-fiber synchrony	
Duration	Spatial (across-fiber) integration	
Rise time	Temporal integration	
Symmetry	Etc.	
Stimulus duration		
Etc.		
Electrode array geometry		
Electrode location		
Electrode-pair orientation		
Electrode size		
Etc.		
Neural array geometry		
Number of functional nerve fibers		
Locations of nerve fibers		
Condition of nerve fibers		
Dendrites present		
Fiber diameters		
Myelination		
Altered functional properties		
Etc.		

discrimination (Pfingst and Rush, 1987), intensity discrimination (Pfingst, Burnett, and Sutton, 1983; Shannon, 1983), gap detection (Shannon, 1986), and other psychophysical functions are all strongly dependent on the level of the stimulus, and these functions are most comparable, not in terms of absolute level, but in terms of level above threshold. Construction of models of these fuctions without an understanding of the state of the auditory nerve response at the level of threshold is particularly difficult. In addition, a biophysical/neural model of threshold could play an important role in the development of psychophysical tests to determine nerve survival patterns in damaged cochleas. We do not, at this time, have a good model of the pattern of activity in the auditory nerve array at the behavioral threshold level, but we do know some characteristics of the behavioral responses of implanted subjects at threshold and have some data on the biophysical and physiological characteristics of the auditory nerve that may help in the formulation of such a model.

Hypotheses

As a basis for discussion of these data, we may consider two alternative hypotheses about the physiological requirements for psychophysical detection. One commonly stated hypothesis, which we will call *hypothesis A,* is that only a single, "most sensitive," auditory nerve fiber is activated at threshold. The "most sensitive" fiber in this model would be determined by both its location with respect to the current fields and its physiological characteristics. An alternative hypothesis, which we will call *hypothesis B,* is that integration of activity from a number of auditory nerve fibers is needed to achieve a detection threshold. A corollary to this hypothesis is that there can be trading between the number of fibers activated and the degree of activation (firing rate) of individual fibers in the array, so that threshold might be achieved by minimal activity in a large number of fibers or high rates of firing in a small number of fibers.

Methods

The psychophysical data shown in Figures 11.1 through 11.7, as well as much of the previously published psychophysical data cited in the text, were collected from nonhuman primate subjects. Adolescent or adult male macaques (*M. mulatta* or *M. radiata*) were used. The subjects were trained psychophysically using positive reinforcement operant conditioning procedures to perform psychophysical tasks that could be used to measure thresholds, dynamic ranges, and various difference limens. The subjects were trained to criterion using acoustic stimuli. They were then deafened in one ear and implanted with a multiple-electrode array in the scala tympani and/or in the cochlear wall. The ear contralateral to the implanted ear was left untreated and was used for additional training and testing with acousitic stimuli. Following implantation, thresholds for electrical stimuli were measured as a function of time until stable, and then a variety of psychophysical data, including thresholds, were collected over a period of several years. Training and data collection sessions lasted 1 to 2 h per day.

During training and testing sessions the subjects sat in double-walled sound-attenuating chambers. A light-display panel faced the subject, a telegraph key was located within reach of either hand, and a tube for delivery of applesauce reinforcers was positioned near the mouth. Sinusoidal stimuli were generated by a Rockland frequency synthesizer which could be gated to start and end at zero phase. Pulsatile stimuli were generated by a pulse generator built in-house. The stimuli were attenuated by a Wilsonics (model PATT) attenuator, gated, when appropriate, by a tone switch and then passed to the earspeaker (Beyer Dynamic DT48, or TDH 49) or to a constant-current stimulator (modified slightly from the design described by Spelman, Pfingst, and Miller, 1978). For electrical stimulation, the output of the constant-current stimulator was connected directly to the implants through a percutaneous connector. IBM PC and AT and DEC PDP11 computers were used to control all experiments and to collect and analyze the data.

Thresholds were measured using a go–no–go procedure in which the subject depressed a telegraph key (observing response) to initiate each trial, held the key during a randomly variable (1 to 6 s) foreperiod, and released the key at stimulus onset if a signal was detected during a 1-s unmarked observation period that followed the variable foreperiod. The stimulus remained on until the subject released the key, or for a maximum of 1 s, except in experiments where fixed-duration stimuli were required. Hits (releases within 1 s of stimulus onset) were reinforced by delivery of 0.2 cc of applesauce to a spout located near the subject's tougue. Stimuli were presented by the method of constant stimuli, and stimulus tables were constructed so as to maintain a relatively constant rate of reinforcement across conditions. Threshold was defined as the level on the psychometric function at which 50% hits were obtained. Catch trials in which no signal occurred were used to assess the guess rate. Releases in the absence of the signal were punished by a brief (5–20 s) time-out from reinforcement. This served to hold the guess rate relatively constant at levels between 5% and 20%. If the guess rate deviated from this range, no data were collected, and the subjects were given additional training until the guess rate was stable within these limits.

Surgery for deafening and implanting the ears was performed under halothane anesthesia using standard sterile operating procedures. After the subject was prepared and draped, a postauricular incision was made exposing the bony external auditory meatus. The peripheral portion of the meatus soft tissue was sutured closed. Soft tissue was then removed from the medial part of the meatus, and the bony meatus was enlarged to provide a wide exposure of the middle ear. The incus was carefully disarticulated from the stapes, and the malleus and incus were removed, leaving the stapes in the oval window. The round window was penetrated with a 30-gage needle, and 50μL of a 10% (w/v) neomycin sulfate solution was slowly injected into the scala tympani. For scalar implants, the round window was then removed and the electrode array was inserted. In some cases, additional electrodes were implanted in holes drilled in the bony wall of the cochlea. Multichannel scalar implants consisted of platinum-iridium electrodes on a silicone rubber carrier about 10 mm in length and approximately half the diameter of the scala tympani (Xue and Pfingst, 1989). These were inserted into the scala tympani, 6 to 10 mm past the round-window niche. Electrodes inserted in the cochlear wall or single electrodes inserted through the round window consisted of spherical platinum-iridium electrodes approximately 0.3 mm in diameter. Wires from all electrodes were led under the skin to a percutaneous connector mounted on the skull.

Results

A number of interesting details are known about the characteristics of psychophysical detection thresholds for electrical stimulation, and these must be accounted for by a biophysical/neural mode. In the following paragraphs we will review some of these data and suggest some implications for the two alternative hypotheses proposed above.

1. The range of detection thresholds across subjects is large. Even when factors such as electrode placement, stimulus waveform, and subject species and training are matched, the range of thresholds across subjects can be as high as 30 dB at low frequencies (below 100 Hz) and 20 dB at high frequencies (above 1kHz) (Figure 11.1). These ranges of thresholds across subjects are equal to or greater than the entire psychophysical dynamic range of any one subject and are much larger than the dynamic ranges of individual auditory nerve fibers.

Studies in monkeys have shown that these threshold levels are inversely correlated with nerve survival patterns, so that low thresholds are associated with relatively good nerve survival and high thresholds are associated with poor nerve survival (Pfingst et al., 1981; Pfingst et al., 1985; Pfingst and Sutton, 1983, 1984). These correlations of thresholds with nerve survival patterns are consistent with hypothesis B, but also could be compatible with hypothesis A if the threshold of the most sensitive fiber is correlated with the nerve survival pattern. High thresholds for the most sensitive fiber could occur in cases of poor nerve survival because the fiber is located far from the electrode array (because fibers near the array have died) or because characteristics of auditory neurons change in cases of pathology, making them less sensitive. To estimate the feasibility of this model, additional data on the biophysics and physiology of the implanted cochlea are needed. Can a 30-dB difference in threshold current be demonstrated between two sites in the cochlea under the conditions of pathology found in deaf ears? For monopolar stimulation, van den Honert and Stypulkowski (1987) found little or no difference in thresholds of auditory neurons innervating the base of the cochlea near the stimulating electrode as compared with neurons innervating the apex of the cochlea. Furthermore, these investigators found that only small changes in level were needed to move from thresholds of responses attributed to activation at the peripheral processes of the auditory nerve, to those attributed to activation at the central processes (van den Honert and Stypulkowski, 1984). In comparing basal to apical neurons, these investigators used Pt-Ir ball electrodes inserted through a slit in the round window into the basal turn of the scala tympani. Merzenich and White (1977) and Hartmann and Klinke (Chapter 10, this volume) found greater selectivity for monopolar stimulation with electrodes housed in silicone rubber carriers inserted in the scala tympani. This greater selectivity could be due to reduced current spread

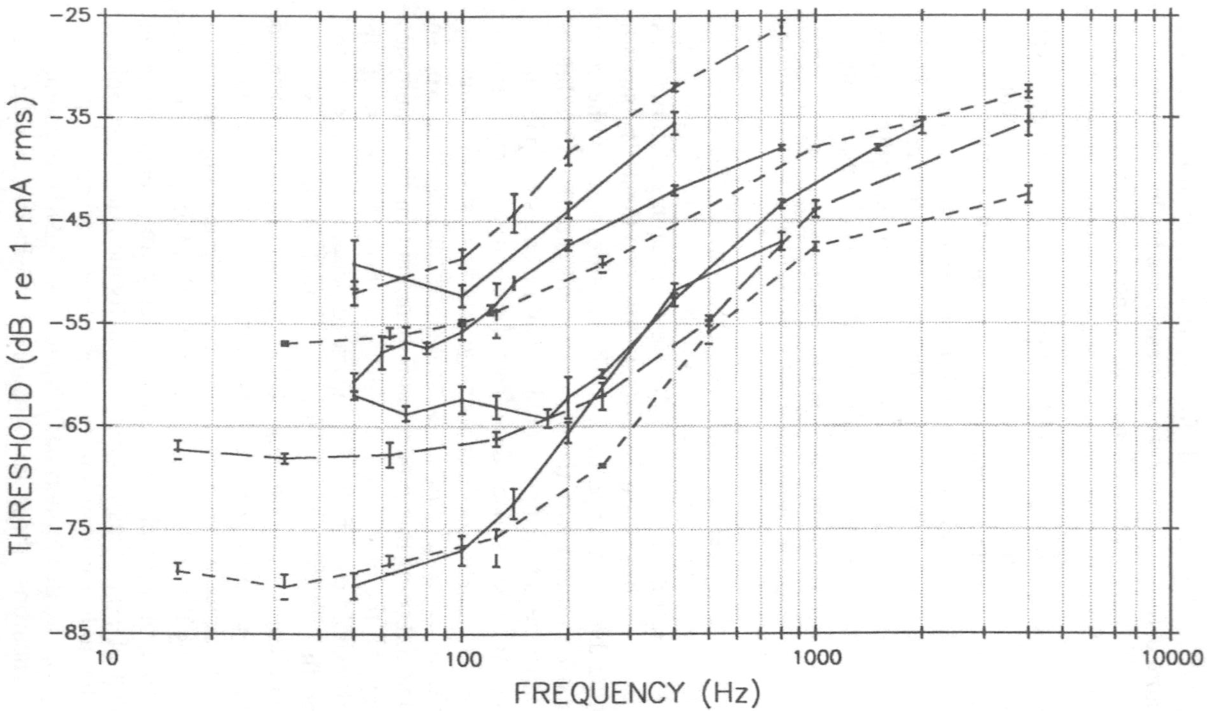

FIGURE 11.1. Psychopysical threshold contours for monopolar sinusoidal electrical stimulation of scala tympani electrodes in neomycin-deafened cochleas of macaque monkeys. Each contour represents a different cochlea. Contours were measured after thresholds had stablized and had remained stable for at least 2 months. Means ±1 SD are shown. The range of thresholds shown here is representative of those seen under comparable conditons in previous studies in 30 monkey subjects and of those reported in the literature for human subjects.

because of a reduction in fluids and closer positioning of the electrodes to the nerve fibers. These considerations apply to the psychophysical experiments as well, and make comparisons of data from the different preparations difficult. Another consideration in comparing the neurophysiological data to the psychophysical data is that the physiological data were collected using short-duration (100 μs) cathodic pulses at higher currents than are required for the lowest behavioral detection thresholds. Whether these results would apply to long-duration pulses for low-frequency sinusoids must be determined. The discrepancy between neural and psychophysical threshold *levels* must also be resolved (see below).

Within populations of auditory nerve fibers, ranges of thresholds as large as 15–30 dB have been seen across fibers (Hartmann, Topp, and Klinke, 1984; van den Honert and Stypulkowski, 1984, 1987). However, there is no evidence to indicate whether or not, when the nerve is damaged, the most sensitive fibers are selectively eliminated. A related question is whether certain fiber types (based, for example, on fiber diameter) are selectively lost in greater numbers when the auditory nerve degenerates.

2. Thresholds for more widely spaced electrode pairs stimulated in a bipolar configuration, or thresholds for monopolar stimulation, are consistently lower than those for bipolar stimulation of more closely spaced electrodes (Pfingst et al., 1979; Figure 11.2). Comparing data from a set of 18 cochleas, Pfingst and Sutton (1984) found that thresholds decreased as a function of electrode separation at an average rate of 3.9 dB/mm for 100-Hz sinusoidal stimuli and 1.7 dB/mm for 1-Hz sinusoids. If increasing electrode separation for bipolar stimulation or stimulation in a monopolar configuration results in greater current spread and stimulation of a greater number of fibers, then these data are consistent with hypothesis B. Some other possible mechanisms, compatible with hypothesis A, must be considered however. It may be, for example, that the optimum electrode configuration for achieving the maximum voltage gradient across the most sensitive neuron is a widely spaced bipolar or a monopolar configuration. Single-fiber recordings by Parkins and Colombo (1987) showed that thresholds for monopolar stimulation on the average were 7 dB lower than those for bipolar stimulation of longitudinal scala tympani electrodes separated by 1.5 mm. Biophysical models, however, indicate that spread of excitation predicts the effects of electrode separation on threshold more closely than does peak current at a single site (Spelman, Soma, and Rubinstein, 1984).

3. Current levels for the most sensitive behavioral thresholds can be very low: as low as 0.1μA rms at frequencies below 100 Hz and as low as 3μA at 1 kHz, for monopolar or widely spaced bipolar stimulation in animals with neomycin-deafened cochleas (Figure 11.1). Even lower thresholds have occasionally been seen in cases where hair cells were

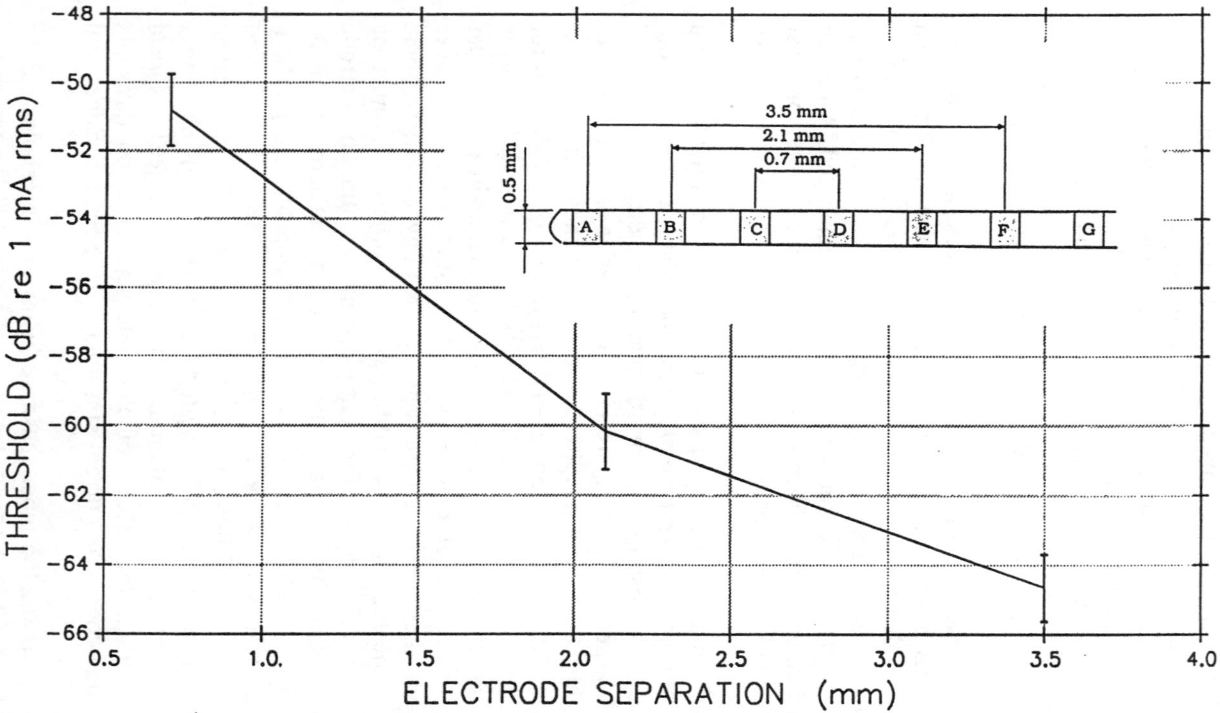

FIGURE 11.2. Psychophysical thresholds as a function of electrode separation for electrical stimulation of bipolar pairs of electrodes in the scala tympani of a neomycin-deafened macaque cochlea. The implant, manufactured by Cochlear Corporation, is depicted schematically in the inset. The platinum-iridium band electrodes (labeled A through G) were stimulated in bipolar pairs for which the separations (center to center) are indicated. Psychophysical thresholds (means ±1 SD) for these three bipolar pairs are shown.

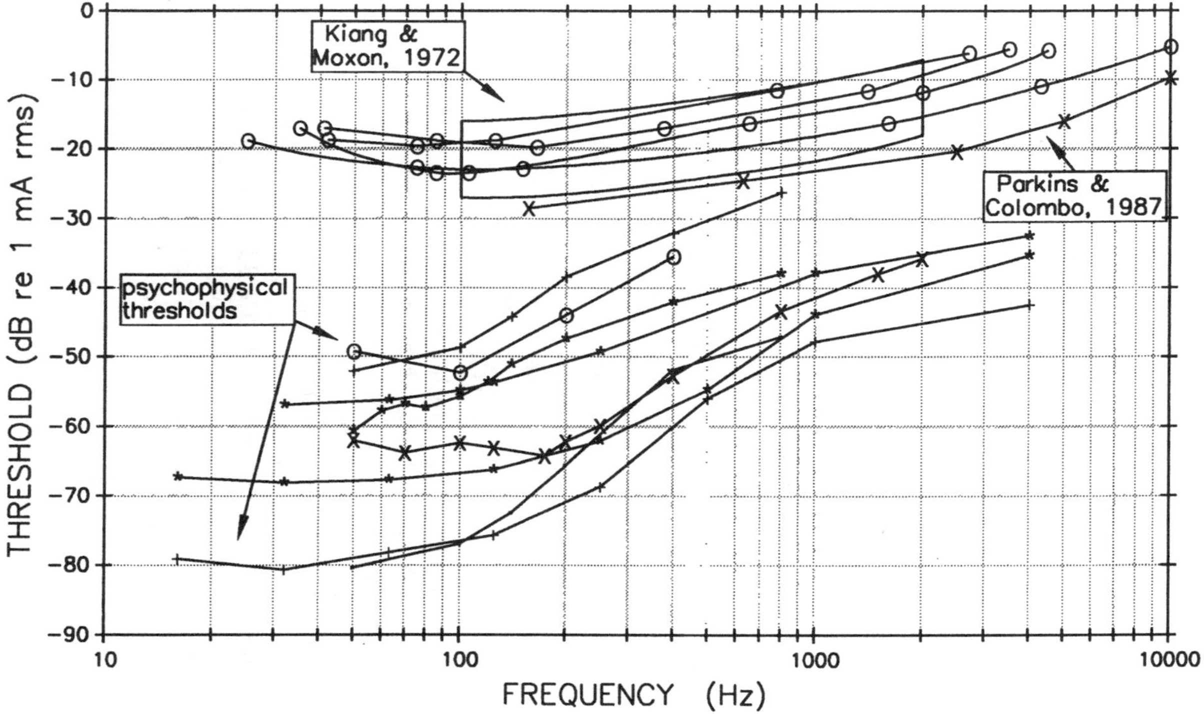

FIGURE 11.3. Psychophysical thresholds for monopolar stimulation of scala tympani electrodes, from Figure 11.1, compared with threshold contours for single auditory nerve fibers from Kiang and Moxon (1972) and Parkins and Colombo (1987). Kiang and Moxon used 30-m bursts of sinusoidal stimulation at frequencies above 100 Hz, and continuous sinusoids for frequencies below 100 Hz, in a neomycin-deafened cat. They stimulated between a cotton-wick electrode on the round window and a stainless-steel electrode placed on the periostium over the apex of the cochlea. Individual curves for 4 fibers and the range of thresholds for 22 fibers (from 100 Hz to 2 kHz) are shown. Parkins and Colombo used continuous and discrete sinusoids and pulses, and after finding no differences in thresholds attributable to the different waveforms, averaged the data from the different waveforms. Their data are from auditory nerve of squirrel monkeys deafened with kanamycin and ethacrynic acid. They used monopolar stimulation of 0.3–0.4-mm-diameter Pt-Ir ball electrodes inserted approximately 3 mm into the scala tympani.

present (Pfingst et al., 1981). These threshold levels are much lower than those typically required to elicit a detectable response in auditory nerve fibers in anesthetized acute animal preparations (Figure 11.3; also see Pfingst, 1988). These data are consistent with the hypothesis that the activity of auditory nerve fibers changes very little at current levels needed for the best behavioral detection thresholds. Thus, it may be necessary to integrate activity from a number of fibers to achieve an amount of activity that is detectable by the brain. If the density of fibers near the electrode is low, more activity in each fiber may be needed for detection; thus thresholds would be higher. However, hypothesis B is not sufficient to account for the large discrepancy between behavioral and neural thresholds since the difference in level between currents that elicit no activity and those that elicit firing on all trials is typically quite small (e.g.,1.5 dB in Parkins and Colombo's experiments).

One potential explanation of the discrepancy between neural and psychophysical thresholds is that the most sensitive neurons have not been sampled in auditory nerve recordings. This explanation would be compatible with hypothesis A or B. There are a number of other potential explanations for the discrepancies between neural and behavioral thresholds, and further study is needed to differentiate among these.

4. Most psychophysical threshold contours differ in *shape* from auditory-nerve-fiber discharge-rate threshold contours. For sinusoids above about 500 Hz–1 kHz, the two sets of contours tend to have similar slopes, roughly 3–4 dB/octave. However, below 1 kHz the slopes of the psycholphysical threshold contours can be much steeper, up to 15 dB/octave (Figures 11.3 and 11.4; see Pfingst, 1984, for more detail regarding psychophysical threshold contours). This is particularly evident in the cases where the psychophysical thresholds are lowest. If we assume that the neural and psychophysical threshold contours were recorded under functionally equivalent conditions, and that the appropriate fibers are being sampled by the recording electrode, then the data suggest that psychophysical thresholds cannot be explained in terms of the discharge rates of a single auditory nerve fiber, at least not using the criteria that are normally used for neural thresholds. Could other criteria applicable to thresholds of single fibers, such as discharge synchronization (Rose et al. 1971), account for the lower psychophysical thresholds at low frequencies? Clopton et al. (1983) tested the effects of disrupting neural synchrony on behavioral thresholds by using narrow-band noise stimuli and found no effect on threshold. Even if stimulus synchrony is completely eliminated by testing with only a single pulse, the slope of the threshold versus pulse-duration contour is steeper than the corresponding neural tuning curve (Figure 11.4). These data suggest that discharge synchrony to the stimulus in single fibers could not account for the lower psychophysical thresholds. One mechanism that could account for the lower psychophysical thresholds is the integration of activity

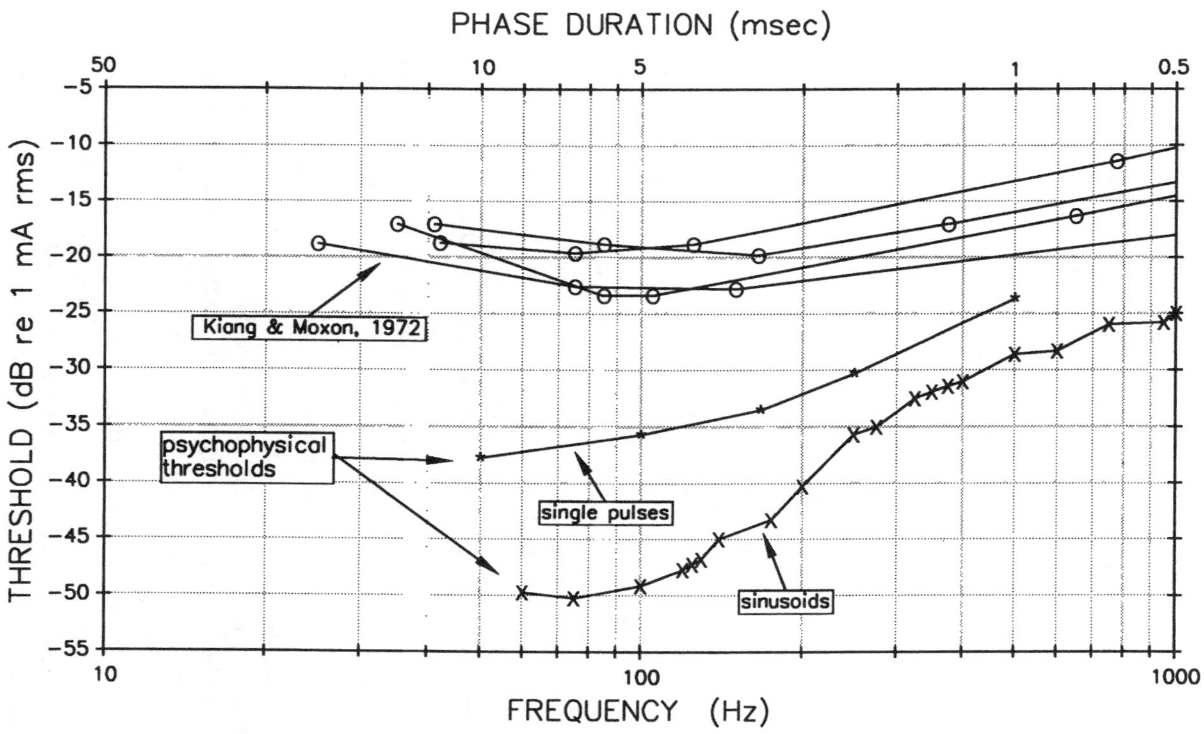

FIGURE 11.4. Psychophysical thresholds for sinusoidal stimulation and single biphasic pulses (one pulse per trial) compared with the neural thresholds from Kiang and Moxon (1972). Thresholds for the single biphasic pulses are plotted as a function of phase duration. The upper abscissa applies to the phase durations of the biphasic pulses and the sinusoids. The lower abscissa applies to the frequency of the sinusoids. The psychophysical thresholds are for bipolar stimulation between an electrode at the round window and one in a hole drilled in the cochlear bone near the apex. Details regarding the neural thresholds are given in the caption to Figure 11.3.

across fibers. A potential mechanism for frequency dependence of across-fiber integration is discussed below.

5. Psychophysical thresholds change over time. Fluctuations of up to 40 dB during the first 2 months after implantation are common. The predominant trend during this period is a decrease in thresholds to some level which then remains stable for many months or years (Eddington et al., 1978; Pfingst, 1989; Pfingst et al., 1979). Later in time, changes occur more rarely and often much more slowly (e.g., Figure 11.5*a*). These changes can be frequency-dependent, the larger changes involving frequencies in the 100-Hz region (Figure 11.5*b*).

Some of the changes in thresholds seen over time in single subjects are of the same general magnitude as those seen across subjects with varying degrees of spiral ganglion cell loss. While the mechanism underlying threshold variation across subjects and across time are not necessarily the same, the changes across time do provide the opportunity to study large threshold differences in the same subject and thus may be useful in determining the mechanisms underpinning detection threshold.

6. When the frequency of a sinusoidal stimulus changes, a number of stimulus features change simultaneously: rate of zero crossings, phase duration (duration of each half cycle of the stimulus), rise times of individual periods of the signal, etc. Effects of these features can be studied separately using pulsatile stimuli.

For pulse trains with fixed frequency, threshold decreases as a function of pulse duration (Figure 11.6, function for single pulses). This effect may be partly accounted for by models based on the Frankenhauser-Huxley equations (e.g., Colombo and Parkins, 1987). However, for long-duration pulses, the slope of this function can be steeper than that predicted by such models.

Psychophysical thresholds for pulse trains having long, fixed-duration pulses (pulse durations greater than 0.5 ms/phase) are more strongly affected by pulse rate (frequency) than are pulse trains having short-duration pulses (Shannon, 1985). Threshold for the long pulses is a nonmonotonic function of frequency in some cases, decreasing as a function of frequency up to about 100–200 Hz and increasing as a function of frequency at higher frequencies (Figure 11.6, function for 200 ms/phase pulses; also see Shannon, 1985). The neural basis for these nonmonotonic functions has not been identified.

It is possible that the effect of phase duration interacts with the effect of frequency to shape the threshold function for sinusoids at low frequencies. Other variables may also play a role in determining the shape and level of the psychophysical threshold contour. These variables and their interactions should be studied further by manipulating different features of pulse trains independently and in concert.

7. Psychophysical thresholds for electrical stimulation show temporal integration, i.e., a decrease in theshold with increasing stimulus duration

for durations less than about 100 ms (Figure 11.7; also see Eddington et al., 1978; Shannon, 1983). Slopes of these functions vary considerably from case to case. They may be dependent on stimulus frequency, as suggested by the data in Figure 11.7, though more data are needed to demonstrate if this relationship is reliable and to determine what other variables influence the slopes of these functions. If temporal integration is frequency-dependent, then this suggests a mechanism to partly account for the discrepancy between the shapes of psychophysical threshold contours and neural threshold contours at low frequencies. If temporal integration occurs at more central stations in the auditory pathway, the signal could conceivably be carried into the CNS by a single auditory nerve fiber. Neurophysiological studies in normal-hearing, acoustically stimulated preparations (Kitzes et al., 1978) have indicated that neural correlates a temporal integration can be seen in peripheral neurons (AVCN) in the auditory pathway. For electrical stimuli, the temporal integration of pulse trains of varying durations has been modeled by Bütikofer and Lawrence (1979). Experiments are needed to establish whether these effects occur in electrically stimulated auditory nerve fibers, and if so, whether they are of the right magnitude to account for the temporal integration measured psychophysically.

Discussion

Taken as a whole, these data are most compatible with hypothesis B, that integration of activity from a number of auditory nerve fibers is needed to achieve a detection threshold, but without further data, neither hypothesis can be disproved.

A key requirement for building a biophysical/neural model of detection threshold is to account for the discrepancies between neural threshold contours and psychophysical threshold contours. Potential explanations of these discrepancies fall into at least two categories: those concerned with differences in the preparations from which the two sets of data were collected and those having to do with central processing of the auditory nerve data. With regard to the first category, there are many differences between the neurophysiological and behavioral experiments that could affect threshold. One concern, based on psychophysical data, is with the chronic versus the acute preparation. In psychophysical studies we typically see large changes in thresholds during the first month or two following the neomycin deafening and subsequent implanting of the cochlea (Pfingst, 1989; Pfingst et al., 1979; Figure 11.5*a*). Early in this period, which may be analogous to the period during which most single-unit data are collected, thresholds can be as much as 40 dB higher than those seen after thresholds have reached a stable level. Because the thresholds are not stable, we have not measured threshold contours

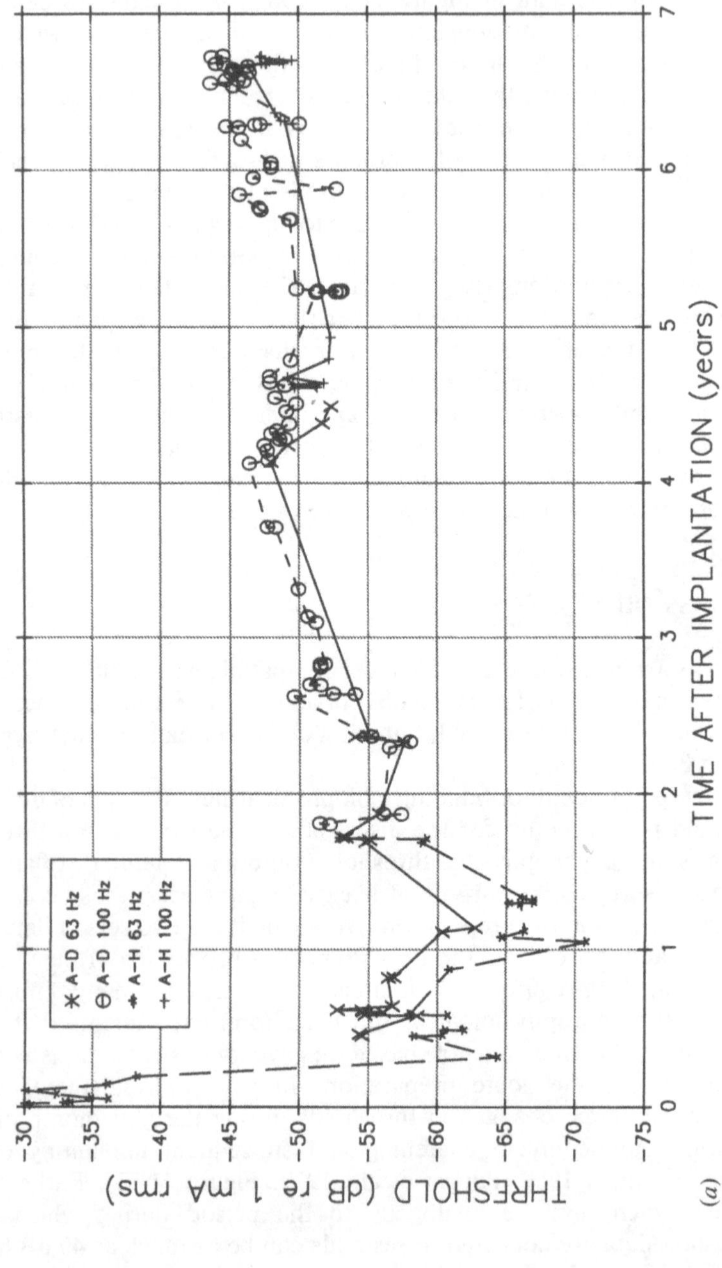
A-D 63 Hz
A-D 100 Hz
A-H 63 Hz
A-H 100 Hz
THRESHOLD (dB re 1 mA rms)
-30
-35
-40
-45
-50
-55
-60
-65
-70
-75
TIME AFTER IMPLANTATION (years)
0
1
2
3
4
5
6
7

(a)

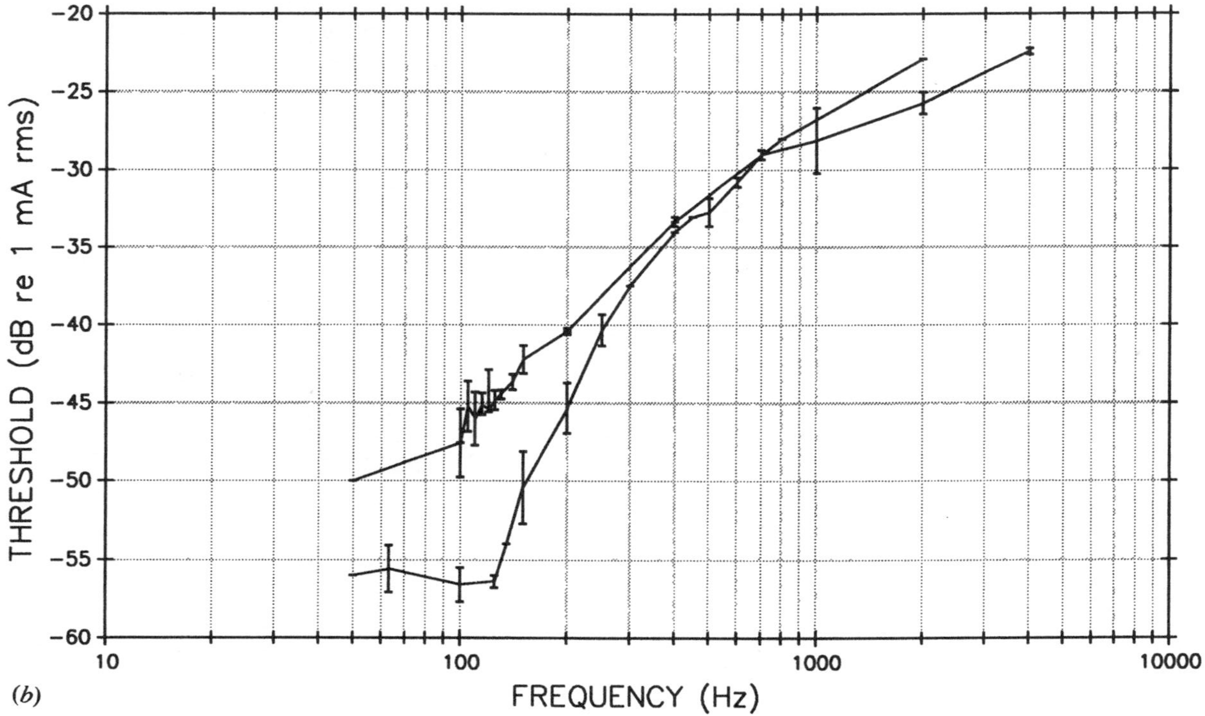

(*b*)

FIGURE 11.5. (*a*) Changes over time in psychophysical thresholds for low-frequency sinusoidal electrical stimulation of a neomycin-deafened macaque cochlea. Thresholds for two electrode pairs and two frequencies are shown. (*b*) Psychophysical thresholds for sinusoidal electrical stimulation measured approximately 4 years apart in a case where low-frequency thresholds have been increasing slowly over time, as shown in part (*a*). The lower curve was measured approximately 2 years after implantation, and the upper curve was measured approximately 4 years later. Means ±1 SD are shown.

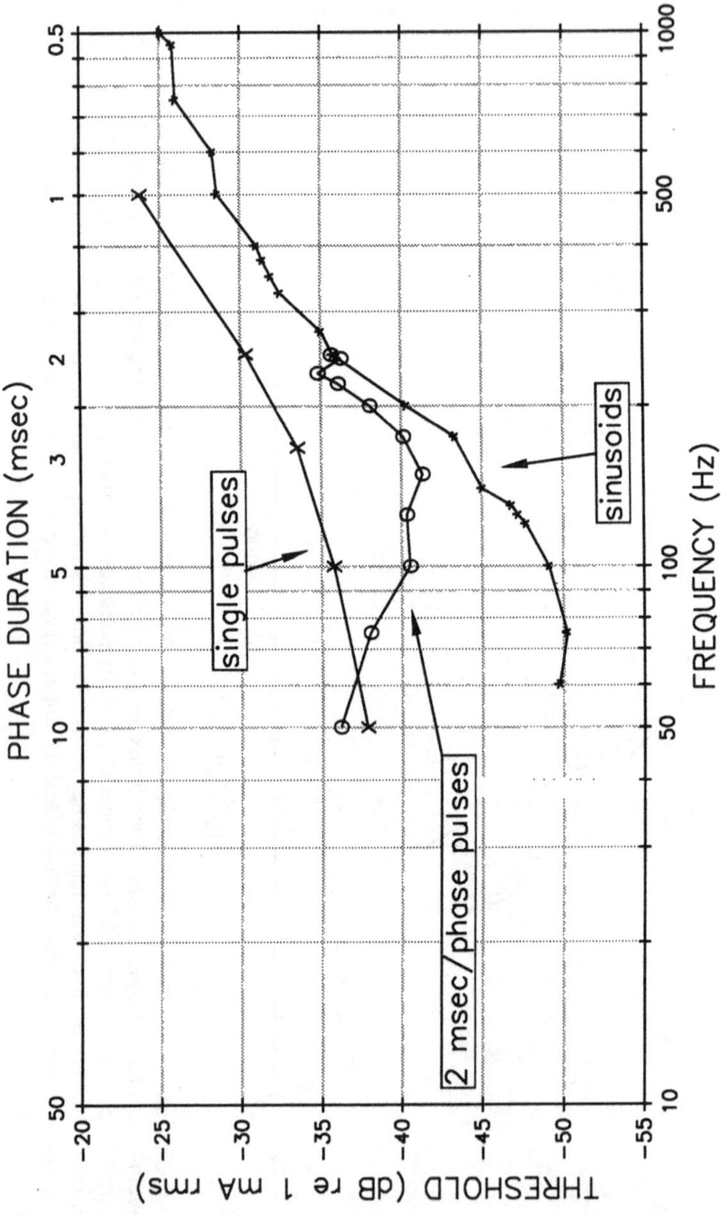

FIGURE 11.6. Psychophysical thresholds for fixed-duration electrical pulses (2 m/phase), as a function of frequency, compared with thresholds for sinusoids and thresholds for single biphasic pulses plotted as a function of phase duration, as in Figure 11.4. The upper abscissa applies to the phase durations of the sinusoids and the single pulses, but not the 2-ms/phase pulses. The lower abscissa applies to the frequency of the sinusoids and the 2-ms/phase pulse trains, but not the single pulses. All three contours were measured in the same subject for the same electrode pair over the same period.

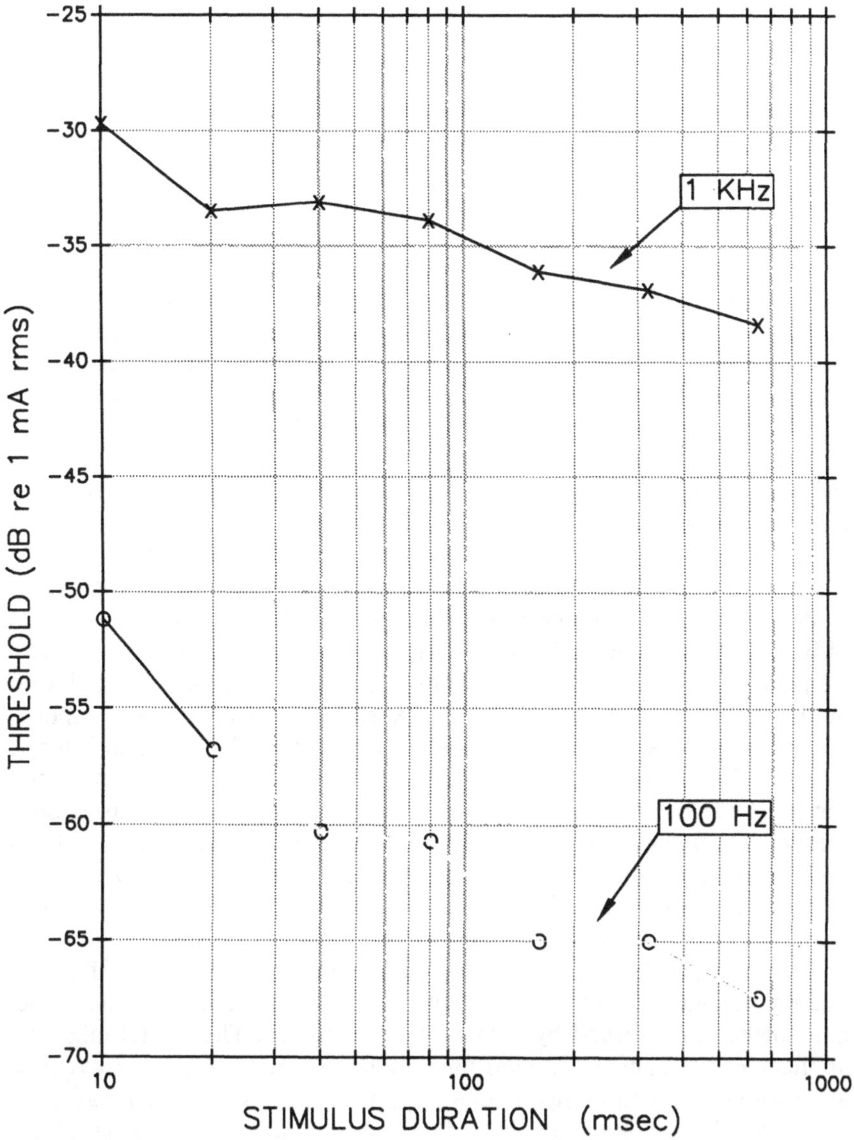

FIGURE 11.7. Thresholds for sinusoidal electrical stimulation at 100 Hz and 1kHz as a function of stimulus duration. The two functions were measured for the same electrode pair over the same period.

during this period. However, from other instances in which thresholds change more slowly (Figure 11.5*b*) and from comparisons of threshold contours across subjects (Figure 11.1), we know that the shape of the psychophysical threshold contour is correlated with threshold level and that psychophysical contours are more similar in shape to the neural threshold contours when the psychophysical thresholds are high than when they are low. These considerations suggest that it would be useful to record neural threshold contours in a chronic preparation, e.g., one that has been deafened, implanted, and stimulated electrically for several months before the single-unit recordings are begun.

Possibilities for central processing of auditory nerve firing patterns include temporal integration of the information carried by single fibers and temporal and spatial integration of the information carried by ensembles of fibers. Techniques for studying ensembles of nerve fibers or peripheral neurons are still being developed (Anderson, Clopton, and Kipke, 1987; Gerstein et al., 1983; Voigt and Young, 1988). Additional information about the integration process might be gained by recording from higher stations in the auditory pathway.

A common feature of much of the data described above is the interaction of stimulus frequency with other variables: nerve loss, electrode separation, and perhaps temporal integration. Furthermore, the difference between neural and behavioral threshold contours seems to be frequency-dependent. This frequency dependence is probably not based in the electrical characteristics of the scala tympani and surrounding tissues since these are largely resistive (Spelman, Clopton, and Pfingst, 1982), so it must lie in the neural elements. Whether it can be accounted for by the membrane properties of a *single* element, or is based on a frequency-dependent integration of activity from a single fiber or from multiple fibers, cannot be resolved at this time. Thresholds derived by the model of Rubinstein and Spelman (1988) for single unmyelinated fibers of 1-μm diameter match closely the psychophysical threshold contours for cases with low thresholds, suggesting mechanisms for single-fiber frequency dependence which were not in previous models, but this model has not been confirmed by single-fiber recordings. The model might be applicable to the small-diameter unmyelinated peripheral processes of the auditory nerve or to demyelinated peripheral processes which may exist in damaged ears. Van den Honert and Stypulkowski (1984) have presented evidence that the site of spike initiation shifts from the peripheral process to the central process with increasing stimulus level. Several studies have shown that when the cochlea is damaged, the peripheral processes of auditory nerve neurons can die, leaving the cell body and central process of the neuron in a seemingly healthy state (Hinojosa and Marion, 1983; Johnsson et al., 1981). Thus, both the changes in psychophysical threshold contour shape associated with nerve loss and the lack of demonstrated physiological threshold contours with high slopes in the low-frequency region might be attributable, in part, to a loss of function in auditory nerve peripheral processes. This hypothesis is supported by the model of Colombo and Parkins (1987). More detailed histological observations of the condition of the myelinated and unmyelinated portions of the auditory nerve peripheral processes in conjunction with psychophysical and neurophysiological data are needed to further test this model.

Another mechanism that might account for the discrepancy between the neural and the behavioral data involves across-fiber integration. If this mechanism is to account for observation that the neural/behavioral discrepancy is greatest at low frequencies, it must be elaborated: i.e., the integration of activity across fibers must be temporally dependent so that responses to low-frequency signals are more effectively integrated than those to high-frequency signals. Dobie and Dillier (1985) attempted to study the temporal characteristics of across-fiber activity by measuring the difference limen for rise time of a trapezoidal waveform. They found that subjects could discriminate rise-time differences as small as 0.08 ms at 250 Hz (rise time/period = 0.02) and 0.17 ms at 1 kHz (rise time/period = 0.17). They postulated that because thresholds of electrically stimulated auditory neurons differ, slow rise times would produce an asynchronous response across fibers which would be discriminable from a synchronous across-fiber response produced by fast rise times. This model implies that a comparison of the across-fiber activity is made at some point in the auditory pathway and thus is compatible with the across-fiber integration model. Thus we suggest that differences in across-fiber synchrony may underlie the hypothesized temporal dependence of across-fiber intergration. Differences in across-fiber synchrony dependent on rise time would apply only to continuous waveforms such as sinusoids where the rise times of the individual cycles vary with frequency. However, the model may be extended to pulsatile waveforms by hypothesizing that pulse duration may also affect across-fiber synchrony. This latter hypothesis has been suggested and modeled by Wilson and Finley (1986).

Electrical sinusoids have many features that change with frequency and that could influence the shape and level of the psychophysical threshold contour. These include the duration of each half cycle of the stimulus, the rise and fall times of each half cycle, rate of zero crossings (frequency), and temporal proximity of zero crossings. These variables can be controlled independently if pulsatile stimuli are used. For example, we can look at the effects of phase duration independent of the other variables by measuring psychophysical thresholds for single biphasic pulses (one pulse per trial) as a function of pulse width (e.g., Figure 11.4). When this is done, we see that the psychophysical threshold contour is more similar in shape to the neural threshold contours than are the psychophysical contours for sinusoids. However, the slopes of the psychophysical threshold contours for pulses in the 5-to-1-ms/phase range are still steeper than those of the neural tuning curves in the 100–500-Hz range. This remaining discrepancy could be accounted for by the hypothesis stated above, that threshold level is influenced by across-fiber synchrony with a low-pass characteristic.

A number of plausible biophysical/neural models of detection threshold may be formulated at this time. The existing data do not constitute a proof of any one model, but taken together they do suggest research directions that may make it possible to differentiate among the alternatives. At this time there are probably more data on detection thresholds than on any other psychophysical measure. Given the relevance of threshold models to most other psychophysical data and to psychophysical measures of nerve survival, a focused effort toward the resolution of this issue is fully justified.

Summary

Models of cochlear prosthesis function serve the purpose of defining the relationship between the physical parameters of electrical stimulation and the psychophysical behavior of the subject. Biophysical/neural models attempt to specify the mechanisms that link the physical stimulus to the behavior. Psychophysics plays the role of specifying values that the model must predict and may help clarify to what extent each of the possible intervening variables influences the behavior.

Psychophysical detection-threshold functions were the focus of this chapter. Models of these fuctions are fundamental because most, if not all, psychophysical performance is dependent on the level of the stimulus re threshold. As a framework for discussion we considered two alternative hypotheses:

A. Only a single "most sensitive" auditory nerve fiber is activated at the psychophysical detection threshold.
B. Integration of activity from a number of auditory nerve fibers is needed to achieve a detection threshold.

The following psychophysical data were considered:

1. The range of detection threshold levels across subjects is large—on the order of 30 dB for 100-Hz sinusoids and 20 dB for 1-KHz sinusoids. The threshold is inversely correlated with the number of spiral ganglion cells in the cochlea.
2. Thresholds for bipolar stimulation are inversely correlated with the distance between the stimulating electrodes.
3. Current levels for the most sensitive behavioral thresholds can be as low as 0.1-μA rms for sinusoids at frequencies below 100 Hz and as low as 3-μA rms at 1 kHz.These threshold levels are much lower than

those typically required to elicit a detectable response in auditory nerve fibers in acute, anesthetized animal preparations.
4. Most psychophysical threshold contours differ in shape from auditory-nerve-fiber discharge-rate threshold contours.
5. Psychophysical thresholds change over time. Fluctuations of up to 40 dB during the first 2 months after implantation are common. Later in time changes also occur, but more rarely. These changes can be frequency-dependent.
6. For pulse trains with fixed frequency, threshold decreases as a function of pulse duration. Threshold for long fixed-duration pulses (pulse durations greater than about 0.5 ms/phase) is a nonmonotonic function of frequency in some cases, decreasing as a function of frequency up to 100 Hz and increasing as a function of frequency above 100 Hz.
7. Psychophysical thresholds for electrical stimulation show temporal integration, i.e., a decrease in threshold with increasing stimulus duration for durations less than about 100 ms. Slopes of these functions may depend on stimulus frequency and other variables.

Taken as a whole, these data are most compatible with hypothesis B, but without further data, neither hypothesis can be disproved. The data indicate directions for additional research that may allow us to choose between these alternatives and develop a plausible biophysical/neural model of detection threshold.

Acknowledgments. The psychophysical experiments on nonhuman primates described in this chapter were supported by NIH Grant NS21440. My thanks to Ben Clopton, Charles Parkins, Jay Rubinstein, and Sandy Spelman for their comments on earlier versions of this chapter and to Daniel Rai, Jed Gardner, and José Nuncio-Cantera for technical assistance.

References

Anderson, D.J., Clopton, B.M., and Kipke, D. (1987). Signal processing of thin film neural recording array data to separate channels of point process information. *Proc. 9th IEEE Eng. Med. Biol. Soc. Conf.* 2:743–744.

Bütikofer, R., and Lawrence, P.D. (1979). Electrocutaneous nerve stimulation—II: Stimulus waveform selection. *IEEE Trans. Biomed. Eng. BME* 26:69–75.

Clopton, B.M., Spelman, F.A., Glass, I., Pfingst, B.E., Miller, J.M., Lawrence, P.D., and Dean, D.P. (1983). Neural encoding of electrical signals. *Ann. N.Y. Acad. Sci.* 405:146–158.

Colombo, J., and Parkins,. C.W. (1987). A model of electrical excitation of the mammalian auditory nerve neuron. *Hearing Res.* 31:287–312.

Dobie, R.A., and Dillier, N. (1985). Some aspects of temporal coding for single-channel electrical stimulation of the cochlea. *Hearing Res.* 18:41–56.

Eddington, D.K., Dobelle, W.H., Brackmann, D.E., Mladejovsky, M.G., and Parkin, J.L. (1978). Auditory prosthesis research with multiple channel intracochlear stimulation in man. *Ann. Otol. Rhinol. Laryngol.* (*St. Louis*) Suppl. 53,87:1–39.

Gerstein, G.L., Bloom, M.J., Espinosa, I.E., and Evanczuk, S. (1983). Design of a laboratory for multineuron studies. *IEEE Trans. Systems Man Cyber. SMC* 13:668–676.

Hartmann, R., Topp, G., and Klinke, R. (1984). Discharge patterns of cat primary auditory fibers with electrical stimulation of the cochlea. *Hearing Res.* 13:47–62.

Hinojosa, R., and Marion, M. (1983). Histopathology of profound sensorineural deafness. *Ann. N.Y. Acad. Sci.* 405:459–484.

Johnsson, L.G., Hawkins, J.E. Jr., Kingsley, T.C., Black, F.O., and Matz, G.J. (1981). Aminoglycoside-induced cochlear pathology in man. *Acta Oto-laryngol.* (*Stockholm*) Suppl. 383 1–19.

Kiang, N.Y.S., and Moxon, E.C. (1972). Physiological considerations in artificial stimulation of the inner ear. *Ann. Otol. Rhinol. Laryngol.* (*St. Louis*) 81:714–730.

Kitzes, L.M., Gibson, M.M., Rose, J.E., and Hind, J.E. (1978). Initial discharge latency and threshold considerations for some neurons in the cochlear nuclear complex of the cat. *J. Neurophysiol.* 41:1165–1182.

Merzenich, M.M., and White, M.W. (1977). Cochlear implant. The interface problem. *Biomedical Engineering and Instrumentation. Funct. Elect. Stim.* 3:321–340.

Parkins, C.W., and Colombo, J. (1987). Auditory-nerve single-neuron thresholds to electrical stimulation from scala tympani electrodes. *Hearing Res.* 31:267–286.

Pfingst, B.E. (1984). Operating ranges and intensity psychophysics for cochlear implants. *Arch. Otol.* 110:140–144.

Pfingst, B.E. (1988). Comparisons of psychophysical and neurophysiological studies of cochlear implants. *Hearing Res.* 34:243–252.

Pfingst, B.E. (1989). Changes over time in thresholds for electrical stimulation of the cochlea. *Abstracts of the 12th Midwinter Research Meeting of the Association for Research in Otolaryngology.* pp. 270–271.

Pfingst, B.E., Burnett, P.A., and Sutton, D. (1983). Intensity discrimination with cochlear implants. *J. Acoust. Soc. Am.* 73:1283–1292.

Pfingst, B.E., Donaldson, J.A., Miller, J.M., and Spelman, F.A. (1979). Psychophysical evaluation of cochlear prostheses in a monkey model. *Ann. Otol. Rhinol. Laryngol.* (*St. Louis*) 88:613–625.

Pfingst B.E., Glass I., Spelman F.A., and Sutton D. (1985). Psychophysical studies of cochlear implants in monkeys: Clinical implications. In *Cochlear Implants,* edited by R.A. Schindler and M.M. Merzenich (New York: Raven Press), pp. 305–321.

Pfingst, B.E., and Rush, N.L. (1987). Discrimination of simultaneous frequency and level changes in electrical stimuli. *Ann. Otol. Rhinol. Laryngol.* (*St. Louis*) Suppl. 128,96:34–37.

Pfingst, B.E., and Sutton, D. (1983). Relation of cochlear implant function to histopathology in monkeys. *Ann. N.Y. Acad. Sci.* 405:224–239.

Pfingst, B.E., and Sutton, D. (1984). Relation of psychophysical thresholds for electrical stimuli to auditory nerve survival: Summary of results for 18 scala tympani implants. *Abstracts of the 7th Midwinter Research Meeting of the Association for Research in Otolaryngology*, p. 10.

Pfingst, B.E., Sutton, D., Miller, J.M., and Bohne, B.A. (1981). Relation of psychophysical data to histopathology in monkeys with cochlear implants. *Acta Oto-laryngol. (Stockholm)* 92:1–13.

Rose, J.E., Hind, J.E., Anderson, D.J., and Brugge, J.F. (1971). Some effects of stimulus intensity on response of auditory nerve fibers in the squirrel monkey. *J. Neurophysiol.* 34:685–699.

Rubinstein, J.T., and Spelman, F.A. (1988). Analytical theory for extracellular electrical stimulation of nerve with focal electrodes. I. Passive unmyelinated axon. *Biophys. J.* 54:975–981.

Shannon, R.V. (1983). Multichannel electrical stimulation of the auditory nerve in man. I. Basic psychophysics. *Hearing Res.* 11:157–189.

Shannon, R.V. (1985). Threshold and loudness functions for pulsatile stimulation of cochlear implants. *Hearing Res.* 11:157–189.

Shannon, R.V. (1986). Temporal processing in cochlear implants. In *Sensorineural Hearing Loss. Mechanisms, Diagnosis, Treatment,* edited by M.J. Collins, T.J. Glattke, and L.A. Harker (Iowa City: University of Iowa), pp. 349–367.

Spelman, F.A., Clopton, B.M. and Pfingst, B.E. (1982). Tissue impedance and current flow in the implanted ear: Implications for the cochlear prosthesis. *Ann. Othol. Rhinol. Laryngol. (St. Louis)* Suppl. 98,91:3–8.

Spelman, F.A., Pfingst, B.E., and Miller, J.M. (1978). A constant-current stimulator for use with chronic cochlear implants. *Proc. San Diego Biomed. Symp.* 17:1–3.

Spelman, F.A., Soma, M., and Rubinstein, J.T. (1984). Electric field models of implanted ear. *Abstracts of the 7th Midwinter Research Meeting of the Association for Research in Otolaryngology*, p. 81.

van den Honert, C., and Stypulkowski, P.H. (1984). Physiological properties of electrically stimulated auditory nerve. II. Single fiber recordings. *Hearing Res.* 14:225–243.

van den Honert, C., and Stypulkowski, P.H. (1987). Single fiber mapping of spatial excitiation patterns in the electrically stimulated auditory nerve. *Hearing Res.* 29:195–206.

Voigt, H.F., and Young, E.D. (1988). Neural correlations in the dorsal cochlear nucleus: Pairs of units with similar response properties. *J. Neurophysiol.* 59:1014–1032.

Wilson, B.S., and Finley, C.C. (1986). Latency fields in electrically evoked hearing. *Abstracts of the 9th Midwinter Research Meeting of the Association for Research in Otolaryngology*. pp. 170–171.

Xue, X., and Pfingst, B.E. (1989). Inner ear implants for experimental electrical stimulation of auditory nerve arrays. *J. Neurosci. Meth.*, 28:189–196.

Bryan E. Pfingst: Discussion

Dr. Shannon: I have a comment on your hypothesis B about threshold as determined by spreading excitation. Certainly there has to be a limitation on the extent of the spread over which you can integrate activity for a threshold sensation, as evidenced by the literature on critical bands. Another experiment that comes to mind is an old experiment with subthreshold noise bands in separate critical bands. If you take subthreshold stimulation in different critical bands and sum them together, it's still subthreshold. So there is some spatial limitation to that kind of integration.

Dr. Pfingst: I think that's really the next step in this process: to try to determine how many fibers must be activated to reach threshold and where they have to be. However, we must demonstrate first whether or not any across-fiber integration is required to reach threshold.

Dr. van den Honert: I have a question about your concern for the threshold changes with time with the chronic implants. In your first graph I thought you mentioned that the threshold actually rises for a few days or weeks and then comes back down. How does the initial threshold compare with the eventual steady-state one? That's the one that's really appropriate to compare with the acute physiological experiments. We don't have data over the low-frequency range, but with 100-μs pulses, our chronic animals didn't show any significant threshold reduction for gross potentials.

Dr. Pfingst: It is a little difficult to detail what is going on immediately after surgery. I only have data on a few animals where we began testing on day 1. Even in these cases we didn't start testing these animals until 24 h after the surgery. In these cases, as soon as we started stimulating, we could see the thresholds rise. This was a very rapid rise. When the thresholds came back down, they seemed to return to the initial level, that is, the 24-h level. However, in most cases we didn't start the animal until several days after the surgery, and in these cases we didn't even see this initial rise.

Dr. Finley: Do you think that learning might account for these threshold changes?

Dr. Pfingst: I don't think so. First, the monkeys are well trained acoustically before they are implanted, and seem to transfer very rapidly to electrical stimulation. Also, there is one case where we didn't start stimulation until about a month after surgery, and in that case the thresholds were stable from the beginning. The fact that some thresholds first rise and then fall also suggests that this is not a learning effect. Finally, there were cases where the thresholds on one electrode pair dropped more rapidly than those on another pair in the same implant. This suggests that maybe there is some kind of local effect.

Dr. Javel: Given that the input-output functions of the auditory nerve fiber response to electrical stimuli are incredibly steep, I don't see how any kind of population summation could drive thresholds down 20 or 30 dB, which you need at these low frequencies to get the data for nerve fiber and behavioral thresholds to correspond. My other concern is that most nerve-fiber recordings are from acutely implanted animals that have a full complement of nerve fibers, while you're recording thresholds in an animal that's been deaf for a good long time. The current paths may be very different. These are two very different preparations and hence could have very different thresholds. Anecdotally, this is supported by the observation that the thresholds to electrical stimulation in normal-hearing people (with ECoG electrodes) always tend to be considerably higher than electrical stimulation thresholds in deaf people that are being considered for implantation.

Dr. Pfingst: I agree with you 100%. The difficulty I have is in applying the neural data that may be from a very different preparation, as you say, than that used for the behavioral experiments. I would like to see some electro-physiological experiments done in cases where the animals are deafened and implanted and then left to sit for a couple of months, maybe with some electrical stimulation during that period, before the electrophysiological experiments are done. I think unless we can get a correspondence in terms of the absolute levels at which we're stimulating, it's difficult to make other correlations between the two sets of data.

12
A Model of Temporal Integration and Forward Masking for Electrical Stimulation of the Auditory Nerve

ROBERT V. SHANNON

Introduction

Cochlear implants provide a unique opportunity to investigate the peripheral determinants of auditory perception. In cochlear implant patients we can stimulate the remaining neurons of the cochlea with electrical currents to produce the sensation of sound. However, the entire spatial-temporal pattern of neural activity is fundamentally different than that produced in the normal cochlea. The normal frequency selectivity of the cochlea is absent, and can only be recreated crudely by placing electrodes at different locations along the cochlea. The temporal discharge characteristics of neurons in response to electrical stimulation are also different than in response to acoustic stimulation. The limited physiological data available (Glass, 1984; Hartmann, Topp, and Klinke, 1984; Javel et al., 1987; Kiang and Moxon, 1972; Merzenich et al., 1973; Moxon, 1971; Stypulkowski and van den Honert, 1984; van den Honert and Stypulkowski, 1984) indicate that an electrical stimulus entrains synchronous firing in all nerves stimulated. Electrically stimulated neurons do not respond stochastically, nor are their responses independent of each other. Since these two aspects of normal cochlear function—the spatial pattern and the temporal microstructure—are quite different in implanted subjects and normal-hearing listeners, we can observe their consequences for perception by measuring quantitative differences in psychophysical measures.

First, let us consider the role of the spatial-temporal pattern of neural activity on auditory perception. Some "primitive" perceptions are probably determined by the global aspects of this pattern, e.g., threshold. Threshold is probably achieved when a small number of auditory neurons respond above their spontaneous rate of discharge (in terms of either rate or synchronized activity). Thus, we can observe the values of the physical electrical stimuli that produce a threshold response. This combination of electrical parameters then specifies the physical electrical stimuli that are effective in activating a single neuron or small group of neurons. These threshold values are probably determined by the biophysical properties of the electrode/neural interface. Shannon (1985) presented a phenomenological model of threshold for biphasic pulsatile stimuli.

However, for more complicated perceptions, more is involved than the biophysics of the electrode/neuron interface. Loudness, for example, probably involves the spread of activity across the neural array (either in rate increases or in synchronization increases.) Pitch appears to be determined by a complex interaction of the place of stimulation, rate of stimulation, and stimulus level (Shannon, 1983; Townshend et al., 1987).

Now let us consider how temporal perception might be related to the neural response to a tone burst. We propose that the temporal envelope of the neural response is the important physiological quantity for tasks which require subjects to detect or discriminate small time intervals, e.g., forward masking. The temporal envelope of the neural response has been extensively studied and quantified (Harris and Dallos, 1979; Smith, 1977, 1979; Smith and Brachman, 1980, 1982; Smith & Zwislocki, 1975; Westerman and Smith, 1984). At the onset of a stimulus, the neural response shows a pronounced peak (or overshoot) in the first 1–2 ms. Following this peak, the neural firing rate decreases exponentially to reach a steady-state firing rate after 50–100 ms. At the offset of the stimulus the neural activity is reduced to levels below its spontaneous rate of firing, after which the firing rate recovers exponentially to the normal spontaneous rate.

Zwislocki (1969) proposed a model of temporal integration using this neural envelope as the input to a central integrator mechanism. Temporal integration data for normal listeners and hearing-impaired listeners could be predicted by this model. If this temporal envelope is indeed the important feature of the neural pattern for temporal integration, then the same approach might also be used to explain other temporal psychophysical performance, such as forward masking. If this approach is valid, we should be able to predict the differences in psychophysical measures between normal and implanted listeners on the basis of differences in the temporal envelope of the neural responses to acoustic and electrical stimulation.

In this paper we will present psychophysical measures of temporal integration and forward masking from cochlear implant patients. The results will be compared with the same psychophysical measures in normal-hearing subjects. A model will be presented (a modification of Zwislocki's model) which will account for these psychophysical results both in normal acoustic stimulation and in electrical stimulation of cochlear implants.

Model

The Model, schematically represented in Figure 12.1, consists of several stages. First the physical stimulus (acoustic or electrical) is transformed at the periphery into a pattern of neural activity. For acoustic stimulation, this process includes cochlear filtering, basilar membrane travel time, and the hair-cell–VIII nerve synapse. This process includes such phenomena as rate saturation, two-tone suppression, combination tone generation, neural adaptation, and recovery from adaptation. For the purposes of this model we will only consider the temporal envelope, i.e., frequency selectivity will be ignored, so that the results will apply only to broadband maskers and signals. We are interested in the quantitative relation between the temporal envelope of the neural response and perception.

In cochlear implants this peripheral transformation is determined by the biophysical characteristics of the electrode/neural interface. There is no frequency selectivity mechanism, no synaptic transmission, and no basilar membrane traveling wave. The neural response is determined by the amplitude and duration of each phase of a biphasic pulse stimulus, by the proximity of the nerve to the electrode, by the diameter of the nerve or dendrite at the point of activation, and by the capacitive properties of the neural membrane-myelin sheath. It is not clear whether or not electrically stimulated nerves show adaptation. Adaptation may not occur in this case if neural adaptation is due to the properties of the synapse. Whatever part of adaptation is due to the inherent properties of the nerve itself (e.g., refractory properties) should still be present with electrical stimulation.

The main part of the model is the same as that proposed by Zwislocki (1969). The initial short-term integrator, called nerual "equilibration" time by Zwiskocki, has not been implemented in the following calculations, but it is assumed to have a very short time constant, on the order of 1–2 ms.

The stimulus intensity is then converted to neural units. This stage is assumed to represent both the neural rate-intensity functions and the loudness growth function, since it is assumed for the purposes of the model that "integrated neural activity . . . is directly proportional to loudness" (Zwiskocki, 1969, p. 433). Thus, even though individual unit responses show a limited dynamic range and rate saturation, the model assumes that the same rate-intensity slope is available somewhere in the excited neural pattern. We will assume, as did Zwislocki, that for acoustic stimulation the relation is described by a power law function; i.e., loudness is proportional to stimulus intensity raised to a power. We will assume that for normal hearing the relationship is compressive (Stevens, 1961).

With electrical stimulation we know that the growth of loudness is an

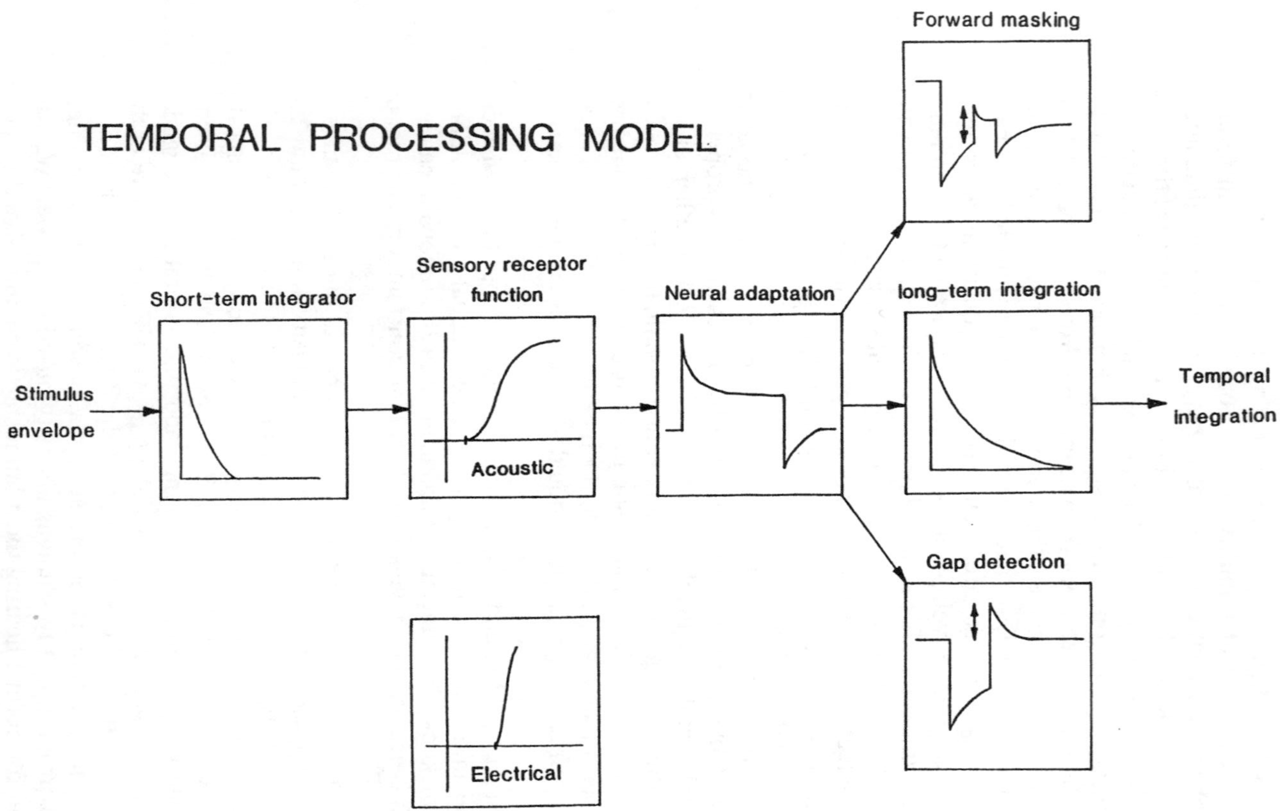

FIGURE 12.1. Block diagram of proposed model of temporal processing. The center path is essentially the model of Zwislocki (1969). The "sensory receptor" function is a simple power function $y = X^p$. The exponent of the power function is less than 1.0 for acoustic stimulation and 2 to 3.5 for electrical stimulation. The neural adaptation function is based on work by Smith and Brachman (1980) and by Harris and Dallos (1979). We assume that the central system can access this neural information directly for tasks such as gap detection or forward masking. The detection of the following signal is presumed to occur at the onset of the second stimulus.

expanding power law function of stimulus amplitude, loudness being proportional to stimulus amplitude raised to an exponent of 2–3 (Müller, 1981, 1983; Shannon, 1983). We also know that the neural rate-intensity functions are very steep compared with acoustic stimulation (Kiang and Moxon, 1972). Thus, for this intensity transformation stage of the model, we assume that the primary difference between acoustic and electrical stimulation is a change in the exponent in the power law function.

This transformed intensity envelope is then the driving stimulus of the neural adaptation mechanism in the model. The neural adaptation consists of three components: a rapid adaptation at the onset of the stimulus, a short-term adaptation, and a steady-state response. Using Zwislocki's terminology, we see that the neural response, $\in(t)$, to a rectangular stimulus envelope is

$$\in(t) = \in_b e^{-\beta t} + \in_c e^{-\Gamma t} + \in_\infty \tag{1}$$

where the first term represents the rapid adaptation component, the second term the short-term adaptation, and the third term the steady-state rate. The two adaptation components are represented as exponentially decaying activity, each with its own time constant, β and Γ, and weighting factor, $\in_b$ and $\in_c$. We know from the extensive work by Smith and colleagues (Smith, 1977, 1979; Smith and Brachman, 1982; Smith and Zwiskocki, 1975; Westerman and Smith, 1984) that the time constants are on the order of 1–2 ms for the rapid adaptation process and on the order of 30–50 ms for the short-term adaptation process. We also know from their work the relation between the firing rates during each of these processes. Figure 12.2 is adapted from Westerman and Smith (1984) and plots the firing rate in the first 1 ms of the neural response (rapid adaptation phase) and the first 10 ms of the neural response (short-term adaptation phase), each as a function of the steady-state firing rate. In Figure 12.2 the short-term adaptation firing rate is a linear function of the steady-state rate. In terms of Equation (1) this means that $\in_c/\in_\infty$ is a constant, which we will call K. However, the rapid adaptation firing rate is a nonlinear function of the steady-state rate, which we will model as the exponential function, $\in_b = \in_\infty^{p2}$. This is an important observation, since it means that the onset response contains more information about the temporal onset of the stimulus than the steady-state response or the short-term adaptation response. As the stimulus level is increased, this onset component of the neural response contains increasingly more information relative to the steady-state response. We will use this fact in our extension of Zwislocki's model to the case of forward masking. Using these two observations from Smith and colleagues' neural recordings, we can simplify Equation (1) as

$$\in(t) = (\in_\infty^{p2})e^{-\beta t} + (K^*\in_\infty)e^{-\Gamma t} + \in_\infty \tag{2}$$

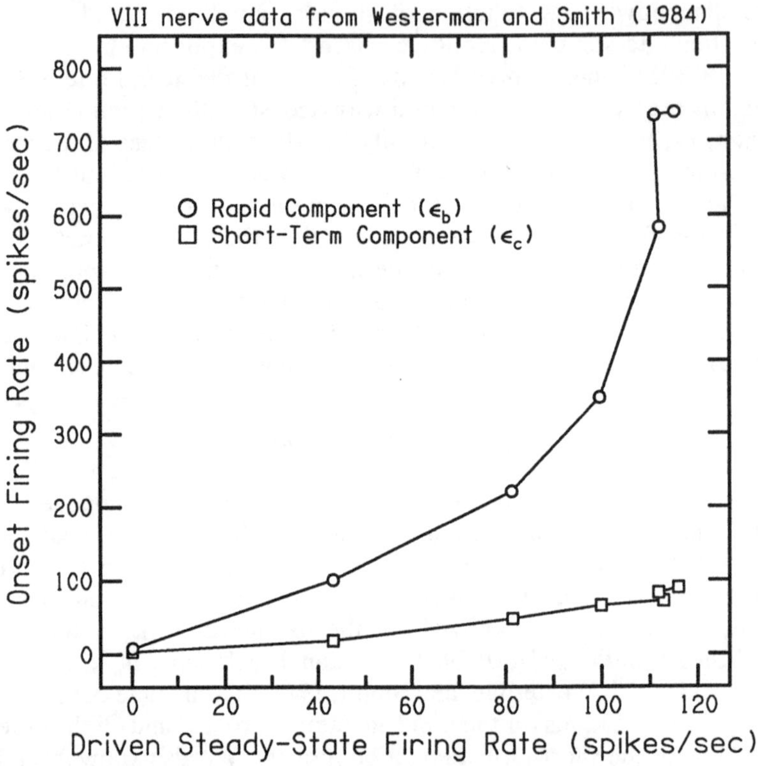

FIGURE 12.2. Comparison of onset response rate as a function of steady-state firing rate, after Westerman and Smith (1984). Note that as stimulus intensity is increased, the rapid adaptation component of the onset response increases faster than the steady-state rate, while the short-term component of the onset response in linearly related to the steady-state rate.

Zwiskocki (1969) then assumes that this neural output is the input to a central, long-term integrator to explain the temporal integration data. We will also make this assumption for temporal integration, but we assume that this central integrator can be bypassed for tasks like forward masking which emphasize quick response times. If the central integrator has a time constant of α, then the total neural output following this integration is specified by the convolution integral

$$\Theta(t) = \int_{-\infty}^{t} \in(\tau)\, e^{-(t-\tau)\alpha}\, d\tau \qquad (3)$$

Modifications in the Model for Electrical Stimulation

Two changes have been made in the model for the case of electrical stimulation: the rate-intensity function is assumed to be steeper for electrical stimulation than for acoustic stimulation, and the rapid-onset component of the neural response is assumed to be missing. These assumptions are consistent with the known differences between electrically stimulated and acoustically stimulated physiological data (Javel et al., 1987; Kiang and Moxon, 1972; Moxon, 1971; van den Honert and Stypulkowski, 1984). The rate-intensity functions are very steep with electrical stimulation, with the firing rate going from spontaneous rate to saturation in only a few decibels.

A model by Smith and Brachman (1982) accurately describes most aspects of the acoustic temporal response pattern. In their model, neural adaptation and its time constants are due to synaptic events, such as ion flow and transmitter depletion. Since this hair cell–VIII nerve synapse is not present in electrical stimulation, we assume that the rapid adaptation component is absent. Unfortunately, there is little physiological data on neural adaptation with electrical stimulation.

Modifications of the Model for Forward Masking

We assume that Zwilocki's model is also applicable to the case of forward masking but that the central integration is bypassed. For forward masking the key features of the neural response are the onset response and its behavior during the recovery from adaptation.

Zwislocki's original model didn't include the effects of the recovery from adaptation following the offset of the stimulus, probably because little was known about this recovery in 1969. Since then, however, this recovery has been extensively studied and quantified (Harris and Dallos, 1979; Smith, 1977; Westerman and Smith, 1984). It has been shown that the driven neural rate and the spontaneous rate recover from adaptation with the same time constant. One feature of the recovery process that is still not well characterized is the behavior of the rapid adaptation component of the rapid onset response during the recovery from adaptation.

Let us consider the possible effect of the recovery from adaptation on the rapid adaptation component of the onset response. As an example, imagine that we have two equal-amplitude stimuli separated by a silent interval, such as would occur in a gap detection experiment. When the silent interval is long, the onset response of the second burst in unaffected by the preceding stimulus. As the silent interval is shortened, both the rapid component and the short-term component of the onset response are reduced by the recovery from adaptation of the first stimulus. As the silent interval is reduced to zero, we know that both onset components must disappear, because in this case the first and second stimulus are contiguous and there is no onset response to the second stimulus. The quantitative effect of the recovery from adaptation on the onset response components has not been well characterized. The rapid and short-term components cannot be reduced by the same amount because they are nonlinearly related. Therefore, the rapid onset component either must recover from adaptation with a different time constant (as suggested by Westerman and Smith, 1984) or must be nonlinearly reduced during adaptation with repect to the short-term adaptation component and steady-state response. We chose the latter possibility for the present model. We will assume that the expanding *exponent* of the rapid onset rate-intensity function [$p2$ in Equation (2)] recovers exponentially following a preceding stimulus. Immediately following a stimulus we assume that there is no rapid adaptation component of the onset response and that it recovers exponentially. This assumption is consistent with the data of Westerman and Smith (1984).

Psychophysical Detection Assumptions

We assume that absolute threshold occurs when the integrated neural output $\theta(t)$ achieves a criterion magnitude. For temporal integration, we compute at each signal duration the signal level necessary to achieve this criterion level in decibels (re threshold for a 1-s duration stimulus).

For forward masking we assume that detection occurs at the leading edge of the signal burst, utilizing the rapid onset reponse component. Since this component provides differentially more information about the onset of the signal than the steady-state rate, it should provide the best and most efficient cue to the presence or absence of the signal. In forward masking the excitation level was computed for masker-alone condition and for the masker-plus-signal condition. Masked threshold was assumed to be achieved at the signal level at which the ratio of the masker-plus-signal to masker exceeded the criterion value.

Method

Subjects

Data from eight listeners are presented in this study. All were adults (25–78 years) with profound, bilateral sensorineural hearing loss. Three subjects were implanted with the Nucleus/Cochlear Corporation 22-electrode device (Clark et al., 1987), four with the Symbion Corporation 6-electrode device (Eddington et al., 1978), and one with the UCSF device (Loeb et al., 1983).

Equipment

For the Symbion patients, stimulus generation and data collection were accomplished using PC AT clone microcomputer. Stimuli were computed digitally, and samples were output at a 10-kHz rate through 12-bit digital-to-analog converters (Data Translation DT2801-A). For sinusoidal stimuli the signal was low-pass-filtered at 5 kHz (6-dB/octave filter slope). This analog signal was then passed through an optically isolated, constant-current source (Vurek et al., 1983) to maintain control over stimulus current and to isolate the patient from electrical continuity with the computer. The output of the optically isolated current source was connected directly to the patient's percutaneous connector (ITT Cannon). The equipment was calibrated, and electrode impedance was measured to assess electrode integrity before each testing session.

The patient was seated in front of a switch that would terminate all connections with the equipment in case of any unpleasant or uncomfortable stimuli. Patients responded on a small hand-held, touch-sensitive tablet (Koala Technologies).

The testing equipment was similiar for the UCSF patient, except a Data General Eclipse computer was used for stimulus generation and response collection and the patient response panel was custom-built.

Nucleus patients were tested through the Nucleus speech processor interface (SPI) under computer control. The Nucleus device allows stimulation with biphasic pulse stimuli only. Custom software controlled presentation of bursts of biphasic pulses to any electrode or combination of electrodes. In presenting data for these subjects, electrodes are indicated as an ordered pair (a,b), where a is the electrode number of the source and b is the number of the ground (or sink) electrode. The electrodes are numbered from 1 at the basal end of the array to 22 at the apical end. Amplitude calibration varied from patient to patient because of impedance variations in the components of the internal portions of each implant device. A table lookup procedure was implemented to deliver the desired amplitude in microamps based on individual calibration curves obtained for each patient from the Nucleus Corporation. Some of these patients were also tested using a custom interface (Shannon et al., 1988). There were no significant differences between any measures using the two interfaces, and the data from both are presented.

Since the implanted portion of the Nucleus implant receives power from the transmitted signal, it is necessary to send several pulses prior to the actual stimulus to power-up the internal receiver. In the present studies, 10 subthreshold pulses were sent at 1000 Hz prior to each stimulus interval.

Procedure

Temporal integration threshold measures were collected using a combination of the method of limits and Bekesy tracking. This procedure, which produces fast and reliable threshold measures, has been described elsewhere (Shannon, 1983). Stimulus bursts of 300-ms duration alternating with 500 ms of silence were presented to the patient. The level of the stimulus was started at a subthreshold level and slowly increased. Patients were instructed to push a button on the response pad as soon as they could hear the pulsing stimulus. The signal level then jumped up in level 2.5 dB (which was clearly audible but not unpleasantly loud) and its level slowly decreased. The patients were instructed to hold the button down until they could no longer hear the stimulus. The duration of the stimulus was then decreased and the procedure repeated. Each threshold estimate represents a single method-of-limits measure, i.e., the average of the ascending and descending response levels.

All forward-masking data were collected using an adaptive, two-interval, forced-choice (2AFC) procedure. A two-down, one-up adaptive strategy was employed to estimate the signal level that could be detected correctly 70.7% of the time (Levitt, 1971). The initial signal level was clearly audible and was decreased 1 dB after two correct responses. After four reversals in level, the step size was reduced to 0.5 dB. These values resulted in rapid convergence, with threshold taken to be the mean of the last eight reversals, discarding the first four. Typical standard deviations of threshold level obtained using this technique were between 0.5 and 1.0 dB.

Results—Fits of Model to Data

Figure 12.3 presents model computations for temporal integration (*a*) as well as temporal integration data from six implanted patients (*b*). The model calculations (*a*) show the changes in the temporal integration functions that can be expected by simply changing the exponent of the power law function that represents the "sensory receptor" function. The model output for an exponent of 0.6 closely matches typical acoustic data from Plomp and Bouman (1959). The slope of the temporal integration function for this normal case indicates that threshold is determined by a constant amount of energy (Garner and Miller, 1947).

Hearing-impaired listeners with loudness recruitment have flatter temporal integration functions than normal-hearing listeners (Fay and Coombs, 1983; Gerken, Gunnarson, and Allen, 1983, Martin and Wofford, 1970; Wright, 1968). This is represented in the model; as the exponent is increased from 0.6 to 3.6, the temporal integration functions get flatter, indicating less apparent integration. In fact, all curves are computed with the same time constant and the same integration. The functions are flatter as the exponent increases, because less intensity increment is needed to compensate for a change of duration. The higher the exponent, the larger the increment in firing rate (or loudness) with level. Another way of describing this effect is to say that the quantity being integrated is related to loudness, rather than to physical intensity. In cases of rapid loudness growth (as in recruitment), less increase in

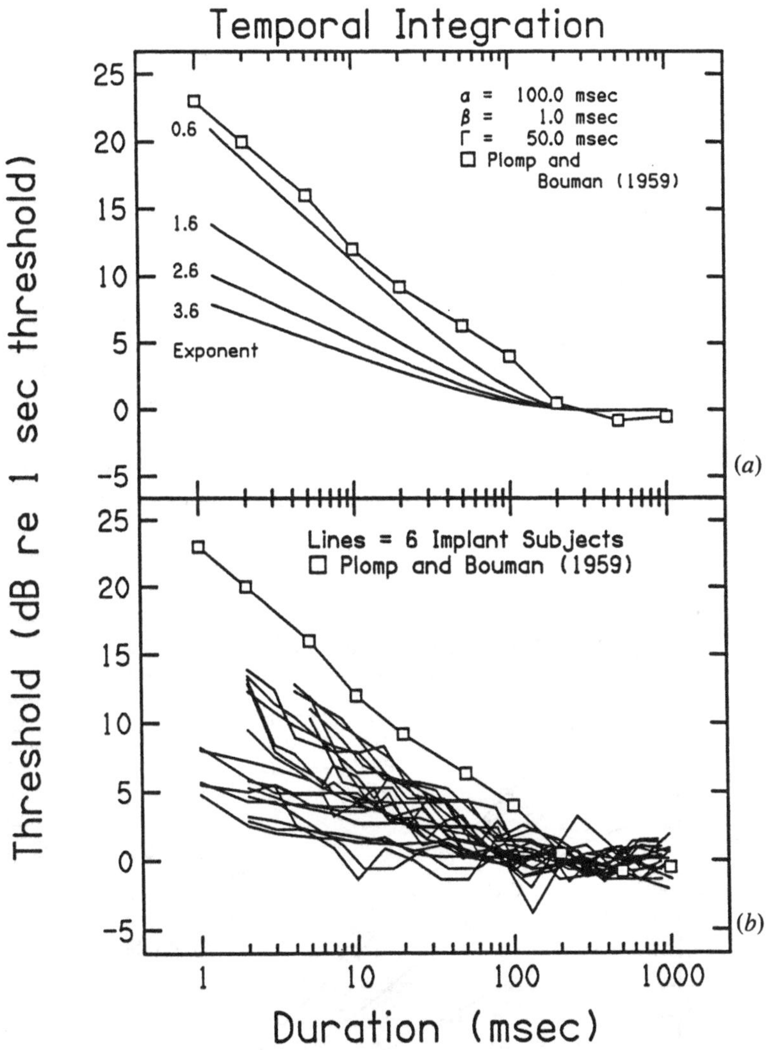

FIGURE 12.3. Comparison of model predictions with data from acoustic and electrical temporal integration. The upper panel (*a*) shows the model predictions for temporal integration with different curves representing different exponents in the power function. Notice that the model predicts shallower slopes as the exponent increases. The open symbols in the upper and lower panels are typical integration data from normal observers (Plomp and Bouman, 1959). The upper panel compares these data with model predictions. The lower panel (*b*) compares these data with temporal integration functions from cochlear implant listeners.

physical intensity is needed to produce the same increment in loudness and thus compensate for a change in duration.

The data from cochlear implant patients (Figure 12.3*b*) show temporal integration functions that range from those that are nearly normal to those that show almost no temporal integration (see also Müller, 1981; Shannon, 1986). This figure presents 22 temporal integration functions from 6 implanted listeners, for stimulation of different cochlear locations and with different electrode configurations. Since we do not have individual loudness functions or rate-intensity functions from these patients, it is not clear if the slope of the temporal integration function is inversely related to the slope of the loudness functions, as is implied by the model. But the range of exponents implied by the range of slopes of the integration functions is consistent with the range of loudness growth exponents observed in cochlear implant patients (Shannon, 1983).

Figure 12.4 presents acoustic forward-masking data from Plomp (1964) along with fits from this model. As can be seen, the model is able to predict the main features of the data quite well: the forward-masking recovery functions on these axes are well represented by a family

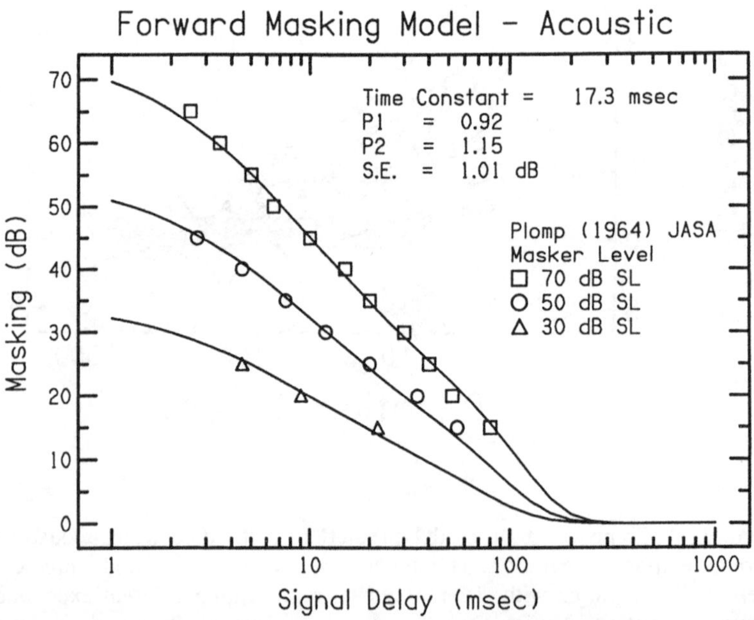

FIGURE 12.4. Forward-masking predictions of the model for normal acoustic stimulation compared with typical acoustic forward-masking data for 30-, 50-, and 70-dB SL maskers (Plomp, 1964). The slope of the data curves and model predictions increases with the masker level.

of converging straight lines. The model parameters that provide the best fit to the data according to a least-squares criterion (standard error = 1.01 dB) are given in the inset of Figure 12.4. The compressive power is only slightly compressive (0.92). The exponent of the rapid onset firing rate is an expanding power of the steady-state rate (1.15). The surprising finding is that the time constant is only 17.3 ms, while the forward-masking effect persists for over 100 ms. This result is due to the fact that, with a compressive nonlinearity followed by an integrator, a short time constant will produce effects at much longer times (Divenyi and Shannon, 1983; Penner, 1978). For a single time constant, more compression will cause the effects to persist longer.

Figure 12.5 presents forward-masking data from four cochlear implant

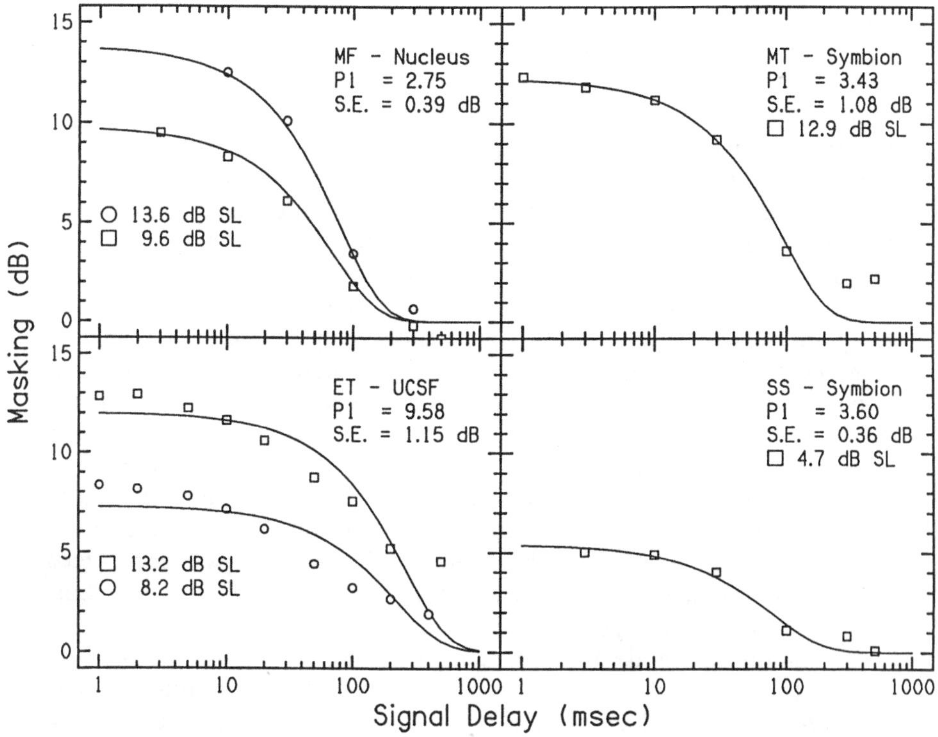

FIGURE 12.5. Forward-masking data and model predictions for electrical stimulation. The same time constant was used to fit these data as was used for the acoustic data in Figure 12.4. The exponent values that provided the best fit of the model to the data were 2.75, 9.58, 3.43, and 3.60 for panels (*a*) to (*d*), respectively. Note that although the curves are different from those obtained with acoustic stimulation, the same time constant of recovery from adaptation was used.

patients along with model fits. These data are similar to previously reported data on forward masking in cochlear implant patients (Dent and Townshend, 1987; Müller, 1981, 1983; Shannon, 1986). The time constant used for the adaptation recovery was the same (17.3 ms) as that used in Figure 12.4 for the acoustic data. The only changes were to eliminate the rapid onset component of the response and to change the exponent of the rate-intensity function. As can be seen, the exponents are considerably larger for the implanted patients than the value 0.92 used for the acoustic data. The exponent differences are in line with the known differences in rate-intensity functions (Kiang and Moxon, 1972) and in loudness functions (Shannon, 1983).

Discussion

The present model demonstrates that it is possible to predict normal and impaired psychophysical temporal processing from a physiologically based model. Figures 12.3 and 12.5 show that the differences between normal and implant psychophysical results are well accounted for by known differences in the physiological response: steeper rate-intensity functions (Kiang and Moxon, 1972) and the lack of a rapid onset component (Javel et al., 1987). The fact that a simple change in the neural response quantitatively predicts the psychophysical changes implies that the central temporal processing is intact, and that implanted patients have no fundamental deficit in temporal processing.

The present model demonstrates that the envelope of the neural temporal response could be the significant stimulus for temporal integration and forward masking. If the model is correct, this implies that the cochlea probably has little influence on these measures. The main differences between measures of temporal resolution in normals and implants can be explained by the differences in the end organ intensity-response functions. The role of the cochlea is important only in its effect on this intensity function. Cochlear processes might introduce additional time delays that would limit the ability of the central system to detect small temporal intervals, and such seems to be the case for gap detection at low frequencies (Florentine and Buus, 1984).

In addition, this model has important implications for implant processor design. If we can make the appropriate intensity translation from acoustic pressure to electrical current, we could deliver the amount of current necessary to produce a temporal neural envelope appropriate for that acoustic level. According to the model this intensity translation should also map loudness correctly from the acoustic to electrical domain. This transformation should make implant temporal processing performance comparable to that of normal listeners.

References

Clark, G.M.,et al. (1987). *The University of Melbourne–Nucleus Multi-electrode Cochlear Implant* (Karger, New York).

Dent, L.J., and Townshend, B.S. (1987). Backward and forward masking for direct electrical stimulation of the VIIIth nerve in two profoundly deaf subjects. *J. Acoust. Soc. Am.* 82(S1), S72(A).

Divenyi, P.L., and Shannon, R.V. (1983). Auditory time constants unified. *J. Acoust. Soc. Am.* 74,S10.

Eddington, D.K., Dobelle, W.H., Brachman, D.E., Mladevosky, M.G., and Parkin, J.L. (1978). Auditory prosthesis research with multiple channel intra-cochlear stimulation in man. *Ann. Otol. Rhinol. Laryngol.* Suppl. 53,87: 1–39.

Fay, R.R., and Coombs, S. (1983). Neural mechanisms in sound detection and temporal summation, *Hearing Res.* 10, 70–90.

Florentine, M., and Buus, S. (1984). Temporal gap detection in sensorineural and simulated hearing impairment. *J. Speech Hearing Res.* 27, 449–455.

Garner, W.R., and Miller, G.A. (1947). The masked threshold of pure tones as a function of duration. *J. Exp. Psychol.* 37,293–303.

Gerken, G.M., Gunnarson, A.D., and Allen, C.M. (1983). Three models of temporal summation evaluated using normal-hearing and hearing-impaired subjects. *J. Speech Hear. Res.* 26,249–256.

Glass, I. (1984). Responses of cochlear nucleus units to electrical stimulation through a cochlear prosthesis: Channel interacton. *Hearing Res.* 17, 115–126.

Harris, D.M., and Dallos, P. (1979). Forward masking of auditory nerve fiber responses. *J. Neurophysiol.* 42,1083–1107.

Hartmann, R., Topp, G., and Klinke, R. (1984). Discharge patterns of cat primary auditory fibers with electrical stimulation of the cochlea. *Hearing Res.* 13, 47–62.

Javel, E., Tong, Y.C., Shepherd, R.K., and Clark, G.M. (1987). Cat auditory nerve fiber responses to biphasic electrical current pulses. *Ann. Otol. Rhinol. Laryngol.* 96, 26–30.

Kiang, N.Y.S., and Moxon, E.C. (1972). Physiological considerations in artificial stimulations of the inner ear. *Ann. Otol. Rhinol. Laryngol. 81,* 714–730.

Levitt, H. (1971) Transformed up-down methods in psychoacoustics, *J. Acoust. Soc. Amer.*, 49,467–477.

Loeb, G.E., Byers. C.L., Rebscher, S.J., Casey, D.E., Fong, M.M., Schindler, R.A., Gray, R.F., and Merzenich, M.M. (1983). Design and fabrication of an experimental cochlear prosthesis. *Med. Bio. Eng. Comput.* 21,241–254.

Martin, F.N., and Wofford, M.J. (1970). Temporal summation of brief tones in normal and cochlear-impaired ears. *J. Aud. Res.* 10, 82–86.

Merzenich, M.M., Michelson, R.P., Petit, C.R., Schindler, R.A., and Ried, M. (1973). Neural encoding of sound sensation evoked by electrical stimulation of the acoustic nerve. *Ann. Otol. Rhinol. Laryngol.* 83,486–503.

Moxon, E.C. (1971). *Neural and Mechanical Responses to Electric Stimulation of the Cat's Inner Ear.* Doctoral dissertation, MIT, Cambridge, Mass.

Müller, C.G. (1981). Survery of cochlear implant work. *J. Acoust. Soc. Am.* 70, S52.

Müller, C.G. (1983). Comparison of percepts found with cochlear implant devices.

In *Cochlear Prostheses: An International Symposioum,* edited by C.W. Parkins and S.W. Anderson, *Annals of the N.Y. Academy of Sciences,* 405: 412–420.

Penner, M.J. (1978). A power law transformation resulting in a class of short-term integrators that produce time-intensity trades for noise bursts. *J. Acoust. Soc. Am.* 63, 195–201.

Plomp, R. (1964). Rate of decay of auditory sensation. *J. Acoust. Soc. Am.* 36, 277–282.

Plomp, R., and Bouman, M.A. (1959). Relation between hearing threshold and duration for tone pulses. *J. Acoust. Soc. Am.* 31, 749–758.

Shannon, R.V. (1983). Multichannel electrical stimulation of the auditory nerve in man: I. Basic psychophysics. *Hearing Res.* 11, 157–189.

Shannon, R.V. (1985). A model of threshold and loudness for pulsatile electrical stimulation of cochlear implants. *Abstracts of the 8th Midwinter Research Meeting of the Association for Research in Otholaryngology,* 107.

Shannon, R.V. (1986). Temporal processing in cochlear implants. In *Sensorineural Hearing Loss: Mechanisms, Diagnosis, and Treatment,* edited by M.J. Collins, T.J. Glattke, and L.A. Harker (Iowa City: University of Iowa Press), pp. 349–368.

Shannon, R.V. (1989). Detection of gaps in sinusoids and biphasic pulse trains by patients with cochlear implants. *J. Acoust. Soc. Am.,* in press.

Shannon, R.V., Adams, D.D., Ferrel, R.L., Palumbo, R.L., and Grandgenett, M. (1988). A computer interface for psychophysical and speech research with the Nucleus cochlear implant. *J. Acoust. Soc. Am.* 83, S16.

Smith, R.L. (1977). Short-term adaptation in auditory nerve fibers: Some post-stimulatory effects. *J. Neurophysiol.* 40, 1098–1112.

Smith, R.L. (1979). Adaptation, saturation, and physiological masking in single auditory nerve fibers. *J. Acoust. Soc. Am.* 65, 166–178.

Smith, R.L., and Brachman, M.L. (1980). Operating range and maximum response of single auditory nerve fibers. *Brain Res.* 184, 499–505.

Smith, R.L., and Brachman, M.L. (1982). Adaptation in auditory-nerve fibers: A revised model. *Biol. Cybern.* 44, 107–120.

Smith, R.L., and Zwislocki, J.J. (1975). Short-term adaptation and incremental responses in single auditory nerve fibers. *Biol. Cybern.* 17, 169–182.

Stevens, S.S. (1961). To honor Fechner and repeal his law. *Science* 133, 80–86.

Stypulkowski, P.H., and van den Honert, C. (1984). Physiological properties of the electrically stimulated auditory nerve: I. Compound action potential recordings. *Hearing Res.* 14, 205–223.

Townshend, B.S., Cotter, N., Van Compernolle, D., and White, R.L. (1987). Pitch perception by cochlear implant subjects. *J. Acoust. Soc. Am.* 82, 106–115.

van den Honert, C., and Stypulkowski, P. (1984). Physiological properties of the electrically stimulated auditory nerve: II. Single fiber recordings. *Hearing Res.* 14, 225–243.

Vurek, L.S., White, M., Fong, M., and Walsh, S.M. (1981). Optoisolated stimulators used for electrically evoked BSER. *Ann. Otol. Rhinol. Laryngol.* Suppl. 82,90: 21–24.

Westerman, L.A., and Smith, R.L. (1984). Rapid and short-term adaptation in auditory nerve responses. *Hearing Res.* 15, 249–260.

Wright, H.N. (1968). The effect of sensor-neural hearing loss on threshold-duration functions. *J. Speech Hear. Res.* 11, 842–852.

Zwislocki, J.J. (1969). Temporal summation of loudness: An analysis. *J. Acoust. Soc. Am.* 46, 431–441.

Robert V. Shannon: Discussion

Dr. Johnstone: Why have you dropped rapid adaptation and kept everything else?

Dr. Shannon: It's because I think the very sharp onset is a different type of adaptation that may not be present in synapses as you go up the system. I think it's a property of the coupling between the hair cell and the first auditory nerve. In other nerve synapses to nerve impulses, there's no AC electrical current in the same sense as there is in the hair cell's first neuron junction. So it's possible in the electrical stimulation case there won't be rapid adaptation, and in fact, I think from what we've seen in the nerve responses to electrical stimulation there may not even be short-term adaptation.

Dr. Wakefield: Have you done modulated transfer functions with your model?

Dr. Shannon: Guido showed modulation transfer functions falling off above 5 Hz. I've had occasion to measure modulation transfer functions in two ways, both as true amplitude modulation and as detection of beats in envelopes. All of the curves that I have show the modulation function dropping off at 100 Hz, looking very similar to the low-frequency component of the absolute threshold curve; which means they're approximately flat up to 100 Hz and then roll off fairly steeply. Not 5 Hz. I don't know what the discrepancy is there.

Dr. Smoorenburg: What carrier frequencies did you use?

Dr. Shannon: I've used 500, 1000, 2000, and 4000 Hz.

Dr. Johnstone: On your adaptation, the models we have suggest both types of adaptation from the synaptic region. If you're going to cut one out, you really shouldn't show favoritism; you should cut the other one out too.

Dr. Shannon: That's no trouble for my model, because the short-term adaptation one is linearly related to the steady state, so it really adds nothing and would detract nothing to take it out. It would just change my scaling factor by one-half. The rapid adaptation component, because it's non-linearly related to the steady-state component, does make a big difference.

Dr. Johnstone: It's very difficult to think in terms of the physiology with reference to your model. There is not a one-to-one match between your boxes and physiological boxes.

Dr. Shannon: It's because the model is of a hybrid. I'm talking about physiological adaptation, but I'm preceding it by a rate-intensity function that has no saturation. I think the way to think about it is that this model represents an aggregate. It's not a model at a single-unit level, but rather as the excitation grows there are always some units that are in the region of increase in rate-intensity function. It's not a true physiological model.

Dr. Spelman: Then this is a conceptual model: a hypothesis.

Dr. Shannon: Right. I think I viewed this model just as a starting point. It's a conceptual model of . . . "is there a way that we can change things about the peripheral physiological response in ways that we know are different and have the perceptual responses follow in the right way." In this simplified view of things, that seems to happen.

Dr. Dent: Getting back to the question of forward masking, in the fall Brent Townshend and I reported that in patients we looked at, the forward-masking time constants were within normal limits for electrical stimulation. We raised the possibility then that all of the forward-masking effects could be supplied centrally. Since then, we did what you suggested, and looked at the growth of loudness, and expressed our time constants in terms of the decline of effective loudness, and we still find normal time constants. You're calling yours abnormal?

Dr. Shannon: No. The time constants I used to fit the cochlear implant data were exactly the same time constants that I used to fit Plomp's acoustic data, and the only thing that changed was the rate-intensity or loudness function, preceding the adaptation.

Dr. Johnstone: In regard to the forward-masking problem, you place great emphasis on the initial segment, or the initial spike, of the very high firing-rate burst. What happens if you lengthen the masker in your model?

Dr. Shannon: It shouldn't have any effect.

Dr. Johnstone: Have you done that in the patients?

Dr. Shannon: Well, the adaptation recovery period following stimulation is not terribly affected by duration of the preceding adapter once it's beyond 100 ms or so. Forward-masking results acoustically show the same phenomenon. If your acoustic maker is more than 100 ms in duration, there is really no difference. But as you shorten the masker duration below 100 ms, then you have an effect.

13
Interim Thoughts on Cochlear Tissues, Neural/Behavioral Models, and Encoding

FRANCIS A. SPELMAN AND JOSEF M. MILLER

Principal questions and challenges facing the field of neural and behavioral modeling of the electrically stimulated ear have been well described by Smoorenburg, van den Honert, Hartmann and Klinke, Pfingst, and Shannon in this volume. There is a clear need for additional data on fundamental issues concerning electrically generated perceptual space and hearing abilities provided by electrical stimulation, the development of this space(s), and the dependency of its characteristics on encoding strategies used to excite eighth nerve fibers, the state of the temporal bone, previous abilities and experiences of the patient, and much more. At a physiological level, we must further define the response features of auditory nerves in the normal and pathological preparation to electrical stimulation, define the dynamic range of function of the system with different stimulation configurations, test strategies for mimicking acoustical response properties with electrical stimuli, and define the important questions to ask high centers of the auditory system regarding the processing of complex signals. As well, issues must be addressed of how we will relate physiological observations to behavioral data, e.g., why the synchrony characteristics of auditory cells observed in response to high-frequency electrical stimuli do not lead to better high-frequency discrimination and pitch perception. As well, we must determine why capabilities to extract information regarding simple signals do not determine discrimination performance of complex signals. Finally and importantly, we must determine how these perceptual abilities and response properties of the system vary with the variety of pathologies that lead to profound deafness.

The models proposed in the papers by Spelman and by Finley, Wilson, and White in this volume may, in part, serve as a theoretical basis for addressing some of these issues, as an interface between concerns for the characteristics of cochlear tissues and issues of neural and behavioral models, and as an avenue to address questions of encoding schemes. Thus, organization of the normal peripheral auditory system suggests that cochlear implants should consist of large numbers of stimulators, each of which excites small numbers of nerve cells. When focused stimuli are used, investigators or therapists can drive localized regions of the auditory nerve to test temporal coding schemes, determine the effects on temporal coding of driving small or large numbers of cells, or develop methods by which patients can be tested. In the last case, specificity of stimuli may lead to determination of pathology and to the modification of a prosthesis to suite a particular patient.

The spatial characteristics of the stimuli produced by an implant are determined by the design of its electrode array, the means by which stimuli are delivered to the array, and the electrical characteristics of the cochlear tissues. Thus, the technique by which a prosthesis could be designed and tested requires a model of the prosthesis and tissues which predicts the system's behavior under changing experimental conditions.

Models describe the system with varying degrees of complexity. Simple models describe small regions of the inner ear with simple mathematical constructs. Such models might include lumped elements arranged to describe an uncoiled cochlear spiral. Complex models include finite-element or finite-difference descriptions of the cochlear tissues. Those descriptions can specify the electrical properties of fluids, membranes, bone, and nerve, and can vary from two-dimensional, cross-sectional models to three-dimensional models of the detailed geometry of the inner ear.

The simple model of Suesserman and Spelman (1988) is a lumped-element model of the first turn of the implanted guinea pig cochlea that shows that potentials can be focused and scanned across the organ of Corti by manipulating electrode current distribution in space.

Two models have been described (Finley, Wilson, & White, Chapter 5) which employ finite-element techniques to predict current flow in the implanted ear. The Girzon and Eddington model reduces the number of modeled tissues to insulating carrier, scalar fluids, bony capsule, neural fibers, and modiolar tissues. This model is a three-dimensional representation of the inner ear. Thus, the model predicts the interaction between electrodes that results from the cochlea's spiral geometry. The Finley model divides cochlear cross sections into a large number of tissue types, but has been represented as either a two-dimensional configuration or as cylindrical blocks whose cross sections are those of single sections. This model predicts the fields along peripheral processes of the auditory nerve up to a point distal to the cell body, and includes neural sensitivity in its estimate of excitation.

Any model, simple or complex, is based on available knowledge of the inner ear, e.g., cochlear anatomy or passive electrical properties of the spiral lamina. The models, though imperfect, suggest experiments to verify the characteristics of specific features of the implanted ear which will describe more precisely the physiology or psychophysics of the implanted ear. Such features also increase the database to make more precise future models. The Eddington-Girzon model predicts that monopolar stimulation with the Symbion array will produce greater potential gradients near apical than basal electrodes; that result is verified in human patients. The Finley model confirms the results of van den Honert and Stypulkowski (1987), that bipolar radial electrodes excite cells in a more localized area and with lower thresholds than either monopolar electrodes or longitudinal bipolar electrodes.

Basic electrophysiological questions are readily definable in terms of predictions of these models and models now in development. These may help us to understand the spatial and temporal gradients that we can generate and control; and these may help us to define the limits of encoding strategies that we may realistically expect to generate and test in the development of the next generation of implants and speech processors.

References

Girzon, G., and Eddington, D.K. (1987). A three-dimensional, electro-anatomical model of the implanted cochlea. *Proc. of the Ninth Annual Conference IEEE-EMBS*, 1904–1905.

Suesserman, M., and Spelman, F.A. (1988). Lumped perameter models for stimulating *in vivo* cochlear stimulation. Abstract 11 MWM Aro 207.

van den Honert, C., and Stypulkowski, P.H. (1987). Single fiber mapping of spatial excitation patterns in the electrically stimulated auditory nerve. *Hearing Research 29*: 195–206.

14
Session II: General Discussion

Dr. Josef Miller: I would like to see if there is a consensus regarding the best general strategy in trying to encode sounds for a prosthesis. Is it really the best bet to try to mimic the function of the normal auditory system?

Dr. Sachs: It is not clear to me that we need to reproduce the temporal aspects of coding. Chris presented a possible way to do it, but I think an important question is: Does the central nervous system use this temporal information? There is no evidence that it does. It might, but it might not. Along those lines, I would like to ask Mike Merzenich, have you ever stimulated at the appropriate place with the appropriate temporal parameters?

Dr. Merzenich: Sure, and no! You can't reconstruct the spatial-temporal distributions of inputs. Blake Wilson has come the closest in attempting to do that, and he may be best to answer that. Unfortunately, the patient that he has studied most is a patient who has a presumptive poor nerve survival.

We have stimulated with sinusoidal stimulation in places that correspond to the representation of that frequency. Is there any systematic relationship between what one perceives with simple stimulation in that form? That is, do you generate the projected pitch? The answer is: Not necessarily. I think the critical feature in representation is that you generate synchronous input from a local sector. From a restricted sector you excite everything more or less simultaneously. Beyond that, my feeling would be: Sure, why not simulate? That's not to say that there aren't handicaps with simulation. As soon as you get to continuous stimuli, the fundamental handicap with simulation is maintaining stimulation isolation between channels. There is no real indication that we have to generate high-frequency inputs because their interaction is unavoidable. I think we have a trade-off between these factors, and the compromise is trying to generate coincident input from the small restricted sector of the auditory nerve. That is the compromise, under conditions where we can avoid interactions. But my view is that it is the time structure in the resonant region that the system is reading, and we create the most faithful simulation if we generate a simulation of the time structure in that resonant region.

Dr. Wilson: We have tried to simulate the accumulation of latencies in the terminal region that are found in normal hearing by using asymmetrical but charge-balanced pulses. The patient we studied has many signs of presumptive poor nerve survival, so we don't know whether we were representing that accumulation of latencies in the terminal region with the asymmetrical pulses or not. The results, when we flipped the polarities of the asymmetrical pulses, putting a tail of latencies on the basal side or a tail on the apical side, were difficult to interpret. The percepts were quite different and were in the direction of high pitch when the tail was on the basal side and low pitch when the tail was on the apical side. The percepts could not be described as sounding more natural in pitch or more pure in tones of quality. So we are looking for a patient who has good signs of nerve survival, and we will repeat the experiment.

Dr. van den Honert: Advocates of simulation are always subjected to the argument that you didn't do it right! There is a degree of perfection that is demanded in simulation. I'm sure there will be people who won't benefit tremendously from attempts to simulate their discharge patterns; but I still believe that you can't go too far wrong attempting to. You must remember that there are still people who hear through hair cells with very few nerves, compared with the number we may be stimulating in some of the profoundly deaf implant patients. Thus, doing it right on a few nerves may be valuable.

Dr. Soli: I think there are several issues here that are easily confused. One is the basic knowledge we are trying to develop of electrical stimulation in the auditory system. From that point, theoretical discussions are important and should be pursued. But the practical side is that more often than not we don't have patients with electrodes in the right places, or there aren't enough electrodes, or enough nerves, etc. So even if this is a theoretically correct point of view, it may not practically lead to optimal performance for a particular patient. This is a distinction that must be remembered.

Dr. Sachs: There are a couple aspects of normal coding that I will talk about tomorrow, but I wonder if people have thought about the fact that in the auditory nerve there is not just one population of nerve fibers, but three, with different thresholds and different characteristics. And in the normal ear we have an efferent system, although we are not sure what it does. What does electrical stimulation do to the efferents?

Dr. Josef Miller: One question raised by Guido Smoorenburg is, when we implant these patients and their perception and performance changes overtime, are they in fact creating for themselves a new perceptual space? Or are they relearning one that existed before? How we view this question in terms of adaptability and plasticity is interesting and important for encoding strategies. How can we test it? How we can find out? Are there features of an old space versus a new space that can be defined behaviorally?

Dr. Rabinowitz: I wanted to ask Mike a question. The plasticity argument is tantalizing. What do you know about experiments on plasticity in the auditory system? I know of a number of studies in vision demonstrating adaptability, but in audition, I think there has only been one experiment where people tried to "reverse ears." It took a long time for people to adapt to that transformation. Do you know of any other?

Dr. Merzenich: A most relevant physiological experiment has been done by Norm Weinberger and colleagues at UC-Irvine. They've looked in auditory areas, before and after an animal has been classically conditioned to a tonal stimulus. What they found in AII and everywhere were changes in tuning curves of neurons, as a result of classical conditioning. There is a cortical area where the tuning curve neurons are sharply tuned, and as a consequence of conditioning with a tonal stimulus, the tuning curves shift to line up their best frequency with the frequency of a applied tonal stimulus. That indicates that over the period of conditioning there is a change in the representation of the conditioning frequency over the period of time of classical conditioning. This can occur in five to seven trials. So there is an indication that there are rapid changes that endure, as long as the animal is conditioned, that are that specific. That is the most direct experiment. But there are lots of auditory behaviors that improve when we practice, which we think are remodeling the auditory system over time.

Also, in regard to Dr. Sachs's question of exciting the three auditory nerve populations, Dr. Leake has made micro-injections into the spiral ganglion, and she has found that there is a typography in representation in the height of the ganglion into the isofrequency dimension of the cochlear nucleus. That is to say, that if she injects into the bottom of the ganglion, she labels fibers in the outer aspect of the isofrequency dimension of the cochlear nucleus. She can make selective lesions in the cochlear nucleus and take out the topmost ganglion cells, the middle stripe, or the bottom ganglion cells. So she has been able to demonstrate a topography in the representation of the height of the ganglion into the cochlea nucleus. She argues on the basis of physiological experiments across the isofrequency dimension that this represents a sorting of input from low and high spontaneous rate fibers. Could you control this excitation? Could you control anything selectively by electrical stimulation? Probably not. The more we understand the details, the more bewildering it becomes. I'm becoming like Merle Lawrence at the first symposium on the cochlear prosthesis, who, understanding the complexities involved, said: ''Never happen!''

Dr. Smoorenburg: I would like to get back to the question of how we can study whether it's a new perceptual world or whether its recovery of the old one. This is hard to do; but the first thing I would do is study the confusions. In speech perception, if we study the confusions between different phonemes, it may give us insight into the dimensions along which people discriminate. And those may be different when they build a new perceptual world.

Dr. Miller: You make me think that it may be useful to compare the results of the tests in an implanted patient who has recently lost his hearing with those of a prelingually deafened implant patient.

Dr. Pfingst: Mike, would you elaborate on the notion of a synchronized input to a local group of nerve fibers? How far would you be willing to carry that? One of the problems with electrical stimulation is that the input is too synchronized, in that it doesn't match the stochasticity of response in the normal system.

Dr. Merzenich: If you take away response representation and the measurement of intervals, you are left with a spatial-temporal cross-correlational process that is looking at the structure of temporal information from the resonant region. I think that's the second most likely possibility. There are conditions in which information will get across these correlators. And obviously those conditions can be idealized. That's what lies behind Blake Wilson's experiments. There's undoubtedly an ideal waveform that creates the spatial-temporal distribution that is most like normal. Presumably that's what the cross-correlator is looking for. But I believe that there must be such correlational mechanisms, and that it is the basis of the independent products that are generated by stimulation of independent channels. That is obviously all the farther I'm going to take that.

Part III Encoding Schemes—Perspectives and Challenges

MURRAY B. SACHS, MODERATOR
WILLIAM M. RABINOWITZ, DISCUSSION LEADER

15
Processing Rate Representation of Complex Stimuli in the Anteroventral Cochlear Nucleus

MURRAY B. SACHS AND C.C. BLACKBURN

The following is a brief synopsis of the paper presented at the Models of the Electrically Stimulated Cochlea International Symposium, Kresge Hearing Research Institute. October 3–5, 1988. Expanded discussion of the issues presented and details of the relevant experimental results can be found in a number of recent publications (Sachs, Blackburn, and Young, 1988; Sachs and Young, 1979).

The general idea of spectral representation in the peripheral auditory system is that peaks of energy in the spectrum (e.g., formant peaks in speech spectra) produce peaks in basilar membrane displacement at corresponding best frequency (BF) places. These peaks in basilar membrane displacement in turn produce peaks of response at corresponding BF places in the population of auditory nerve fibers. Two measures have been used to characterize responses in the auditory nerve: average firing rate and phase-locked rate (Carney and Geisler, 1986; Delgutte and Kiang, 1984; Sachs and Young, 1979; Young and Sachs, 1979). A temporal (phase-locked) measure has been shown to provide a very precise spectral representation, and more emphasis has been placed on this measure. In this paper, on the other hand, we were concerned solely with rate representations. Specifically we considered "rate profiles" for steady-state vowels in the auditory nerve and anteroventral cochlear nucleus (AVCN). A rate profile is a plot of discharge rate versus BF across a population of auditory nerve fibers or AVCN cells.

An important aspect of auditory nerve representation is that auditory nerve fibers can be classified by their spontaneous rates (SR) into three groups. Low-SR (less than 1 spike/s) fibers have high thresholds; high-SR (greater than 18 spikes/s) fibers have low thresholds (Liberman, 1978). In considering auditory nerve representation we must take into account possible differences between these populations. For example, rate profiles for the high-SR populations provide a good representation of spectral peaks at low stimulus levels (Sachs and Young, 1979). However, this representation deteriorates with an increase in sound level or in the presence of background noise (Sachs, Voigt, and Young, 1983). This deterioration is the result of rate saturation and two-tone suppression. Because of their high thresholds and relatively wide dynamic ranges (Schalk and Sachs, 1980), rate profiles for low-SR fibers maintain a representation of spectral peaks at high stimulus levels where the high-SR fibers are saturated.

This difference in behavior between the low-SR and high-SR auditory nerve population suggests that a rate representation which is robust over stimulus level could be provided by a weighted sum of the rates of low-, medium-, and high-SR fibers. The rates of high-SR (low-threshold) fibers should be given greatest weight at low sound levels and the rates of low-SR fibers should be weighted more heavily at high sound levels. That is, the central nervous system should "listen" to its high-SR inputs at low sound levels and to its low-SR inputs at high sound levels.

The cochlear nucleus is the first level in the CNS where the auditory nerve representation is processed. Stellate cells are one morphologically defined principal cell type in the AVCN which give promise of being able to carry out this "selective listening" function. They receive a large number of small bouton inputs on their dendritic trees, and in some cases on their cell bodies (Cant and Morest, 1984). They produce chopper response patterns to BF tones (Rhode, Oertel, and Smith, 1983), their spike trains are very regular, and the number of spikes is quite constant from one stimulus presentation to the next. Their complex dendritic structure could produce significant processing of rate representations in a way that might preserve or even sharpen rate profiles over a wide range of stimulus levels. Recently we have shown that at low stimulus levels rate profiles for one type of AVCN chopper unit, the ChT units (or transient choppers; Young, Robert, and Shofner, 1988), are similar to those for the high-SR auditory nerve population; at higher sound levels the ChT profiles are similar to those for low- and medium-SR fibers and very different from those of the high-SR fibers. Specifically, at high sound levels the ChT profiles clearly reflect peaks in the stimulus spectrum, whereas these peaks disappear from the high-SR auditory nerve profiles at high levels.

These results are consistent with the hypothesis that ChT units weight high-SR inputs heavily at low sound levels and low-SR inputs at high levels. Interestingly, virtually all the ChT units in the population studied had little or no spontaneous activity, so that one might question whether these units receive any high-SR auditory nerve inputs. There is some preliminary evidence on this point. Young and Sachs (1988) have recorded simultaneously from auditory nerve and cochlear nucleus units. Using cross-correlation analysis they have found evidence consistent with excitatory interactions between auditory nerve fibers with high SR and AVCN ChT units with little or no spontaneous activity.

Acknowledgments. This work was supported by Grants RO1NS12112 and T32NS07283 from the National Institute of Neurological and Communicative Disorders and Stroke. C.C. Blackburn was a National Research Service Award postdoctoral fellow. M.B. Sachs is a Javits Neuroscience Investigator.

References

Cant, N.B., and Morest, D.K. (1984). The structural basis for stimulus coding in the cochlear nucleus of the cat. In *Hearing Science,* edited by C.I. Berlin (San Diego: College-Hill Press), pp. 374–422.

Carney, L.H., and Geisler, C.D. (1986). A temporal analysis of auditory-nerve fiber responses to spoken stop consonant-vowel syllables. *J. Acoust. Soc. Am.* 79:1896–1914.

Delgutte, B., and Kiang, N.Y.S. (1984). Speech coding in the auditory nerve: I. Vowel-like sounds. *J. Acoust. Soc. Am.* 75:866–878.

Liberman, M.C. (1978). Auditory-nerve response from cats raised in a low-noise chamber. *J.Acoust. Soc. Am.* 63:422–455.

Rhode, W.S., Oertel, D., and Smith, P.H. (1983). Physiological response properties of cells labeled intracellularly with horseradish peroxidase in the cat ventral cochlear nucleus. *J. Comp. Neurol.* 213:448–463.

Sachs, M.B., Blackburn, C.C., and Young, E.D. (1988). Rate-place and temporal-place representatives of vowels in the auditory nerve and anteroventral cochlear nucleus. *J. Phonetics* 16:37–53.

Sachs, M.B., Voigt, H.F., and Young, E.D. (1983). Auditory nerve representation of vowels in background noise. *J. Neurophysiol.* 50:27–45.

Sachs, M.B., and Young, E.D. (1979). Encoding of steady-state vowels in the auditory nerve: Representation in terms of discharge rate. *J. Acoust. Soc. Am.* 66:470–479.

Schalk, T.B. and Sachs, M.B. (1980). Nonlinearities in auditory-nerve fiber responses to bandlimited noise. *J. Acoust. Soc. Am.* 67:903–913.

Young, E.D., Robert, J.M., and Shofner, W.P. (1988). Regularity and latency of units in ventral cochlear nucleus: Implications for unit classification and generation of response properties. *J. Neurophysiol.* 60:1–29.

Young, E.D., and Sachs, M.B. (1979). Representation of steady-state vowels in the temporal aspects of the discharge patterns of populations of auditory-nerve fibers. *J. Acoust. Soc. Am.* 66:1381–1403.

Young, E.D., and Sachs, M.B. (1988). Interactions of auditory nerve fibers and ventral cochlear nucleus cells studied with crosscorrelation. Abstract, 18th Annual Meeting, Society for Neuroscience, Toronto, Ontario, Canada.

16
Neural Processing of Complex Electric and Acoustic Stimuli

BEN M. CLOPTON, JAMES A. WILER, AND PATRICIA M. BACKOFF

Introduction

One aspect of deafness, the loss of sound awareness, is largely alleviated by cochlear implants now available if sufficient primary afferents survive. However, the loss of speech discrimination ability, which is of greater functional importance for integrating the patient into a "hearing" world, has not been satisfactorily resolved by current prosthetic designs. This chapter examines two classes of neurophysiological mechanisms on which successful encoding of speech and other complex sounds as acoustic or electrical stimuli depend: the peripheral transduction process and central processing. Acoustic and electrical transduction are inherently different, but each is selective in the stimulus information it passes. They can be compared when both are treated in equivalent stimulus terms. Central processing mechanisms accept and act on acoustic input much more readily than electrical input for reasons which are only partially known. We contrast the processing of electrical and acoustic inputs for comparable stimulus parameters and suggest ways to enhance or replace the processing now available with implants.

Our viewpoint is that central mechanisms selectively parse incoming acoustic patterns over subpopulations of neurons. In the cochlear nuclei these are associated with distinct anatomical cell types, individually and in networks, which may differ in their connectivities, membrane biophysics, and biochemistry. The design of cochlear prostheses has stressed the role of tonotopic organization, the consequence of an orderly projection from the cochlea. This well-known correlate of sound analysis into its component frequencies has promoted the design of electrode arrays which selectively access subgroups of spiral ganglion cells. We will describe measures of central processing which indicate that the control of additional parameters of the electrical stimulus is required if the normal parsing operations are to function. Specific directions of research are indicated to clarify how peripheral and central mechanisms can be better matched for information transfer and utilization. If gains are to be made in prosthetic effectiveness, our knowledge of central processing capacities should motivate the design of electrodes and processors.

Transduction

Peripheral transduction of electrical stimuli limits information transfer to central auditory structures. Can we specify properties of electrical stimuli which are, in any sense, optimal? Attempts to characterize the transduction of electrical stimuli using sinusoids have yielded only limited insight into the process (Clopton et al., 1983). Below we discuss choices of parameters and describe techniques using pulse and noise stimuli.

Charge Utilization

There is experimental evidence for an efficient use of charge with electrical stimulation of the cochlea over brief phase durations. The threshold for neural and behavioral responses, expressed as charge delivered during one phase of a pulse, decreases with phase duration up to a few hundred microseconds (Clopton and Bosma, 1982; Pfingst, 1984; Pfingst et al., 1979). This indicates that charge is integrated efficiently over this period. Behavioral observations indicate that charge utilization is also relatively constant in the 3–10-ms range (Parkins and Colombo, 1987; Shannon, 1985). This may reflect the integration of activity across the neural population more than properties of individual neurons because it does not appear in neurophysiological measurements on single neurons (Parkins and Colombo, 1987; Wiler, Clopton, and Mikhail, 1988, 1989).

Electrical Tuning

Determinations of the threshold for evoking neural responses using electrical sinusoids show "tuning" for neural membranes across diverse species when expressed in terms of current. Tuning is predicted from the nonlinear differential equations approximating membrane dynamics derived from voltage clamp experiments (Clopton et al., 1983; Colombo and Parkins, 1987; McNeal, 1976; Motz and Rattay, 1986; Reilly, Freeman, and Larkin, 1985). Spike generation in squid axon (Guttman and Hachmeister, 1971), frog (Backoff, Clopton, and Bledsoe, 1988; Frankenhaeuser and Huxley, 1964), and cochlear afferents (Hartmann, Topp, and Klinke, 1984; Moxon, 1971; van den Honert and Stypulkowski, 1984, 1987[a,b]) has been observed to have qualitatively similar frequency response characteristics. Figure 16.1 is an illustration of tuning curves for spike generation in myelinated nerve of the lateral line organ of *Xenopus laevis*. These axons were stimulated with sinusoids delivered through bipolar electrodes near the isolated nerve bundle. In Figure 16.1*a*,

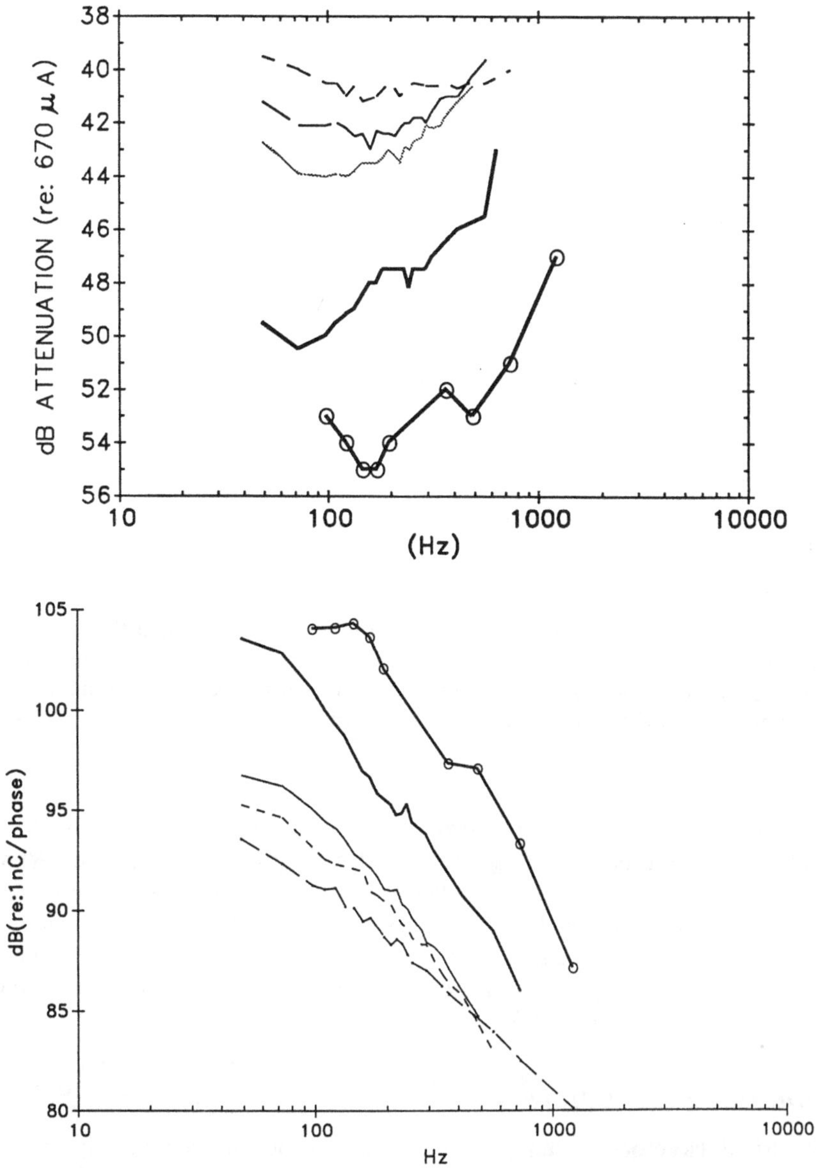

FIGURE 16.1. Electrical threshold curves for five axons in the lateral-line organ of *Xenopus laevis*. This nerve and lateral-line stitch were excised and maintained in frog Ringer solution. Stimulation was through bipolar platinum-iridium electrodes spaced 1 mm along the nerve trunk, which had been surgically isolated from the stitch (*a*) Threshold expressed in terms of current, where 0 dB = 670 μA; (*b*) threshold expressed as charge delivered per phase of the stimulating sinusoid.

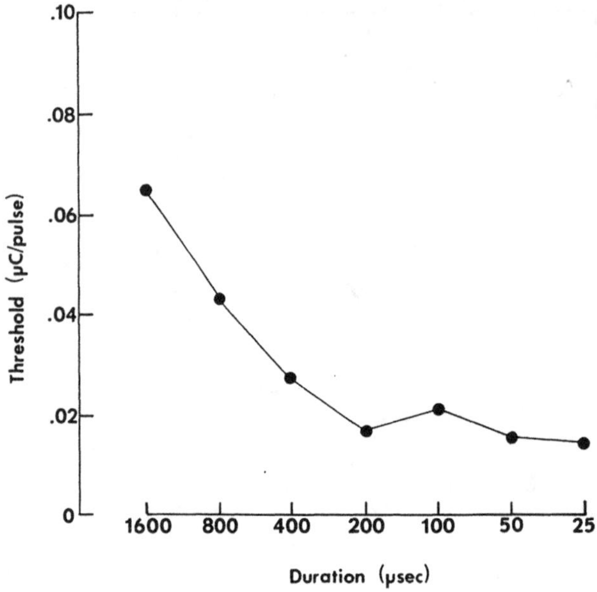

FIGURE 16.2. Threshold for evoking a criterion-evoked potential at the brachium of the inferior colliculus in the guinea pig using monophasic square pulses delivered to the cochlea. Charge utilization is most efficient for pulses with durations of less than 200 μs (Clopton and Bosma, 1982).

threshold response levels are expressed in terms of current, while in 16.1*b* they are shown as the charge delivered during one pulse phase. What appears as "tuning" in part (*a*) is better described as increasingly efficient charge utilization in part (*b*). As illustrated in Figure 16.2, the charge-utilization curve for cochlear stimulation in mammalian afferents appears to be minimal for phase durations below about 200 μs (Clopton and Bosma, 1982; Parkins, 1987).

Optimal Parameters

Electrical waveforms used to stimulate the cochlea are generally biphasic, charge-balanced, and constant current. Symmetrical phase durations and intensities are commonly used since they meet these conditions, but alternative waveforms which may have more desirable characteristics have not been examined. In general, useful stimulus properties include:

- Charge balance (to minimize the generation of chemical by-products; Brummer and Robblee, 1983)
- Constant current (to counter time variation in tissue and electrode impedances)

- Minimal charge transfer per phase (to lessen the chance of tissue damage; Duckert and Miller, 1982)
- Minimal duration per phase (to lessen damage, permit high rates of information transfer, and allow multiplexing on multicontact electrode arrays)
- Maximal spike count per pulse (for greatest control over afferent activity)

Waveshape for Biphasic Square Pulses

We explored different electrical waveshapes for pulses to determine which ones might best meet these criteria. It is not apparent a priori that all of the criteria are compatible. In order to restrict the range of possible waveshapes, we used charge-balanced biphasic square pulses delivered through a voltage-to-constant-current stimulator (Spelman, Pfingst, and Miller, 1978).

For charge-balanced pulses, the parameters which define a waveshape, shown in Figure 16.3, are its initial polarity (p), its charge transfer per phase (C), and the durations of its two phases (t_1, t_2). In order to see if pulse shape is influential, we explored a large set of them with a fixed-charge transfer per phase and electrode arrangement. Since $C = I_1t_1 = I_2t_2$, currents I_1 and I_2 are inversely related to the phase durations for a constant-charge transfer.

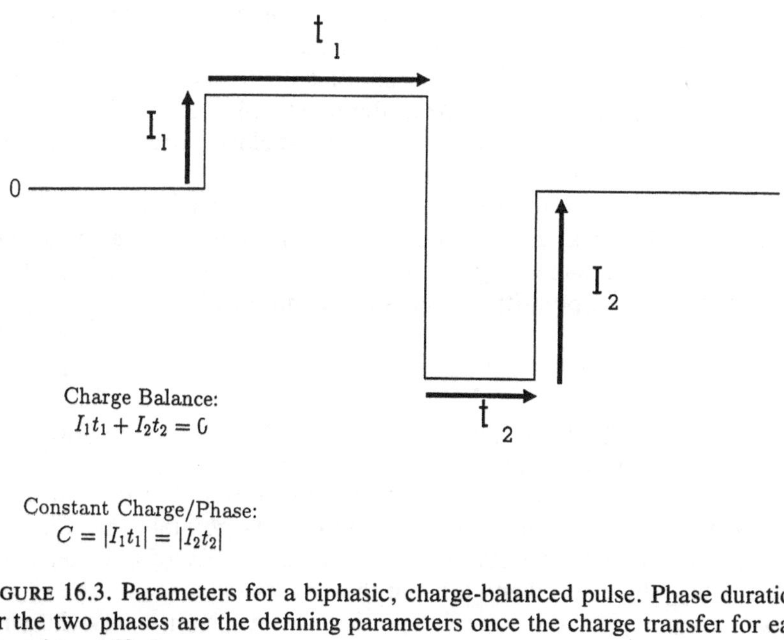

FIGURE 16.3. Parameters for a biphasic, charge-balanced pulse. Phase durations for the two phases are the defining parameters once the charge transfer for each phase is specified.

The response measure was not the threshold stimulus level; rather, it was the number of spikes evoked as a function of the durations of the first and second phases of the pulse. This provides a more direct indication of spike generation for fixed-pulse parameters. Since charge transfer was held constant for a given set of phase durations, it was an indicant of pulse efficiency for different pulse shapes.

In the acute guinea pig preparation, we recorded from single units in the anteroventral cochlear nucleus (AVCN) using glass micropipettes. Cochlear stimulation was accomplished through two 5-mil platinum-iridium wires spaced about 1 mm apart passing through the lateral wall of the cochlea in the scala tympani. Preparations included those with intact hair cells and with hair cell destruction due to topical administration of neomycin sulfate solution. No difference was observed in the results due to hair cell presence or absence.

Although some variation was seen from unit to unit, distinctive pulse shapes were observed to evoke the highest spike counts, dependent on their initial polarity. Examples of spike counts evoked by 200 presentations of many different pulse shapes are shown in Figure 16.4.

While it has been shown that the cathodal electrode is the more effective in eliciting spikes (Clopton and Bosma, 1982; Parkins and Colombo, 1988; van den Honert and Stypulkowski, 1984, 1987a,b), in the pulse-duration study it was not known which electrode was nearest the site of stimulation during its cathodal phase. Assuming that lower thresholds were associated with an initial phase which was effectively cathodal at the site of stimulation, some differences could tentatively be associated with pulse shape and initial polarity. For low rates of pulse delivery (50/s), initially cathodal phases of 200–300 μs followed by a brief anodal phase of 100–200 μs evoked the most spikes for each pulse. For higher pulse rates, where an anodal phase must closely precede a cathodal phase, an initially anodal phase of long duration, 50 μs or more, followed by a brief cathodal phase of 100 μs or less was highly effective in evoking spikes. In both cases, asymmetrical phase durations are indicated, with approximately the same degree of asymmetry. The asymmetry of the pulse, not its initial polarity, appears to be more salient.

Implications of Pulse Shape

These results suggest that pulse shape is an important consideration for cochlear stimulation. Asymmetrical pulse shapes are especially efficient when their phase durations are appropriately chosen, but it is uncertain what aspect of the asymmetry is effective. It is possible that the brief second phase is the effective one, and that the utility of a longer initial phase is to reduce its magnitude and thereby its influence on the second phase, assuming that charge integration decays over a few hundred microseconds. Both initially cathodal and anodal pulses evoked spikes

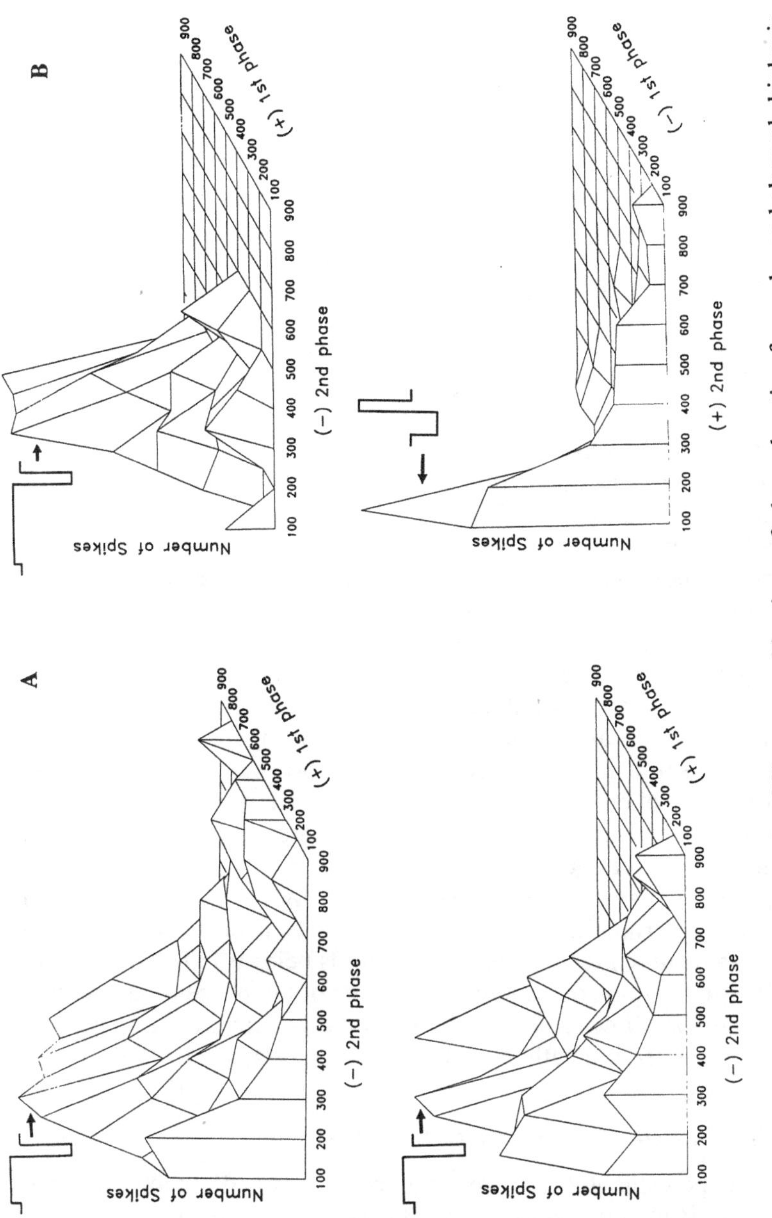

FIGURE 16.4. Spike-count surfaces for different combinations of phase duration for a charge-balanced, biphasic pulse. (*a*) Two different units in AVCN responding to initially positive pulses to the reference electrode; maximum spike counts associated with pulses having asymmetrical shapes. (*b*) Responses from one unit showing both initial polarities.

with about the same minimal latencies, so some support exists for an equivalence of the pulse shapes regardless of the initial polarity.

Estimation with Noise Stimuli

The exhaustive search of biphasic pulse shapes described above could not determine the effectiveness of waveshapes outside that class. However, it is possible to estimate the waveshape-evoking spikes using more general stimuli (Wiler and Clopton, 1989). Specifically, we have used digitally synthesized wideband noises, delivered as constant-current waveforms for electrical stimulation, to estimate the waveshape which tends to precede spike occurrence under the same conditions of the pulse experiments. The procedure used was *reverse correlation* as described by de Boer and de Jongh (1978), except for the alternative of replacing acoustic stimuli with electrical. It provides an estimate of the linear, first-order transfer function relating stimulus waveform and the probability of spike occurrence, commonly known as the "impulse" or weighting function for the relationship.

A set of 16 independent, periodic noises were synthesized containing frequencies from 300 to 12,500 Hz at equal amplitudes and random phase. Each had a period of 163.84 ms, and could be presented without transients. A period histogram for unit firing in the AVCN was collected for each noise presented for 200 periods. These histograms were used to weight the noise waveform immediately preceding a 40-μs bin by the probability of a spike occurring in that bin. This gave an "average" waveform immediately preceding spike occurrence. Estimations of this waveform for electrical stimulation are shown in Figure 16.5.

For comparison a reverse-correlation waveform for acoustic stimulation of a phase-locked unit in AVCN is shown in Figure 16.6.

While some variations were observed across units with electrical stimulation, the waveshape estimated with the reverse-correlation technique had distinctive features. It was essentially triphasic with a total duration ranging from 1.2 to 1.96 ms. The phases decreased in duration with decreasing time precedence, the durations being 0.76 to 1.12, 0.24 to 0.6, and 0.2 to 0.24 ms, respectively. The sign of the phases was inverted for some units, as shown in Figure 16.5*b*, corresponding, we assume, to a reversal in the effective cathode (Clopton and Glass, 1984).

Implications of Reverse Correlation

The waveshape estimated with reverse correlation had obvious similarities to the most effective pulse shape determined in the earlier study. A brief phase of about 200-μs duration immediately preceded a spike, which was, in turn, preceded by a longer phase of roughly 300 to 600-μs duration. Beyond these similarities, reverse correlation suggested that more than two phases are effective. At least three phases of increasing duration and decreasing magnitude were indicated. In practical terms, however, the results corroborate the utility of asymmetrical pulse shapes of the type described.

The reason for the specific waveshape observed with reverse correlation is not known. It is likely determined by membrane dynamics at the site of electrical stimulation. The possibility, expressed earlier, that spike occurrence depends only on part of the waveshape, such as the effective cathodal phase, is not supported by this result. The entire waveshape appears to be contributory to spike occurrence since the expected value for an ineffective segment of the waveshape would be zero. This does not exclude the possibility that features of higher order, such as first and higher derivatives, at least partially determine the shape estimation.

Central Processing

Peripheral electrical excitation of the cochlea is only effective insofar as it can produce a range of responses in neurons of the cochlear nuclei and other central auditory structures. Discriminative responses to speech and other biological sounds cannot occur without a mapping from elements of the electrical code to distinctive neural activities. Central processing is normally matched to a precise temporal and spatial code arising from acoustic features passed through the analytical and transduction mechanisms of the cochlea. The success of an electrical encoding strategy appears to depend on matching the range of acceptance for these processing mechanisms to that available for crudely presented electrical stimuli. We now address some of the complexities of central processing in terms of acoustic features which are normally extracted, as compared with the situation which holds for electrical stimulation.

Background

Strategies for the encoding of acoustic features in electrical form have been based on traditional theories of acoustic encoding. The view that spike rate and synchrony specific to anatomical place are the primary indicators of stimulus content in central activity is well represented in these strategies. Electrodes have been assessed for their spatial selectivity in activating cochlear afferents (van den Honert and Stypulkowski, 1987a) and for the persistence of temporal detail in neural activity, such as phase locking at high frequencies, with electrical stimulation (Glass, 1984; Hartmann, Topp, and Klinke, 1984; van den Honert and Stypulkowski, 1987a,b). While these are undoubtedly important to information processing in the auditory system, their implications for schemes of electrical

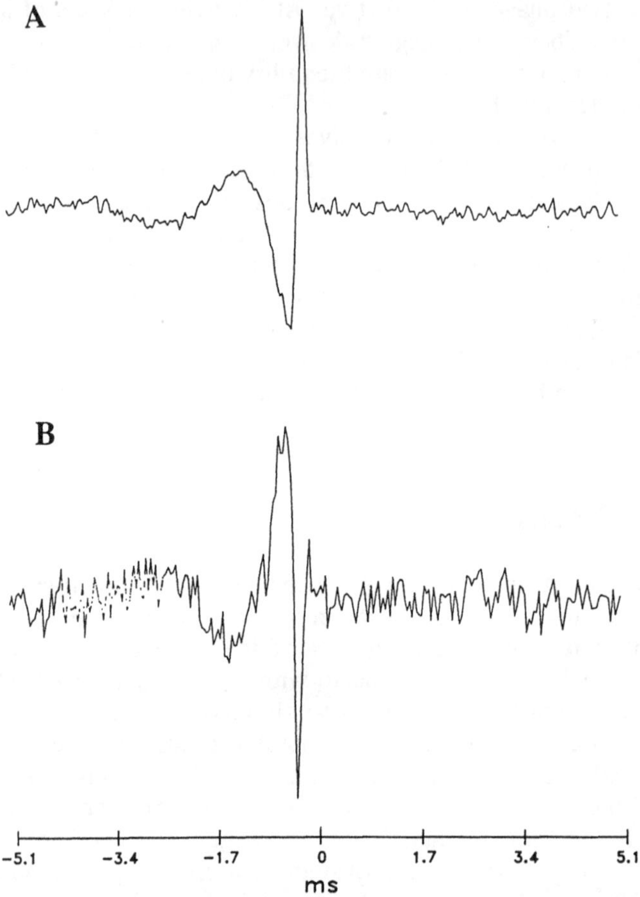

FIGURE 16.5. Reverse-correlation functions for three neurons in the AVCN obtained with constant-current stimulation of the cochlea using noise waveforms. Spike occurrence was at $t = 0$. Parts (*a*) and (*b*) show two different neurons having different polarities for their functions. Part (*c*) illustrates details of an expanded function for another unit. At least three phases over about 1.5 ms are observed to precede spike occurrence.

encoding are obscure because we don't know how rate and synchrony codes are utilized in central auditory structures. More generally, the rules of combination and exclusion for elements of auditory information progressing through neuronal pathways and within groups of neurons are not known; traditional approaches for the characterization of the relationship between stimuli and neuronal responses offer no obvious base for discovering them.

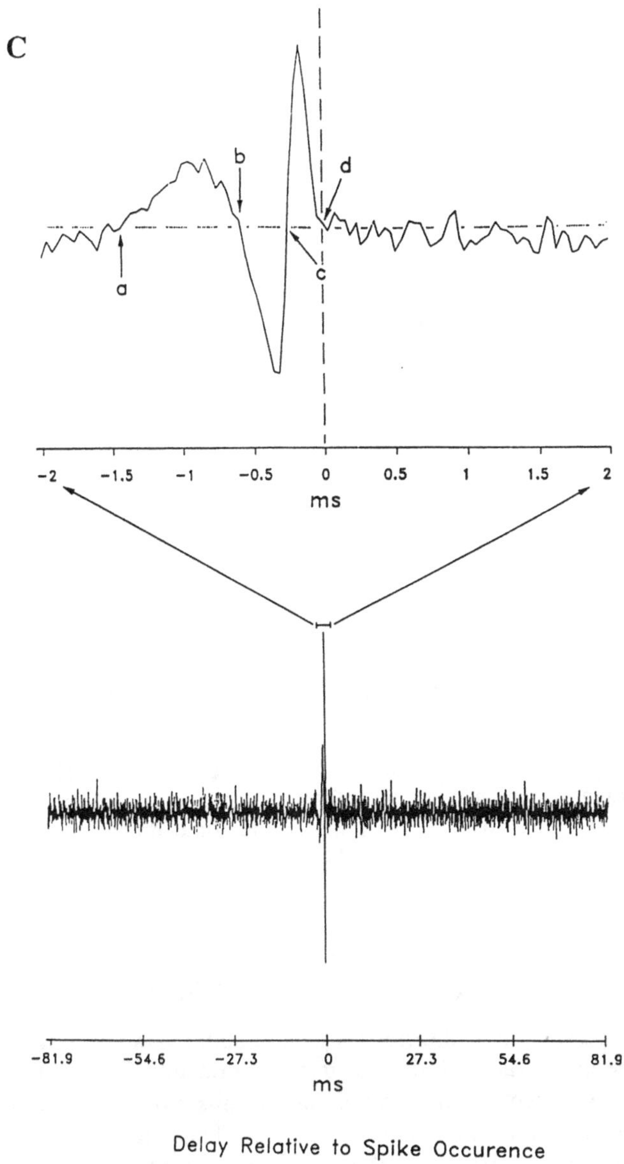

FIGURE 16.5. *Continued*

In this section, we consider an alternative approach to the representation of sounds in spike patterns of acoustically and electrically stimulated neurons. It is intended to clarify the nature of the disparity in information between these two modes of stimulation which exists under present schemes and to suggest new strategies for the processing and delivery of sound information by electrical means.

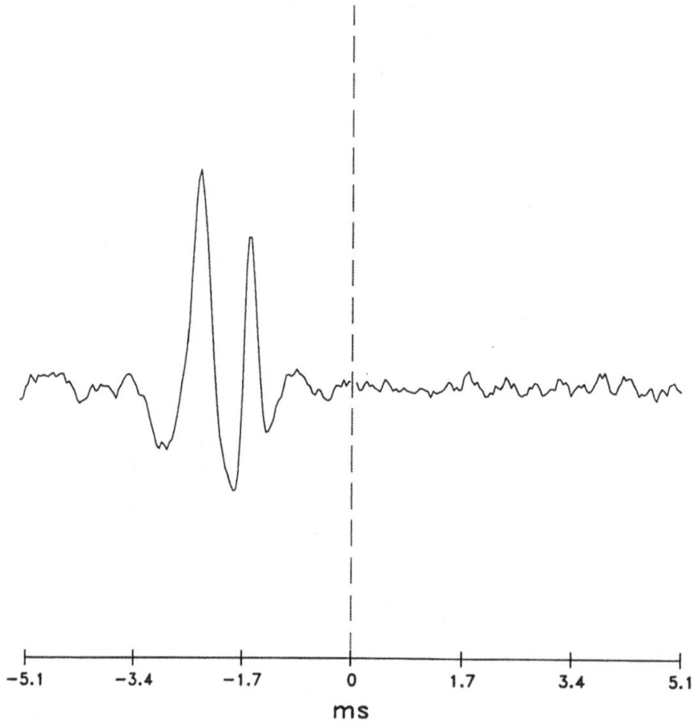

FIGURE 16.6. A reverse-correlation function for a neuron in AVCN obtained with acoustic stimulation using noise waveforms. This neuron was phase-locked to tones near its CF of 1565 Hz. Note the greater time precedence for acoustic stimulation.

Spectrotemporal Representation of Sounds

The display of speech and other biological sounds as sonogram patterns has long been an accepted and useful procedure (Flanagan, 1972). Features are apparent in sonograms that are obscured in the original time waveform or in standard frequency analyses. These features are heuristic for auditory theory because they are presumably analogous to the time-varying spike activity over the array of axons of the auditory nerve. However, the sonogram is limited as an accurate representation of complex sounds. It is obtained using arbitrary filter parameters for the bank of filters from which it is generated, and these will invariably distort sound features in comparison with the activity of auditory afferents.

More general mathematical expressions for representations of energy fluctuations over time and frequency in sounds are available (Cohen,

1966; Rihaczek, 1968). Such expressions, in general, can be viewed as partitions of the total energy in a sound over time and frequency, a *spectrotemporal* pattern of the energy fluctuation in the sound. Figure 16.7 illustrates such a display for the word "cowboy."

By representing acoustic and electrical stimuli in this way, it is possible to estimate what patterns precede spike occurrence, just as with the reverse-correlation procedure described earlier which used the stimulus waveform. In the following, we will contrast the manner in which neurons of the CN respond to features in complex acoustic and electrical stimuli when they are represented as patterns of energy in time and frequency.

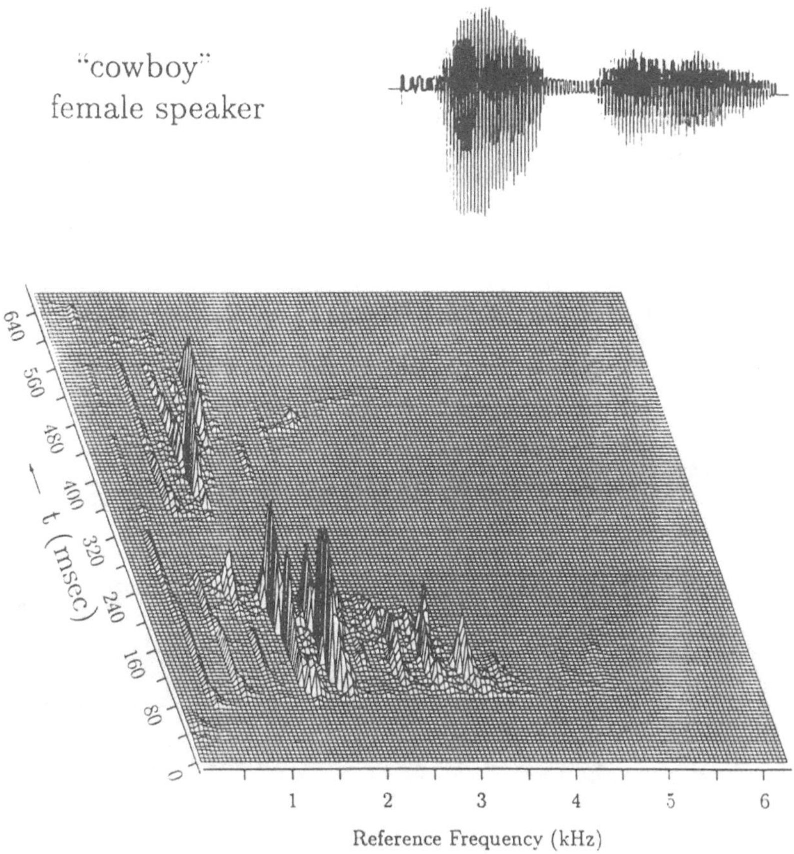

FIGURE 16.7. Energy variation in the word "cowboy" expressed as a function of time and frequency. While similar to a sonogram, this display more accurately represents the energy fluctuations in time and frequency present in the original waveform.

General Stimuli

In order to determine what features in sounds might excite a neuron in the CN, it is necessary to use a class of stimuli chosen to probabilistically contain all possible features up to a certain level of complexity. These features appear as variations on the energy surface in time and frequency. The features of interest are peaks and valleys, i.e., a relative excess or lack of energy associated with specific times and frequencies. Noises, generated in a specific way, approximate such general stimuli. Figure 16.8 illustrates the time-frequency surface for such a noise. It is periodic; that is, it repeats with a period equal to the time segment shown. And it is bandlimited; that is, it has energy only over a range of frequencies. It has equal power for all frequency components within that range (although the instantaneous energy varies because of the interaction of frequency components), and the starting phase of each component is random. Most importantly, the chance of a peak or trough in energy at any point on the surface is random, within limits, so that an independent set of such noises provides a sample of the variety of features that can occur in time and frequency.

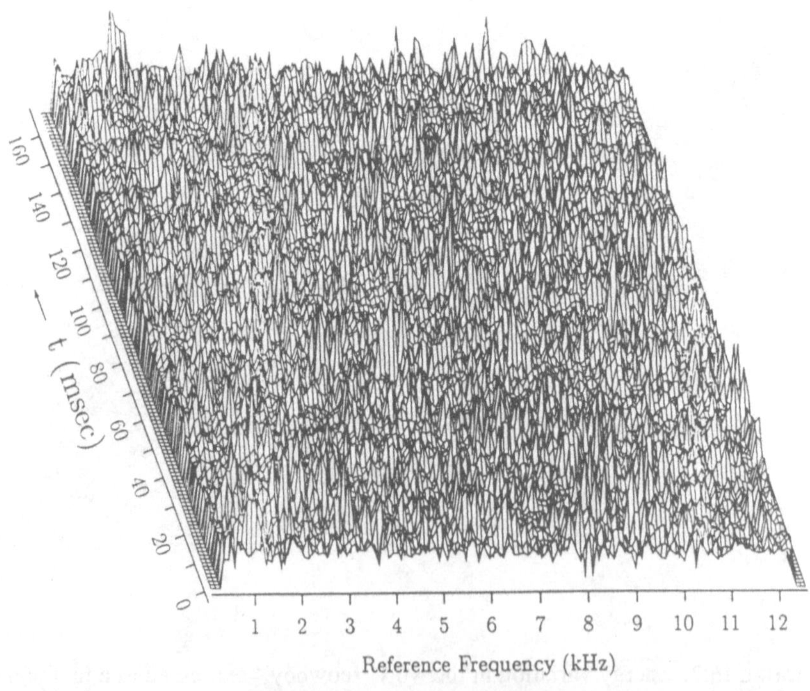

FIGURE 16.8. Energy variation in a periodic noise as a function of time and frequency. Within the bandlimits of this noise the magnitudes of frequency components are equal and their phases are random. Interactions between components cause the instantaneous energy to fluctuate.

Hypothesis

We postulate that an orderly relationship exists between an energy surface for a stimulus and the neural response that it evokes. Specifically, if $I(t, f_R)$ is an energy value on the stimulus surface at time t and reference frequency f_R, it affects the probability of spike occurrence $s(t)$ after scaling by a weighting function $U(\tau, f_R)$, where τ is *time precedence* relative to the present time t when $s(t)$ is estimated. This can be expressed as

$$s(t) = \iint I(t - \tau, f_R) U(\tau, f_R) d\tau df_R$$

Figure 16.9 graphically summarizes this relationship. The selectivity of the neuron for features in the stimulus is characterized by the weighting surface $U(\tau, f_R)$. Each neuron will have a unique weighting surface which describes the information it extracts from stimuli. This surface can be estimated by determining if peaks or troughs of energy tend to precede spike generation. Practically this requires that a histogram, approximating $s(t)$, be collected over many periods of the noise and then be used to weight $I(t, f_R)$ in a reverse-correlation algorithm (de Boer and de Jongh, 1978) relative to τ using $I(t, f_R)$ instead of the original waveform $x(t)$. The

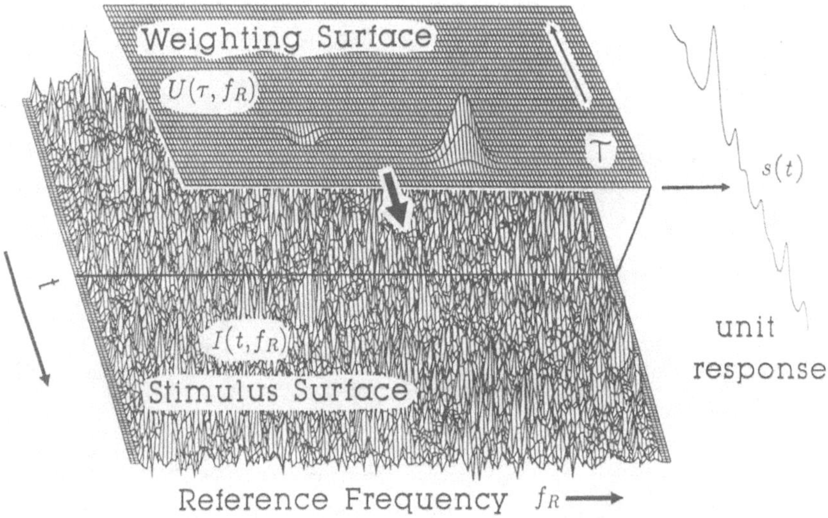

FIGURE 16.9. Functional relationship postulated to relate stimulus energy fluctuations in time and frequency, $I(t, f_R)$, and the probability of a neural spike occurring $s(t)$. The neuron's activity is characterized by the weighting surface $U(\tau, f_R)$, which determines the relative influence of past values of $I(t-\tau, f_R)$ on its response. The weighting surface or *spectrotemporal receptive field* is zero over most of its extent, but can have positive and negative regions (peaks and troughs, respectively) which are distinctive for a neuron.

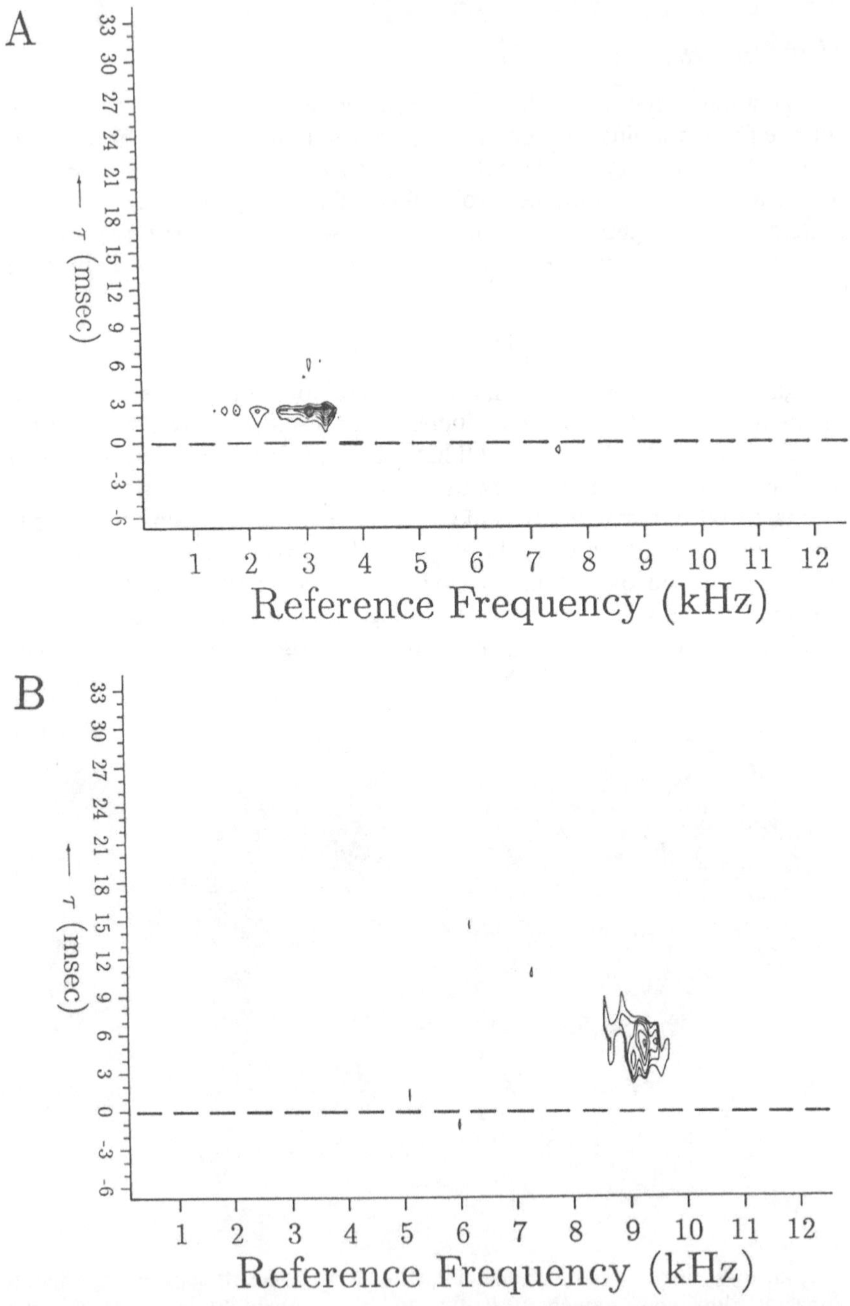

FIGURE 16.10. STRFs shown as contour plots for acoustic stimuli from three units in CN. (*a*) A unit in the ventral part of CN having a primarylike response to tone bursts (CF=3144 Hz). (*b*) DCN unit having a pauser-type response to tone bursts (CF=9034 Hz). (*c*) DCN unit having a chopper-type response (CF=3026 Hz). Arrows indicate troughs in the STRF. Resolution for these contour plots is 1.28 ms by 97.66 Hz.

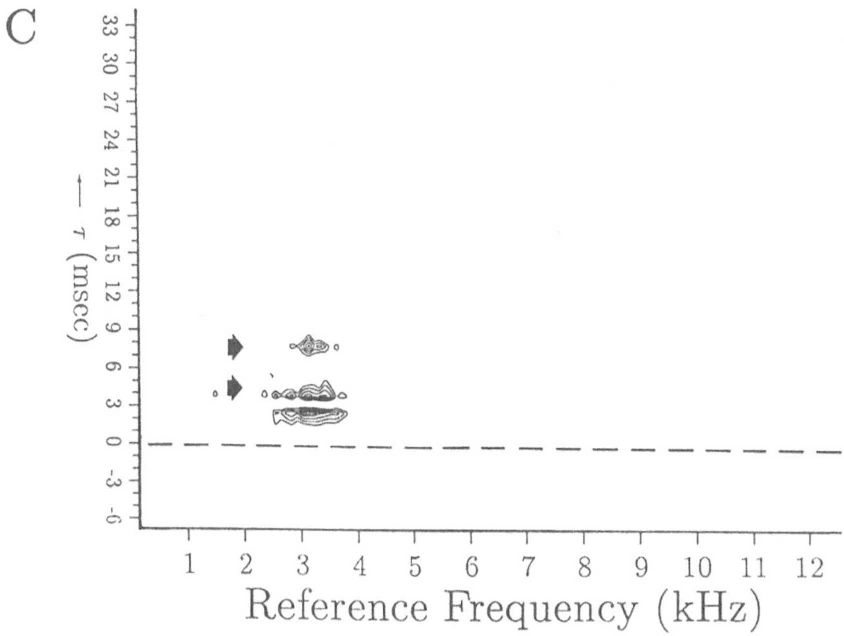

FIGURE 16.10. *Continued*

result is a *spectrotemporal receptive field* (STRF), which illustrates how the unit "sees" the stimulus (Hermes et al., 1981). It is expected to be flat if there is no stimulus influence on unit activity; otherwise, it will contain features which, on the average, occur before the neuron generates a spike.

Acoustic Stimulation

The procedure described was applied with acoustic noises presented to guinea pigs and spikes recorded extracellularly in the CN. Examples of $U(\tau,f_R)$ estimated for some units are shown in Figure 16.10. They range from the simplest pattern, observed for VIIIth nerve fibers and primary-like units of AVCN (16.10*a*), to patterns having a number of peaks and troughs seen for units in DCN (16.10*c*). These surfaces indicate processing in the CN at varying levels of complexity. We interpreted elevations on the surfaces to correlate with excitatory inputs to the neuron and troughs with inhibitory inputs. To the extent that a pattern of energy fluctuation in the stimulus corresponds to a unit's STRF weighting surface, the probability of that unit generating a spike is increased. A unit's STRF is presumably determined by its connectivity and the biophysical properties of its membrane in conjunction with the nature of its synaptic inputs and morphology.

Electrical Stimulation

Analogously to the acoustic presentation of the noise stimuli, we presented them electrically as constant-current waveforms through bipolar platinum-iridium electrodes in the scala tympani of guinea pigs. Spike histograms from neurons in the CN were used to estimate the STRFs, summarizing the relationship between the electrical stimuli and neural spike generation. Examples are shown in Figure 16.11. It is apparent that the stimulus patterns in the electrical stimuli which tended to evoke spikes were not as detailed as those observed with acoustic stimulation.

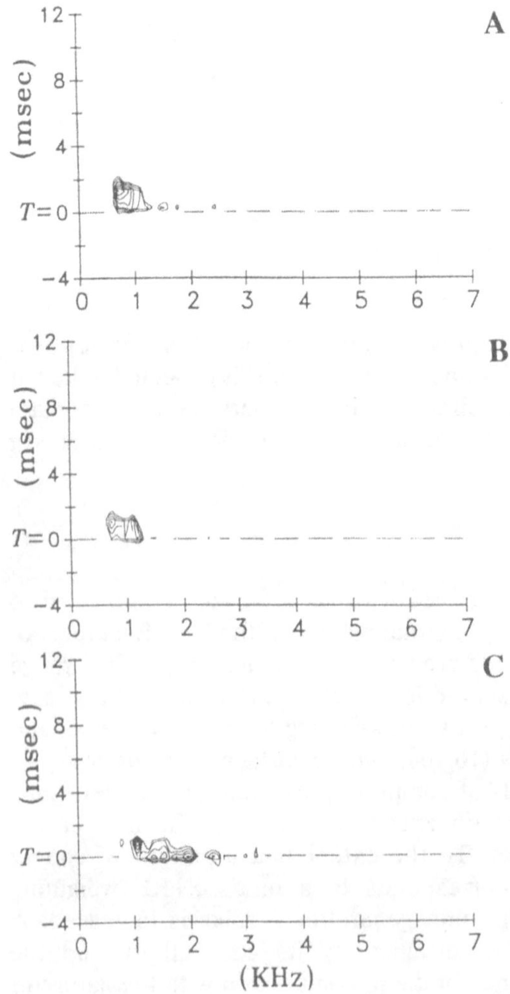

FIGURE 16.11. STRFs for electrical stimuli observed for three units in VCN. These units are activated by frequencies in the range from 500 to 2000 Hz with relatively short time precedence. All neurons observed to date in the CN have relatively simple STRFs for electrical stimuli. The time and frequency resolution are the same as in Figure 16.10.

This held even for the few neurons recorded in the DCN, whereas more complex STRFs predominated for acoustic stimulation. The electrical cases were restricted to lower-frequency response areas, generally less than 4 kHz, and the time between a peak in the stimulus energy and the spike was quite short, often less than the 1.28-ms time resolution of our method. This agrees with the results from reverse correlation with the original stimulus waveform. No troughs in the surfaces were observed, and a lack of features involving multiple peaks was ubiquitous. These and earlier results agree in suggesting a relatively uniform mechanism for electrical stimulation; however they differ from estimates for frequency response for electrical stimulation using sinusoids (Clopton et al., 1983). Continuous electrical stimulation with multispectral noise waveforms is mediated thorough frequency components in the range of 700 to 2000 Hz. Spikes are locked to temporal components in these stimuli, and these are uniform. A very restricted aspect of complex electrical waveforms is signaled with great temporal precision.

Implications

These observations indicate that electrical stimulation, as it is presently implemented, does not selectively activate some neural circuits of the CN as do comparable sounds. While not surprising, this measure stresses the disparity between acoustic and electrical stimuli in terms of neuronal processing. A lack of cochlear frequency analysis, excessive current spread from the electrodes, and other inadequacies of implant operation can be cited. It is perhaps more productive to assess present capacities and discuss strategies which bridge the gap between limited informational transfer in the electrical case and in acoustic stimulation.

Three strategies are apparent. Each has been considered previously in relation to prosthetic development. We examine them below within the context of neural processing supported by our observations.

Transduction and Processing

It was originally planned that cochlear prostheses should replace normal cochlear function to the greatest extent possible. If this were fully accomplished, central processing mechanisms would operate normally since afferent patterns of activity in the auditory nerve would be indistinguishable, whether evoked acoustically or electrically. Central neurons would, in effect, be fed acoustic information which they were configured to process. This is clearly impractical because of restrictions on the number and size of electrodes which can be introduced into the inner ear by the physics of current spread which governs their spatial selectivity, and the intricacy of normal cochlear function. Perhaps the most important limitation is our present ignorance about the encoding necessary to match peripheral encoding and central processing. Current strategies have been successful primarily because humans are able to extract temporal cues from speech, even with minimal processing. A greater knowledge of the mechanisms which account for acoustic feature selectivity in auditory neurons may enable us to better approximate cochlear function and enhance implant operation.

Single-unit data from the guinea pig point to an unsuccessful match between the transduction of electrical stimuli and the requirements of more intricate processing mechanisms in the CN. Numerous postulates for this failure can be advanced, but their resolution depends as much on increased knowledge about processing for acoustic as for electrical stimuli. Solving this mismatch for the CN may go a long way toward resolving the entire problem of electrical encoding.

Alternate Processing

As a result of the limitations of replacing cochlear function with an implant, greater emphasis is being placed on preprocessing acoustic information before delivery as an electrical waveform. However, the optimal form of this preprocessing is not apparent. The extraction of speech features is a common goal, but these tend to be ad hoc at best. Implementations commonly enhance temporal information, which electrical stimulation seems to convey well. In short, the choice of a preprocessing algorithm is pragmatic and guided, if at all, by the view that linguistic categories are effective indicators for acoustic features. The correspondence between linguistic features and the processing logic of the central auditory system is now known. Presenting sound components extracted from speech to the cochlear nuclei may not tap the processing capacities of those nuclein or their subsequent projection sites.

We suggest that identifying the naturally occurring selectivities of central processing will constrain designs for external devices which preprocess sound information. If the cochlear nucleus provides a necessary transformation of incoming acoustic patterns for higher processing, it seems logical that preprocessing should be aimed at accomplishing this in the pathological case.

Plasticity

Evidence for adaptive processes in the central auditory pathways of mammals exists although major periods of plasticity may be restricted to sensitive periods in early development (e.g., Clopton and Silverman, 1977). However, there is no good evidence bearing on the plasticity of pattern selectivities as discussed here. Obviously the adaptive reorganization of processing would be important for prosthesis and processor design strategies because it could help resolve differences between central processing capacity and the limits of electrical encoding. This area of research is of significant clinical importance because of the large number of children who are candidates for the implantation of a cochlear prosthesis. Unfortunately, it has proved difficult to examine plasticity in central auditory mechanisms for processing complex sounds and patterns of neural activity from a cochlear implant. As with other questions about implant function, clinical evidence from children implanted from an early age may precede experimental evidence bearing on the mechanisms of plasticity.

Summary

In this chapter we attempted to more precisely designate "central processing" as it relates to the operation of cochlear prostheses. Estimates of the complex acoustic features processed by neurons of the cochlear nuclei have been examined for both acoustic and electrical modes of activation. Both peripheral transduction and central processing mechanisms are responsible for the loss of information for electrical stimulation as opposed to acoustic. A lack of cochlear analysis is thought to produce a mismatch between acceptable inputs to central processing at the cochlear nuclei. Understanding this disparity and its sequelae at the cochlear nuclei can help resolve many problematic aspects of encoding complex sounds for presentation through a cochlear implant. Obtaining a better match between electrically induced afferent activity and that which is processable, incorporating some processing in an external device, and utilizing adaptive plasticities of the auditory system are possible routes for improving implant function.

Acknowledgments. Dr. Sandy Bledsoe collaborated in research on the lateral line of *Xenopus*. We thank Daryl Kipke for software development, which made much of the data collection possible, and Mike Mikhail for his assistance in the pulse studies. This research was supported by grants from the NIH and the NSF.

References

Backoff, P.M., Clopton, B.M., and Bledsoe, S.C. (1988). Responses of peripheral amphibian nerve (*Xenopus laevis*) to electrical stimulation. *Soc. Neurosci. Abstr.* 14:492.

Brummer, S.B., and Robblee, L.S. (1983). Criteria for selecting electrodes for electrical stimulation: Theoretical and practical considerations. *Ann. N.Y. Acad. Sci.* 40:159–171.

Clopton, B.M., and Bosma, M.A. (1982). Effectiveness of middle ear electrical stimulation for activating central auditory pathways. *Ann. Otol. Rhinol. Laryngol.* 91:285–291.

Clopton, B.M., and Glass, I. (1984). Unit responses at cochlear nucleus to electrical stimulation through a cochlear prosthesis. *Hearing Res.* 14:1–14.

Clopton, B.M., and Silverman, M.S. (1977). Plasticity of binaural interaction. II. Critical period and changes in midline response. *J. Neurophysiol.* 40:1081–1089.

Clopton, B.M., Spelman, F.A., Glass, I., Pfingst, B.E., Miller, J.M., Lawrence, P.D., and Dean, D.P. (1983). Neural encoding of electrical signals. *Ann. N.Y. Acad. Sci.* 40:146–158.

Cohen, L. (1966). Generalized phase-space distribution functions. *J. Math. Phys.* 7:781–786.

Columbo, J., and Parkins, C.W. (1987). A model of electrical excitation of the mammalian auditory-nerve neuron. *Hearing Res.* 31:287–312.

de Boer, E., and de Jongh, H.R. (1978). On cochlear encoding: Potentialities and limitations of the reserve correlation technique. *J. Acoust. Soc. Am.* 63:115–135.

Duckert, L.G., and Miller, J.M. (1982). Acute morphological changes in guinea pig cochlea following electrical stimulation. *Ann. Otol. Rhinol. Laryngol.* 91:33–40.

Flanagan, J.L. (1972). *Speech Analysis, Synthesis, and Perception* (New York: Springer-Verlag).

Frankenhaeuser, B., and Huxley, A.F. (1964). The action potential in the myelinated nerve fibre of *Xenopus laevis* as computed on the basis of voltage clamp data. *J. Physiol.* 171:302–315.

Glass, I. (1984). Phase-locked responses of cochlear nucleus units to electrical stimulation through a cochlear implant. *Exp. Brain Res.* 55:386–390.

Guttman, R., and Hachmeister, L. (1971). Effect of calcium, temperature, and polarizing current upon alternating current excitation of space-clamped squid axon. *J. Gen. Physiol.* 58:304–321.

Hartmann, R., Topp, G., and Klinke, R. (1984). Discharge patterns of cat primary auditory fibers with electrical stimulation of the cochlea. *Hearing Res.* 13: 47–62.

Hermes, D.J., Aersten, A.M.H.J., Johannesma, P.I.M., and Eggermont, J.J. (1981). Spectro-temporal characteristics of single units in the auditory midbrain of the lightly anaesthetised grass frog (*Rana temporaria L.*) investigated with noise stimuli. *Hearing Res.* 5:147–178.

McNeal, D.R. (1976). Analysis of a model for excitation of myelinated nerve. *IEEE BME*-23:329–337.

Motz, H., and Rattay, F. (1986). A study of the application of the Hodgkin-Huxley and the Frankenhaeuser-Huxley model for electrostimulation of the acoustic nerve. *Neuroscience* 18:699–712.

Moxon, E.C. (1971). Neural and mechanical responses to electrical stimulation of the cat's inner ear. Doctoral dissertation, MIT, Cambridge, Mass.

Parkins, C.W. (1987). Single auditory neuron response patterns to different implant stimulus wave forms. *Ann. Otol. Rhinol. Laryngol.* Suppl. 128, 96:41–42.

Parkins, C.W., and Colombo, J. (1987). Auditory-nerve single-neuron thresholds to electrical stimulation from scala tympani electrodes. *Hearing Res.* 31:267–286.

Pfingst, B.E. (1984). Operating range and intensity psychophysics for cochlear implants. *Arch. Otolaryngol.* 110:140–144.

Pfingst, B.E., Miller, J.M., Donaldson, J.A., and Spelman, F.A. (1979). Psychophysical evaluation of cochlear prostheses in a monkey model. *Ann. Otol. Rhinol. Laryngol.* 88:613–625.

Reilly, J.P., Freeman, V.T., and Larkin, W.D. (1985). Sensory effects of transient electrical stimulation: Evaluation with a neuroelectrical model. *IEEE BME*-32:1001–1011.

Rihaczek, W. (1968) Signal energy distribution in time and frequency. *IEEE Trans. Info. Theory IT*-14:369–374.

Shannon, R.V. (1985). Threshold and loudness functions for pulsatile stimulation of cochlear implants. *Hearing Res.* 18:135–143.

Spelman, F.A., Pfingst, B.E., and Miller, J.M. (1978). A constant current stimulator for use with chronic cochlear implants. In *Proc. San Diego Biomed. Symp.*,1–3.

van den Honert, C., and Stypulkowski, P.H. (1984). Physiological properties of the electrically stimulated auditory nerve. II. Single fiber recordings. *Hearing Res.* 14:225–243.

van den Honert, C., and Stypulkowski, P.H. (1987a). Single fiber mapping of spatial excitation patterns in the electrically stimulated auditory nerve. *Hearing Res.* 29, 195–206.

van den Honert, C., and Stypulkowski, P.H. (1987b). Temporal response patterns of single auditory nerve fibers elicited by periodic electrical stimuli. *Hearing Res.* 29:207–222.

Wiler, J.A., and Clopton, B.M. (1989). Single-unit responses in guinea pig AVCN to pulse and continuous electrical stimulation of the cochlea. *A.R.O. Abstr.*, XII Midwinter Meeting, p. 57.

Wiler, J.A., Clopton, B.M., and Mikhail, M.A. (1988). Single-unit responses in cochlear nucleus to electrical stimulation of the cochlea with biphasic pulses of variable shape. *Soc. Neurosci. Abstr.* 14:646.

Wiler, J.A., Clopton, B.M., and Mikhail, M.A. (1989). Effect of electrical pulse shape on AVCN unit responses to cochlear stimulation. *Hearing Res.*, in press.

Ben M. Clopton: Discussion

Dr. Javel: Do you have any explanation for why those surfaces for the different stimuli were so complex? One would think they would be slightly more predictable in simplified physical terms, and yet they look very complex.

Dr. Clopton: If you look at the details, a lot of those contours were low contours, and we put them in there simply to have a complete representation. The peaks over on the edge, which were the greatest, are quite high. For example, some of those were

180 spike counts out of 200 presentations, whereas a lot of the lower contours were below 40. So it's a good indication of the nonlinearity of the system. In many cases, a specific pulse shape is much more efficient than other similar pulse shapes.

Dr. Spelman: If you change the total charge delivered per phase, do you find that the shapes are invariant or do you find that the shapes of the contours vary substantially?

Dr. Clopton: We have varied intensity in some cases, but since this profile takes a very long time to complete, we haven't looked at a lot of intensities. The dynamic range isn't large, so that limits the intensity range available. The answer is that it doesn't seem to change.

Dr. van den Honert: I am fascinated by the dimples or troughs. The implication is that the absence of some spectral component is helpful in getting this cell to fire. I wonder if you would speculate on how you think that might come about. When we routinely think of any kind of stimulus as being unilaterally excitatory, it's very hard to stop neurons with electrical currents. Do you think this relates somehow to turning on another cell which is inhibiting this one? And when you don't turn it on, release it from inhibition?

Dr. Clopton: We don't tend to see energy troughs for STRF surfaces in the VCN. When we do see them for acoustic stimuli, the most reasonable interpretation is that inhibition is effective.

Dr. Pfingst: If I understand your experiment, you have shown (1) that there is an optimal pulse shape for each neuron, for which charge/phase at threshold is minimum; and (2) that this charge is often similar to the minimum psychophysical threshold charge/pulse for sinusoids. My question is, In a typical case where these charges are similar, how do the phase durations and peak currents of the two waveforms compare?

Dr. Clopton: The peak currents for psychophysical thresholds are slightly lower, but sinusoidal thresholds, when measured for current values in psychophysical tasks, tend to be best at low frequencies in contrast to lower thresholds for somewhat higher frequency components in the pulses when measured in terms of charge/phase.

17
Acoustic and Electrical Encoding of Temporal Information

ERIC JAVEL

Introduction

A well-known, well-studied phenomenon in auditory pshysiology is phase locking, which refers to synchroniziation of neuronal discharges to stimulus waveform cycles for frequencies <5 kHz. Since its discovery in cat by Galambos and Davis (1943), synchronization has been studied in considerable detail in several animal species. Although strikingly close correspondences exist between phase-locked activity patterns in peripheral auditory nuclei of animals and perceptual performance of human listeners on certain tasks, there is still no clear evidence that the human brain actually bases perceptual decisions on temporally encoded information.

Many features of neural synchronization are retained in auditory-nerve-fiber responses to sinusoidal and pulsatile electrical stimuli of the type used in cochlear implants, but some important differences between electrical and acoustic responses nonetheless exist. These include (1) a lack of nonlinear behavior in electrically elicited responses to multifrequency stimuli, (2) a loss of statistical independence among responses elicited in different electrically stimulated neurons, and (3) large differences in the degree of synchronization and entrainment. Despite the differences, physiological data obtained with electrical stimulation of cochlear implants suggest that those perceptual processes using synchronized neural activity receive generally appropriate inputs. Indeed, one can argue that the superior synchronization of responses to electrical stimuli should produce even better performance on some psychophysical tasks than that observed in their acoustic counterparts.

Although similarities exist with respect to trends in psychophysical performance of electrically stimulated versus acoustically stimulated ears, absolute performance levels differ. That is, implantees do not perform as well as normal-hearing listeners on most tasks requiring temporal processing. Rather than indicating that implantees do not use temporally encoded information, the failure to perform as well as normal-hearing listeners is more likely due to the generally smaller number of stimulable auditory nerve fibers and a smaller number of available perceptual channels.

This paper proceeds from a description of the basic features of neuronal discharge synchronization observed in acoustic stimulation to a consideration of some aspects of acoustic stimulus coding. Following that is a discussion of physiological mechanisms underlying two perceptual tasks that might use temporally encoded information. These are, in increasing order of degree of temporal resolution required, the pitch of complex tones and pure-tone frequency discrimination. The focus then shifts to an examination of auditory-nerve-fiber responses to electrical stimuli, with particular emphasis on describing temporal response features. Finally, the discussion section attempts to relate the physiological data to the general issue of temporal information processing in hearing.

Elements of Discharge Synchronization in Auditory Neurons

The basic phenomenon of phase locking is depicted in Figure 17.1*a*, which shows a snippet of 200 Hz acoustic sinusoid and several overlaid traces of action potentials (spikes) generated in response to that waveform. Synchronization, defined as the tendency of the spikes to cluster at a particular point in the waveform cycle, is apparent in this response. A useful way to quantify the degree of synchronization was developed by Goldberg and Brown (1969), who expressed the waveform cycle as a unit circle, plotted the position of stimulus-elicited spikes as unit-length vectors on the circle, and computed the length of the mean vector. This value, called vector strength or synchronization index, ranges from 0, implying an even distribution of spikes in the waveform cycle, to 1, implying perfect synchronization with all spikes occurring at precisely the same point in the waveform cycle. As will be discussed later, the same result is obtained mathematically by taking the forward Fourier transform of a period histogram and normalizing the result by dividing the amplitude of the response at the fundamental by the DC term.

The synchronization of auditory-nerve-fiber discharges to acoustic stimuli is a simple outgrowth of the fact that hair cells are excited only when their stereocilia move toward the kinocilium, or longest sterocilium (Hudspeth and Corey, 1977). In other words, hair cell depolarization occurs when the basilar membrane moves in an upward direction (Russell, Richardson, and Cody, 1986). Since hair cells drive the auditory nerve, phase-locked neurotransmitter release at the hair cell/auditory nerve synapse will lead to synchronization of stimulus-elicited spikes in afferent fibers.

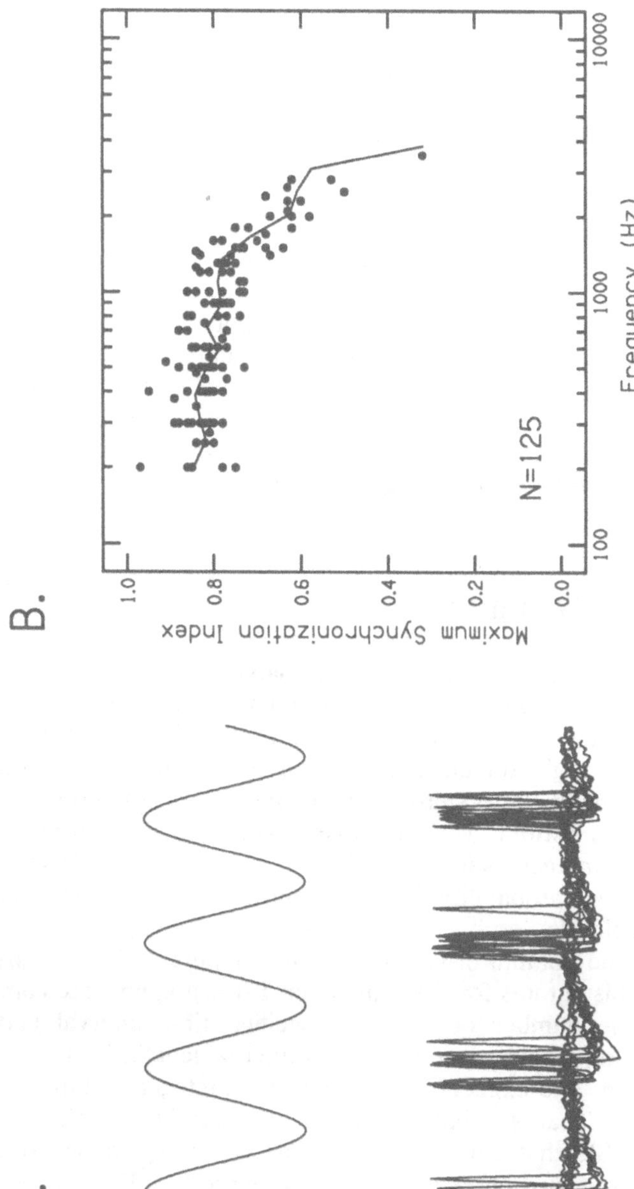

FIGURE 17.1. (*a*) Synchronization of cat-auditory-nerve-fiber discharges to a 200-Hz tone. (*b*) Maximum synchronization index of cat auditory nerve fibers as a function of frequency.

Acoustically, the ability of auditory nerve fibers to synchronize their discharges to individual waveform cycles is a frequency-dependent variable. Figure 17.1*b*, shows a graph of the maximum value obtained for the synchronization index plotted as a function of stimulus frequency. These data were obtained from cats. The solid line represents a moving-window average. Sychronization is relatively constant at approximately 0.82 for frequencies below 1.2 kHz, decreases at higher frequencies, and is lost above 4–5 kHz. The values obtained below 1.2 kHz are slightly higher than the synchronization index associated with a half-wave-rectified sinusoid, namely $\pi/4$, or 0.78. That value is what one expects if discharge probability were a linear function of instantaneous waveform amplitude.

Synchronization of auditory-nerve-fiber responses of acoustic signals possesses a dynamic range in just the same manner that discharge rate possesses a dynamic range. Dynamic range is the intensity range over which a variable, synchronization or discharge rate in this case, changes from a minimum to a maximum value. For both discharge rate and synchronization, the dynamic range is 20–30 dB.

Analytical Techniques

In Figure 17.2 are shown examples of the analytical tools most often used to assess synchronized activity. At the left is a column of period histograms, which are plots of discharge probability as a function of waveform phase angle, obtained in response to an acoustic pure tone. The column is arraged in 10-dB steps, with low intensities at the top and high intensities at the bottom. The half-sinusoidal shape of the period histograms at higher intensities indicates that (1) the response is phase-locked and (2) discharge probability is a montonic function of instantaneous waveform amplitude.

The right-hand column of graphs shown in Figure 17.2 are interspike interval (ISI) histograms for the same data. ISI histograms are compiled by plotting the number of times a specified time interval between successive spikes occurs, as a function of interval length. If the response is phase locked, one expects ISIs to cluster at integer multiples of the stimulus period. That is, spikes occurring on successive waveform cycles will produce ISIs that cluster at times corresponding to one stimulus periods; spikes occurring on every other cycle produce ISIs clustering at two stimulus periods; and so on. The exponential decay of the ISI histogram envelope is characteristic of auditory-nerve-fiber responses to acoustic stimuli. It indicates that ISIs obey Poisson-process rules; more precisely, the rules are obeyed for ISIs exceeding the 0.5m absolute refractory period.

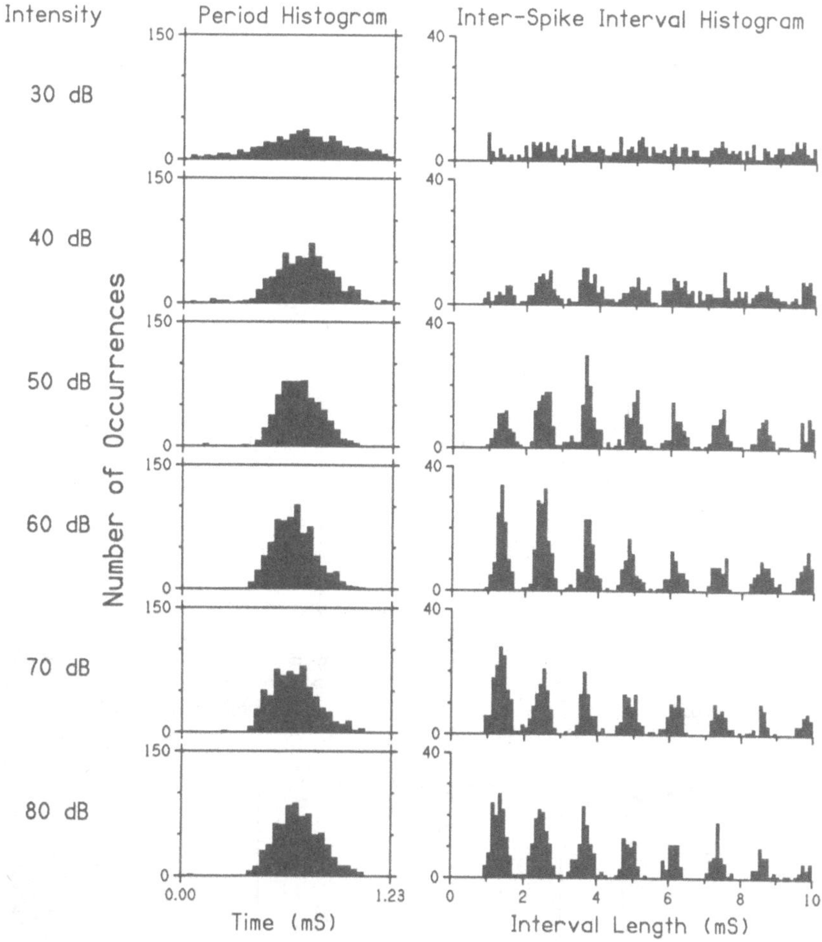

FIGURE 17.2. Period and ISI histograms obtained in response to an 800-Hz tone presented at several intensities.

In Figure 17.3 are shown examples of how one can use period and ISI histograms to extract temporally encoded frequency information. One way to do this is to take the Fourier transform of the period or ISI histogram. This technique provides estimates of the frequency content of the histogram "waveform," expressed as integer multiples of the waveform fundamental. In the case of period histograms, the stimulus period is equal to the period of the fundamental, and a priori we would expect Fourier magnitudes to be greatest at that frequency.

The top displays in Figure 17.3 show a period histogram and its normalized Fourier transform or synchronization spectrum. The normalization is performed by dividing the amplitude of each harmonic by the

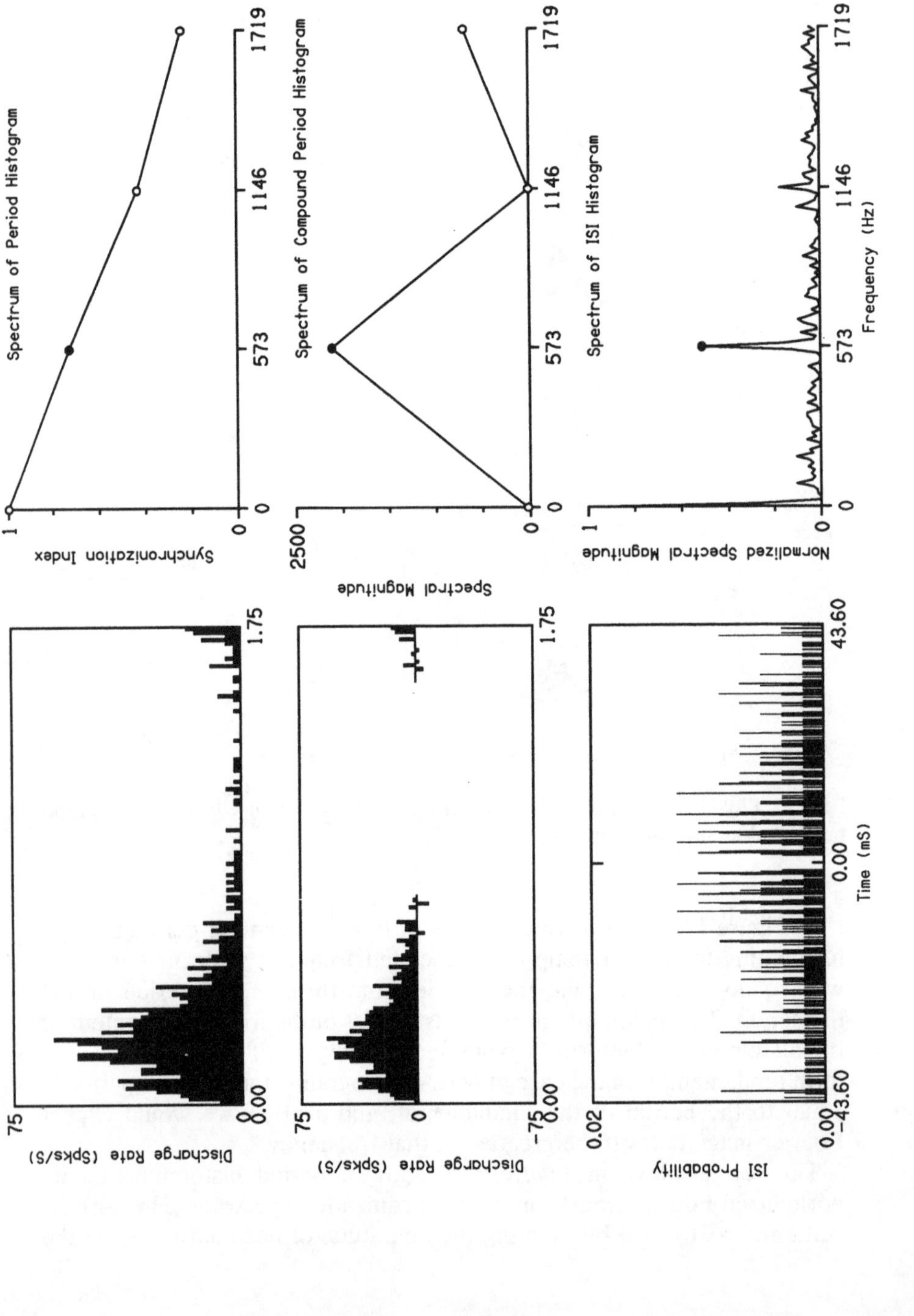
Spectrum of Period Histogram
Synchronization Index
Spectrum of Compound Period Histogram
Spectral Magnitude
Spectrum of ISI Histogram
Normalized Spectral Magnitude
Frequency (Hz)
Discharge Rate (Spks/S)
ISI Probability
Time (mS)
0
573
1146
1719
1.75
0.00
43.60
−43.60
75
−75
2500
0.02

DC amplitude. It removes the effects of overall discharge rate, leaving only the degree of synchronization. The filled symbol in the Fourier spectrum indicates the degree of synchronization to the frequency actually presented, and the open symbols indicate synchronization at multiples of the fundamental, which of course were not present in the tone. There is a substantial response at stimulus harmonics. In addition, a response at DC (0 Hz) exists because standard period histograms do not contain a negative-going half cycle.

Responses at stimulus harmonics are introduced by two factors. One of these is half-wave rectification of the input histogram, and the other is the departure of the the period histogram from a perfect half sinusoid.

Harmonic distortion caused by half-wave rectification can be eliminated by forming and analyzing a compound period histogram. In this technique a tone is presented and a period histogram determined from the response to that tone. This will resemble a half-wave-rectified sinusoid. Then the tone is presented again, this time 180° out of phase, and another period histogram is computed. All things being equal, the fiber should now respond at precisely the opposite point(s) on the waveform cycle. The compound period histogram is formed by bin-by-bin subtraction of the "phase-inverted" period histogram from the original period histogram. Since the compound period histogram is no longer half-wave-rectified, the Fourier transform should no longer be contaminated by rectification distortion effects. The outcome of this procedure is shown is the middle row of Figure 17.3. The Fourier transform indicated little energy at DC, and responses at harmonics are much reduced.

In a commonsense approach to interpreting the frequency content of period histograms, one can usually safely disregard Fourier components at frequencies other than those actually present in the signal. The only time that caution must be applied is when signal bandwidth exceeds one octave.

Yet another way to determine the temporally encoded frequency content of a neuron's response is to take the ISI histogram as a waveform and perform a Fourier transform on it. Johnson (1974) has shown

FIGURE 17.3. Uses of period histograms and Fourier transforms to assess temporal-frequency content of phase-locked responses. *Top:* Period histogram and its normalized Fourier transform. Note the responses at DC and at integer multiples of the 573-Hz stimulus frequency. *Middle:* Compound period histogram and its Fourier transform. Note the absence of response at DC and twice the stimulus frequency. *Bottom:* ISI histogram reflected around $t = 0$, and its normalized Fourier transform. Note the addition of information at frequencies other than multiples of the stimulus frequency.

mathematically that the Fourier transform of an ISI histogram should behave as the square of the transform of a period histogram. Thus, transforms of period and ISI histograms both provide the same information.

A useful step in analyzing the frequency content of ISI histograms is to create a mirror image of the histogram by duplicating it in "negative time," and perform the Fourier transform on the double-length histogram. This is shown at the lower left of Figure 17.3. Doubling the length of the histogram halves its fundamental frequency, hence doubling the resolution of the Fourier spectrum, but it does not affect the magnitudes of the components. The result of such a manipulation is shown at the lower right of Figure 17.3. Note that the resolution of individual frequencies is much sharper than was the case for period histograms (Figure 17.2). This is a simple outgrowth of the fact that a typical ISI histogram encompasses many stimulus periods, or, stated another way, its fundamental frequency is much lower. This gives us an indication of responses, if any, at frequencies between the harmonics of the stimulus. As can be seen, there is essentially no response at any frequencies other than that of the stimulus and its harmonics. For reasons described earlier, responses at harmonics arise because ISI histograms are half-wave-rectified.

Nonlinear Aspects of Temporal-Frequency Coding

We can get an idea of the power of the aforementioned analytical techniques by using them to examine responses to stimuli possessing more than one frequency. An example of this, for an auditory nerve fiber's response to an acoustic two-tone complex, is shown in Figure 17.4. The complex contained energy at 500 and 700 Hz. At the left of Figure 17.4 are two period histograms. The upper histogram was obtained by resetting the histogram bin pointer at every period of the 500 Hz tone, and the lower histogram was obtained by resetting at every period of the 700 Hz tone. Even though the actual fundamental frequency of the complex is 100 Hz, corresponding to a period of 10 ms, it is both possible and mathematically acceptable to compile period histograms that are based on other periods, so long as the stimulus duration is a multiple of the desired period. The peaks in the period histograms indicate synchronization at both 500 and 700 Hz. At the upper right is the corresponding ISI histogram, and at the lower right is its normalized Fourier transform. The peaks at 500 and 700 Hz in the Fourier transform indicate that both frequencies are present in the temporal response.

The data shown in Figure 17.4 are part of a larger data set. This set was selected for presentation here because it demonstrates one of the principal features of temporal-frequency coding in the auditory nerve, namely synchrony suppression. Synchrony suppression refers to the ability of a

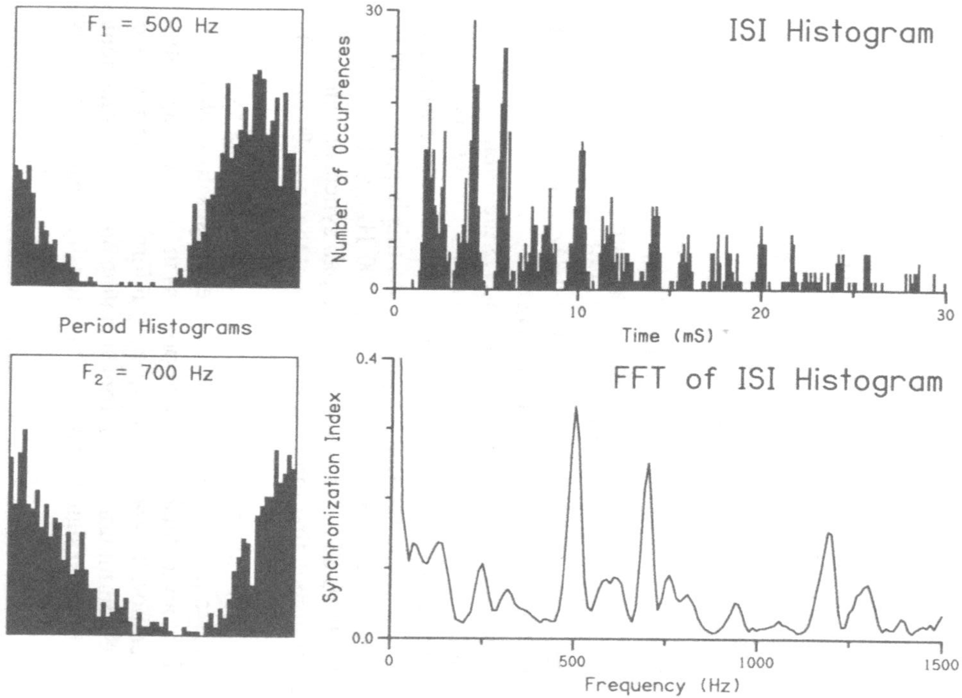

FIGURE 17.4. Temporal analysis of an auditory nerve fiber's response to a two-tone complex consisting of 500 and 700 Hz. *Left:* Period histograms obtained by basing the recycling period of the histogram of periods corresponding to 500 Hz (*top*) and 700 Hz (*bottom*). *Right:* ISI histogram (*top*) for these same data, and its normalized Fourier transform (*bottom*). The degree of synchronization to 500 Hz is slightly greater than to 700 Hz, but the neuron responds to both tones simultaneously.

tone at one frequency to reduce responses to tones at other excitatory frequencies. This response nonlinearity has been studied in considerable detail (e.g., Arthur, 1976; Javel, 1981). Although some of synchrony suppression arises as a result of nonlinear cochlear mechanics, most of it is due to the hair cell's inability to code accurately waveforms whose components possess greatly disparate amplitudes.

The full data set is shown in Figure 17.5. Two-tone stimuli were used to obtain these data, and the auditory nerve fiber was capable of responding to either tone. One tone was set to 700 Hz and fixed in intensity at 80-dB SPL. The other tone was set to 500 Hz and was varied in intensity from 70 dB SPL to 100 dB SPL in 5 dB steps. The uppermost row of Figure 17.5 shows responses obtained when the 500-Hz tone was set to 70-dB SPL. From left to right, the displays are (1) the period histogram based on the period of the 500-Hz tone, (2) the period histogram based on the 700 Hz tone, (3) the ISI histogram, and (4) the normalized Fourier transform of the ISI histogram. In the first condition the 700 Hz tone is more intense than the 500 Hz tone. The period histograms indicate no obvious synchronization to 500 Hz and excellent synchronization to 700 Hz. Likewise, the ISI histogram exhibits peaks only at multiples of 1.43 ms, which is the period of the 700 Hz tone, and the Fourier transform of the ISI histogram exhibits energy at 700 Hz (and, because of rectification, at its harmonics) but not at 500 Hz.

For the second and subsequent rows in Figure 17.5 the intensity of the 500 Hz tone was increased in 5 dB steps. Gazing down the left-hand side of the figure, one can see a response to the 500 Hz tone emerge, a evidenced by synchronization to that frequency. As this happens there is a corresponding decrease in synchronization at 700 Hz. At the highest intensity, namely 100 dB SPL for the 500 Hz tone, all synchronizaiton to 700 Hz is lost, even though that tone is still present at the same 80 dB SPL intensity.

The point made in Figures 17.4 and 17.5 is that the response to a complex tone is not equal to the sum of the responses to each of its components. Rather, an intrinsic nonlinear process in the cochlea creates variations in the temporally encoded frequency information. In the case shown the response continuum ranges from signaling only one component of the two-tone complex to signaling both. The intensity range over which

FIGURE 17.5. Nonlinearity of temporal response to a two-tone complex. The stimulus consisted of tones at 500 and 700 Hz. The intensity of the 700-Hz tone was fixed at 80 dB SPL, and the intensity of the 500 Hz tone was varied in 5-dB steps from 70 dB (*top*) to 100 dB (*bottom*). Reading left to right, displays include period histograms based on the periods of the 500 and 700 Hz tones, the corresponding ISI histogram, and the normalized Fourier transform of the ISI histogram. Over the 30 dB interaction range, the temporal information content of the response changes from signaling only 700 Hz to signaling only 500 Hz.

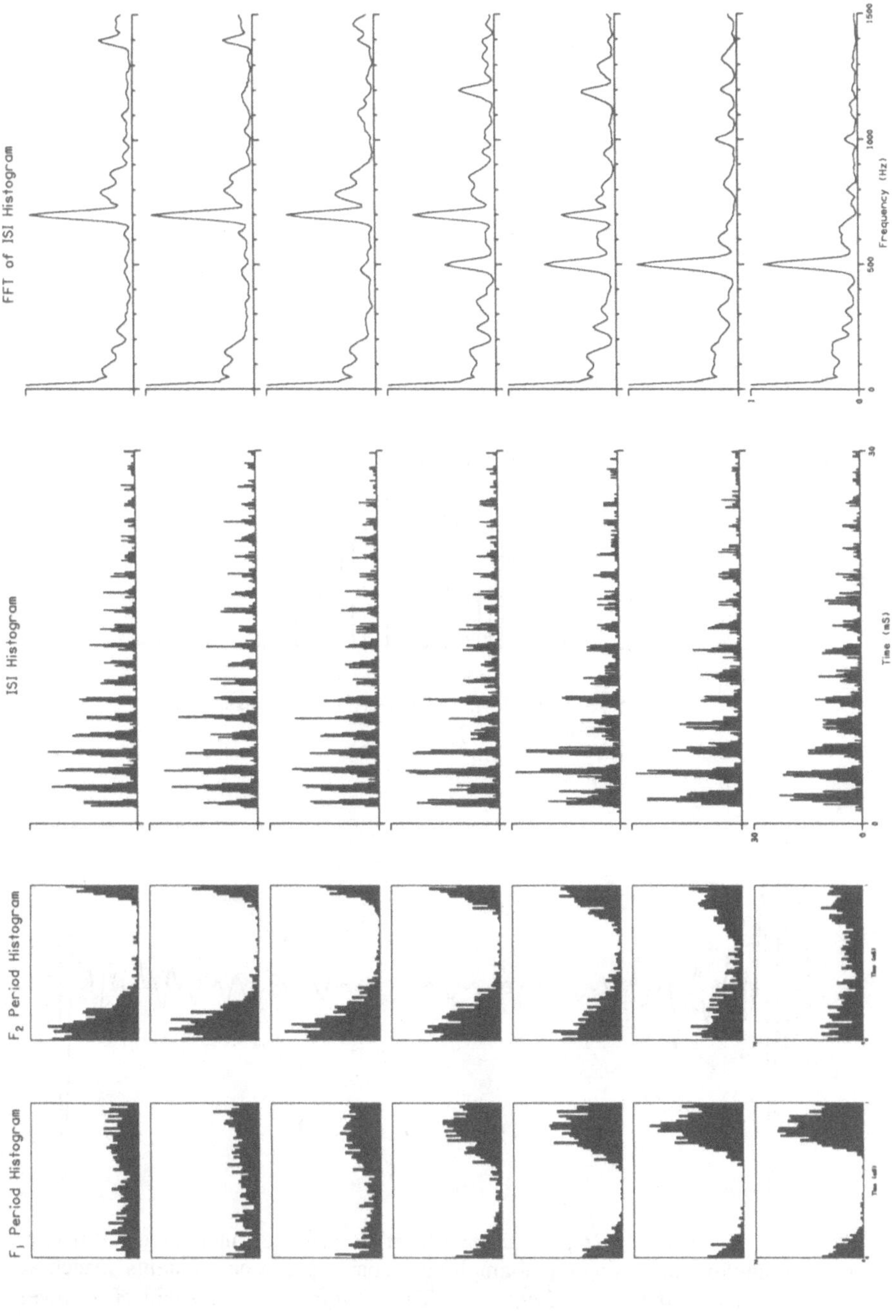
FFT of ISI Histogram
Frequency (Hz)
ISI Histogram
Time (mS)
F_2 Period Histogram
F_1 Period Histogram

the response contains both frequencies is relatively limited. Contemporary speech processing strategies for cochlear implants make no provision for this kind of nonlinear frequency coding.

Another example of nonlinear processing of the frequency content of complex tones is shown in Figures 17.6–17.8. Figure 17.6 shows a spectrum and waveform of an octave-bandwidth harmonic complex. This signal possesses energy at evenly spaced frequencies, and each component has the same amplitude. The corresponding waveform, shown in the lower panel of the figure, is periodic and rather peaked. The harmonic complex's waveform is reminiscent of a vowel waveform, which is not surprising because a vowel is nothing more than a filtered, wideband harmonic complex. For a vowel, the spacing betweeen adjacent harmon-

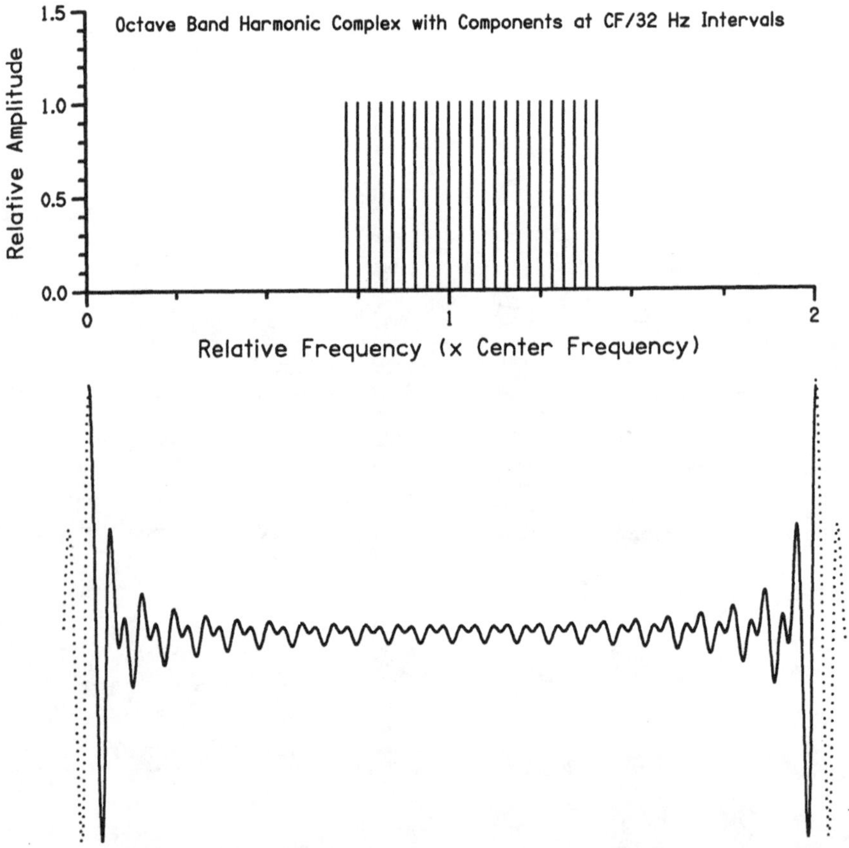

FIGURE 17.6. Spectrum (*top*) and waveform (*bottom*) of an octave-width harmonic complex possessing equal-amplitude, cosine-phase components spaced at 1/32 multiples of the center frequency. The waveform, reminiscent of a vowel waveform, is periodic and possesses a high crest-to-trough ratio.

ics is the glottal pulse rate or voice pitch frequency. Responses of auditory nerve fibers to harmonic complexes were studied extensively by Horst, Javel and Farley (1985, 1986).

The data shown in Figure 17.7 represent an application of the analytical techniques described earlier. The acoustic stimulus used to obtain the data shown in the upper row was a pure tone at 884 Hz. On the left is the ISI histogram, reflected around $t = 0$ in the same manner introduced earlier in Figure 17.3. At the right is the normalized Fourier transform of the ISI histogram. Not surprisingly, it shows energy principally at the stimulus frequency and its multiples. In the lower row are shown the ISI histogram and related Fourier transform obtained when the stimulus was an octave-band harmonic complex centered at 884 Hz. The complex contained five components, each space 100.5 Hz apart, and each component possessed the same intensity. Although the discharge rate elicited by this signal was approximately the same as that elicited by the pure tone, the distribution of ISIs is very different. Likewise, the Fourier transform shows that not all components are represented to the same degree in the temporal response. Rather, the response to the central component (884 Hz) is strongest, and the strength of the response to the other components decreases as the frequency difference between a given component and the central component increases. In the case shown in Figure 17.7 the five-component complex was centered on the fiber's characteristic frequency (i.e., the frequency to which the neuron is most sensitive). It is reasonable to expect, then, that the response to the central component would be greatest. In fact the responses to the other components are almost exactly what one would expect if the harmonic complex were passed through a filter shaped like the fiber's tuning curve. Thus, for the data shown in Figure 17.7 the frequency content of the temporal response is a simple, linearly filtered version of the input.

Figure 17.8 shows what happens when another type of harmonic complex is presented at very different intensities. In this case the stimulus was a 17-component harmonic complex. Each frequency component possessed the same intensity, except for the central component which was either 2 (top row), 4 (middle row), or 6 (bottom row) dB more intense than the others. This situation is reminiscent of the formant structure of a vowel, which exhibits spectral peaks that depend on the size and shape of the vocal tract cavities.

Signal spectra are shown in the left-hand column of Figure 17.8. The central components of these signals were slightly lower than the fiber's characteristic frequency. At low intensities (middle column) the temporally encoded frequency content of the response is what one expects from linear filtering through a tuning curve. That is, the shape of the tuning curve is evident, and the higher-intensity central component is somewhat more prominent in the response. Synchronization to the central component of the signal is greatest because its intensity is greatest.

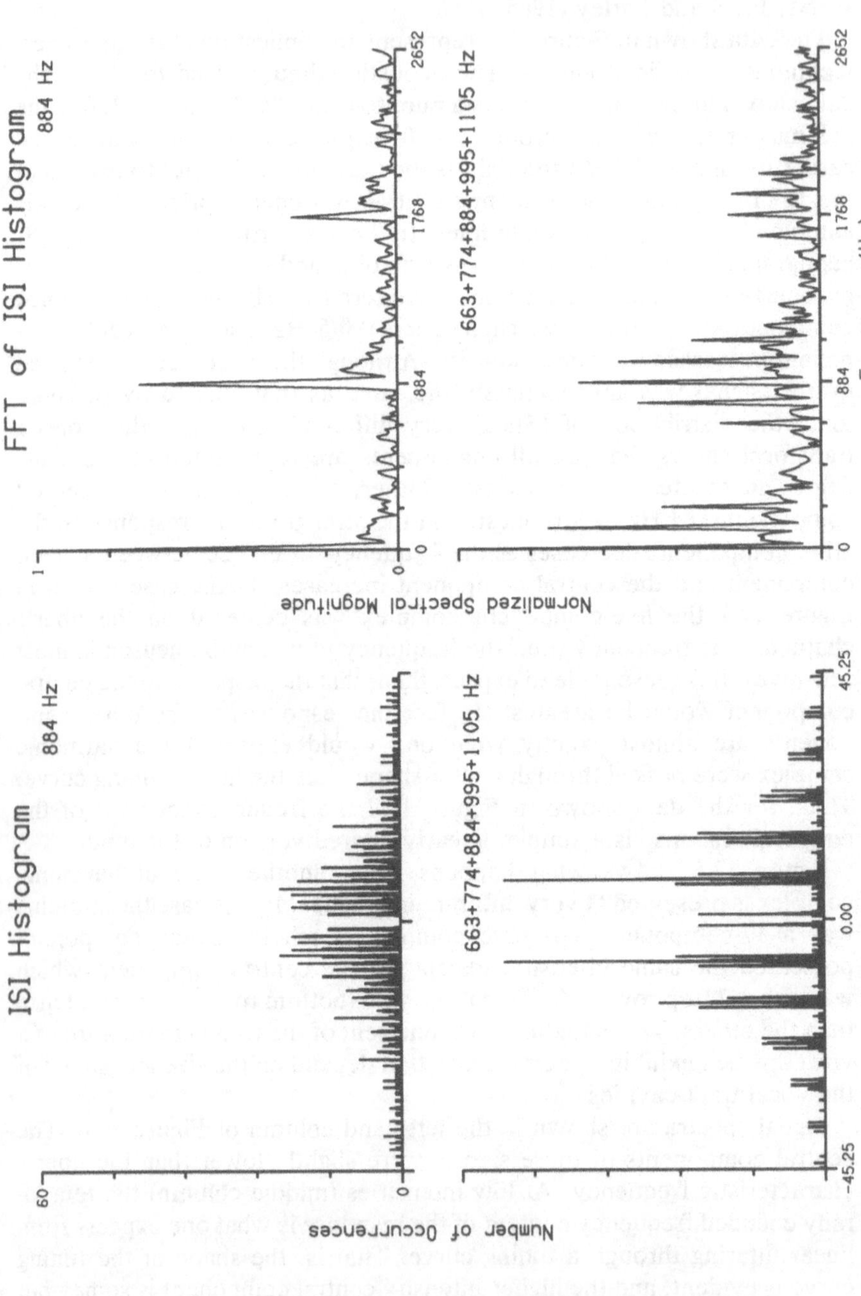
ISI Histogram
884 Hz
Number of Occurrences
60
0
663+774+884+995+1105 Hz
-45.25
0.00
45.25
Time (mS)
FFT of ISI Histogram
884 Hz
Normalized Spectral Magnitude
1
0
663+774+884+995+1105 Hz
0
884
1768
2652
Frequency (Hz)

The situation is markedly different at high intensities (right column). No longer is the response a linearly filtered version of the input. Rather, the temporal response is completely dominated by the central component, to the extent that none of the other components is represented in the response. Equally notable is the fact that one component need only be 2 dB higher in intensity than the others to dominate the response at high intensities. As Javel, Horst, and Farley (1987a) and Greenwood (1988) have shown, this kind of response behavior is caused by the hair cell's compressive or saturating input-output function.

Responses of cochlear nucleus neurons to electrical two-tone complexes were obtained by Clopton and Glass (1984). Their data, while limited in scope, suggest that a cell's response is basically a linear function of instantaneous waveform amplitude at all intensities. In contrast, neural responses to acoustic two-tone stimuli (Brugge et al., 1969; Rose et al., 1974) are linear functions of waveform amplitude only over a narrow intensity range, and that range depends on overall intensity. Also, response nonlinearities associated with discharge rate saturation (Figure 17.8) apparently don't occur when electrical stimuli are used.

The data shown in Figures 17.4 to 17.8 demonstrate that the temporal response of the cochlea to multifrequency tones is strongly nonlinear. Although the behavior of the nonlinearities has been studied thoroughly, contemporary cochlear implants do not attempt to make provisions for them in the speech processing strategies they employ. Whether such an attempt is either warranted or feasible, however, is open to debate.

Perceptual Phenomena and Temporal Physiological Correlates

A considerable amount of speculation has been forwarded on the issue of frequency coding in the temporal domain. For example, de Boer (1956), Schouten, Ritsma, and Cardozo (1962), and others have proposed that the characteristic low pitch of complex tones is extracted by monitoring high-amplitude peaks in the temporal fine structure of stimulus wave-

FIGURE 17.7. Temporal analysis of responses of an auditory nerve fiber to a pure tone (*top*) and an octave-width harmonic complex possessing five equal-amplitude, cosine-phase frequency components centered on 884 Hz, which was the fiber's CF (*bottom*). On the left are shown ISI histograms, reflected around $t = 0$, and on the right are the normalized Fourier tranforms of the ISI histograms. The response to the pure tone exhibits energy only at the signal frequency and, owing to rectification distortion, its integer multiples. The response to the harmonic complex exhibits energy at each of the frequencies in the complex, appropriately filtered by the fiber's tuning curve.

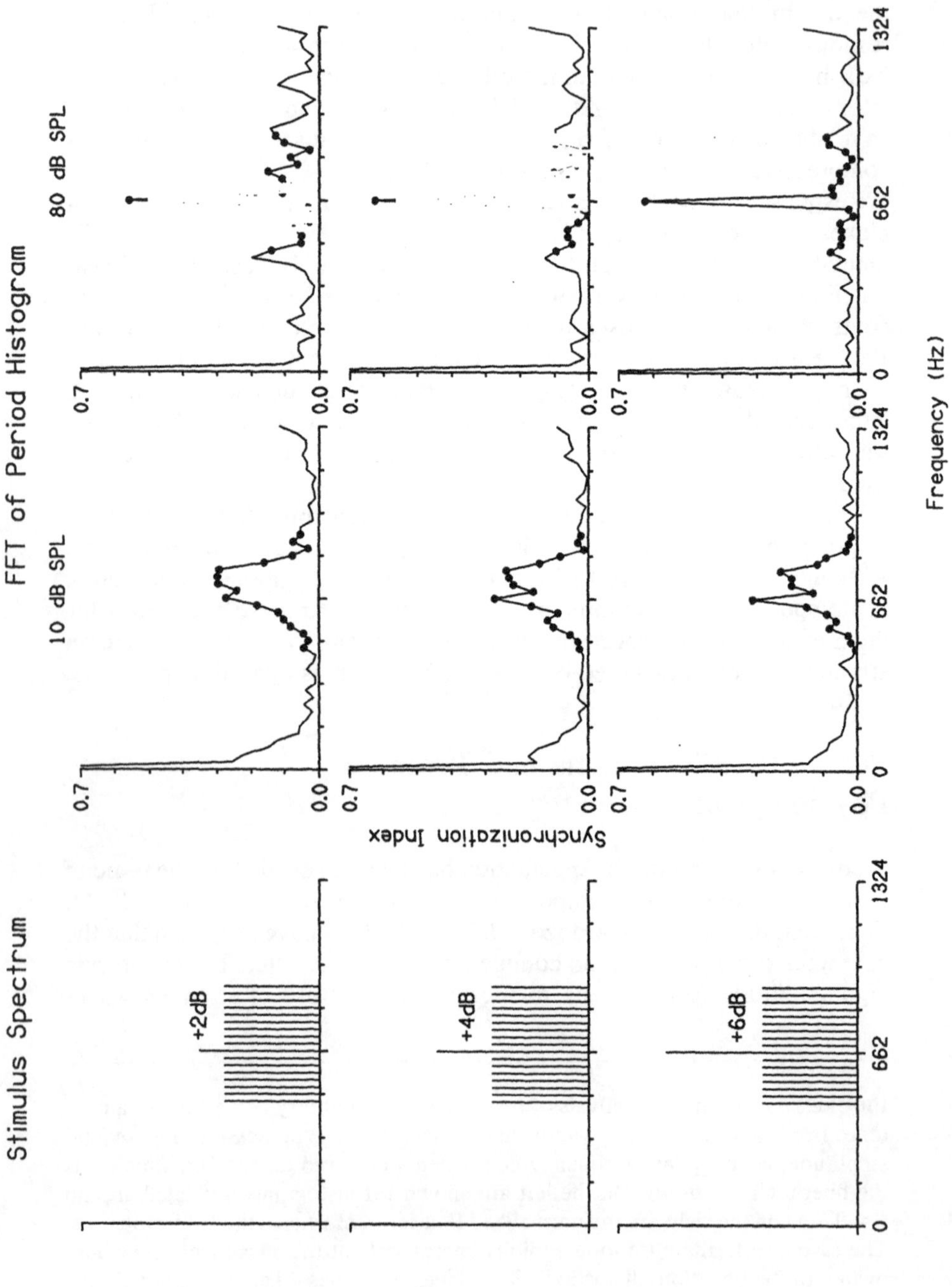
Stimulus Spectrum
FFT of Period Histogram
10 dB SPL
80 dB SPL
+2dB
+4dB
+6dB
Synchronization Index
0.7
0.0
0
662
1324
Frequency (Hz)

forms. In another vein, Siebert (1970), Luce and Green (1974), and Goldstein and Srulovicz (1977) employed mathematical approaches to predict the degree to which neural synchronization can account for perceptual frequency discrimination. All concluded that the frequency information provided by optimal processing of phase-locked responses more than accounts for human perceptual performance.

Young and Sachs (1979), Delgutte and Kiang (1984), and others have analyzed the temporal structure of responses to synthesized speech sounds. They found that temporal coding of vowel formant frequency is robust (in the sense that it resists degradation by masking noise) and that synchronization-based meaures maintain representations of vowel formant frequencies in cochlear space better than rate-based measures at all but near-threshold intensities. Despite a wealth of knowledge about possible perceptual correlates of phase-locked neural activity, the degree to which the brain actually uses that information is still unclear.

Pitch of Complex Tones

Harmonic complexes possess a dominant low pitch when the signal comprises frequencies below 5 kHz and frequency spacings below 1 kHz (Ritsman, 1962). Even though the signal contains only higher frequencies, the dominant pitch resembles that of a low-frequency tone. Schouten (1940) demonstrated that this pitch, of which a telephone dial tone is but one example, cannot arise as a result of distortion in the middle or inner ears. De Boer (1956) extended Schouten's findings and proposed that the perceived pitch is extracted by monitoring temporal aspects of the complex waveform, in particular the high-amplitude fine-structure peaks. This approach is known as the temporal fine structure (TFS) theory, and the way it operates is illustrated in Figure 17.9. Pitch is determined by examining time intervals present in the waveform fine structure and weighting each of the intervals by its prominence in the waveform. Thus, the time interval denoted by T_1 in Figure 17.9 receives greatest weight, T_2 receives less weight, and so on. The dominant pitch is simply the interval with the greatest overall weight.

In physiological terms, the TFS theory assumes that neuronal discharge probability is proportional to instantaneous waveform amplitude; hence,

FIGURE 17.8. Normalized Fourier transforms of period histograms obtained from a cat auditory nerve fiber in response to octave-band harmonic complexes consisting of 16 equally spaced, cosine-phase components centered at fiber CF (662 Hz). The center frequency was 2 (*top*), 4 (*middle*), or 6 (*bottom*) dB more intense than the other components. Waveform spectra are shown at the left. In the center are Fourier transforms obtained at a low (10 dB SPL) intensity, and at the right are Fourier transforms obtained at a high (80 dB SPL) intensity. The response is linear at low intensities but is highly nonlinear at high intensities.

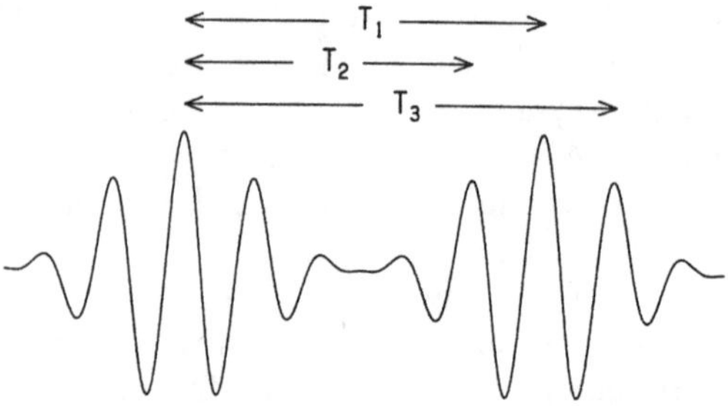

FIGURE 17.9. Basic operation of the temporal fine structure theory for determining pitch of complex tones. The theory presumes that the number of ISIs arising from spike initiation during high-amplitude waveform peaks (T_1) exceeds the number arising during lower-amplitude peaks (T_2 and T_3), and that pitch and timbre are assigned on the basis of temporal information provided by the ISIs.

the time interval between adjacent high-amplitude waveform peaks becomes the dominant ISI in the neural response. As the fine structure of the waveform changes, so do the probabilities of occurence of the intervals, and this can change the pitch of the signal. An important aspect of TFS theory is that even though neurons excited by the complex tone might normally respond to frequencies much higher than any contained in the signal, the temporal code transmitted by active neurons resembles that elicited by a sound of considerably lower frequency.

Alternatives to the TFS theory of pitch extraction also exist. Most prominent of these are the pattern recognition theories proposed by Licklider (1951), Wightman (1973), Goldstein (1973), Tarhardt, Stoll, and Seewann (1982), and Patterson (1987). These were developed in part to reconcile Mathes and Miller's (1947) observation that the pitch of complex tones is relatively insensitive to variations in component starting phase, and to account for the pitch of inharmonic complexes. The theories assume that the CNS performs an internal analysis, such as autocorrelation or harmonic pattern matching, on central excitation patterns estabished by components of a complex tone. Pitch estimates are arrived at by determining times of coincidence of temporal peaks in the excitation patterns or by fitting spectra to the internal representation of the signal.

Schouten, Ritsma and Cardozo (1962) investigated the low pitch of amplitude-modulated (AM) tones. AM tones are defined as a carrier frequency F_c varied in amplitude by a modulating frequency F_m. When F_c and F_m are pure tones, the complex possesses energy at three frequencies, namely F_c-F_m,F_c, and F_c+F_m. Javel (1980) and others have shown that ISIs arising in response to AM tones occur at times predicted by the TFS theory, and at low to moderate intensities the ISIs occur in approximately the correct proportions.

Figure 17.10 consists of ISI histograms obtained as the carrier frequency F_c of an AM tone was increased stepwise from a harmonic situation (i.e., F_c/F_m as an integer, 4 in this case) to various inharmonics situations (i.e., F_c/F_m is not an integer). The modulating frequency F_m was held constant. Subjective pitch shifts upward in these conditions, and the amount of pitch shift is a nearly linear function of F_c/F_m (de Boer, 1956). The arrows in Figure 17.10 indicate multiples of the period of the pitch frequency. These data show that neural ISIs cluster at the correct values predicted by TFS theory, and as carrier frequency changes, the ISIs change as the theory predicts. Thus, the correct input for a TFS analysis of pitch is present at the level of the auditory nerve.

TFS theory presents a parsimonious way of explaining perceptual findings. It can account for some of the changes and ambiguities in pitch when signal components are inharmonically related and when they undergo phase shifts. Although pattern recognition models in many cases achieve similar results, they require the existence of CNS mechanisms that have yet to be demonstrated physiologically. The strong correspondences between neural synchronization and the perceived pitch of complex tones suggest that the two are linked. Since vowel sounds are also complex tones of the same type discussed here, one would also expect, by inference, that temporal-frequency coding is important in speech processing as well.

Frequency Discrimination

An issue of long-standing interest among auditory theorists concerns the ability to discriminate small changes in frequency. Data related to this phenomenon are shown in the top panel of Figure 17.11. These were reported by Wier, Jesteadt, and Green (1977) for human listeners and by Elliott, Stein, and Harrison (1960) for cats. The index shown here is the Weber fractions, defined as the just-noticeable frequency difference (jnd) divided by the frequency in question. Both sets of data indicate that relative performance varies with frequency, being best at 1–2 kHz and poorer at lower and higher frequencies. Studies involving human subjects have shown that frequency discrimination performance improves with increasing intensity (Wier, Jesteadt, and Green, 1977) and duration (Moore, 1973). Dye and Hafter (1980) demonstrated qualitative differences in frequency-discrimination performance in the presence of masking noise. They showed that at constant signal-to-masker levels performance improves with masker level at low frequencies but declines with masker level at high frequencies. The principal issues in determining the physiological basis of frequency discrimination are how to account for the shape of the frequency-performance curve, how to account for the absolute size of the jnd, and how to account for the frequency-dependent behavior of performance in the presence of masking noise.

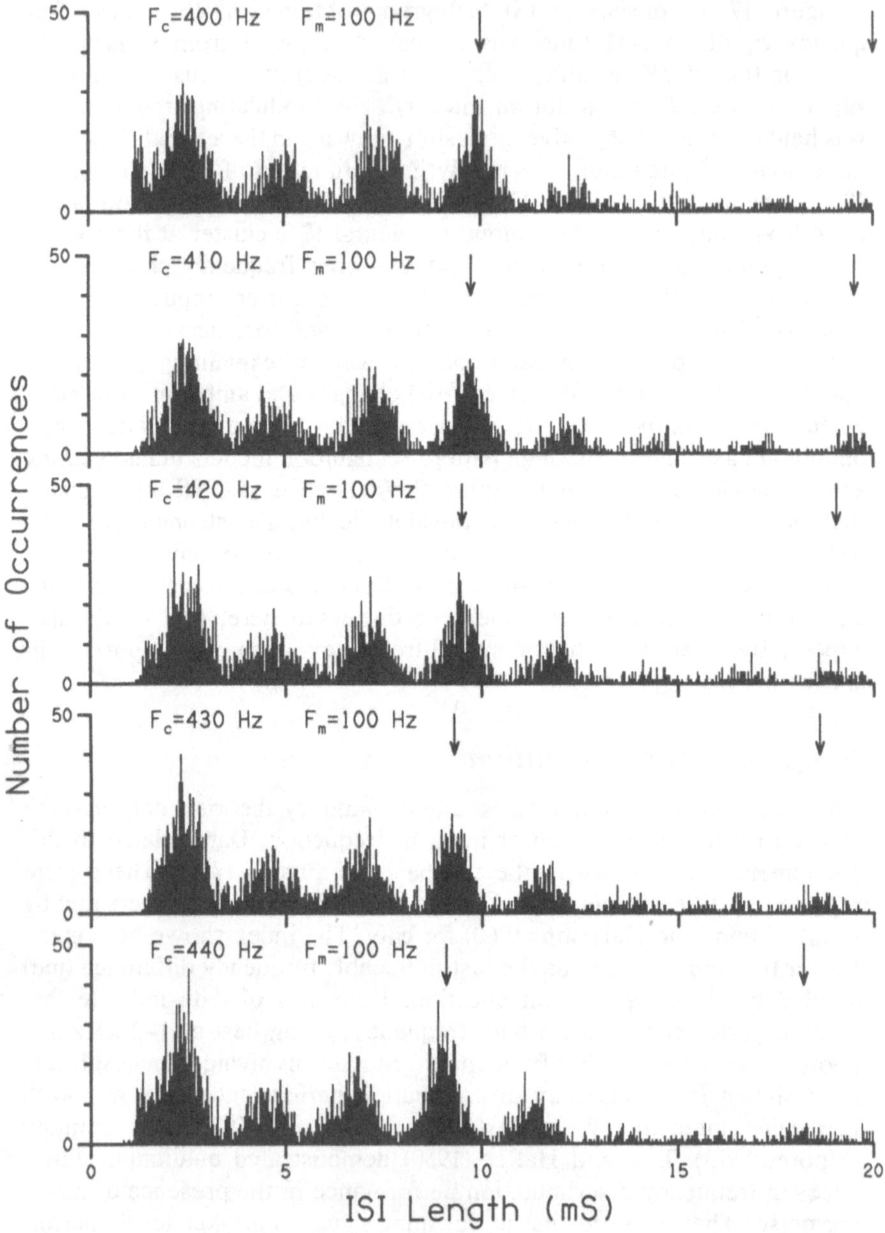

FIGURE 17.10. ISI histograms obtained from a cat auditory nerve fiber in response to AM tones of variable carrier frequency. Carrier frequency F_c was varied from 400 to 440 Hz, modulation frequency F_m was fixed at 100 Hz, and modulation depth was fixed at 100%. Arrows indicate times corresponding to integer multiples of the period of the dominant perceived pitch.

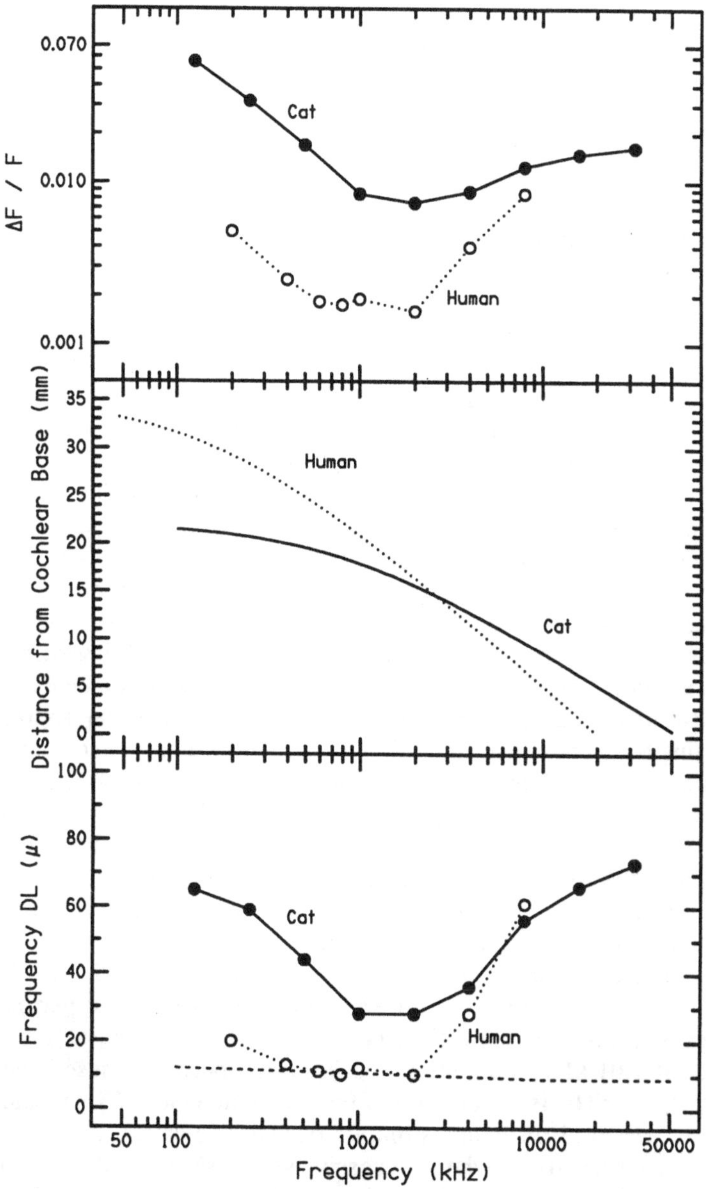

FIGURE 17.11. *Top:* Performance of humans (filled symbols connected by solid lines) and cats (open symbols connected by dotted lines) on a pure-tone frequency-discrimination task. Findings from human listeners considered signals of 0.5-s duration presented at a 40-dB sensation level, and findings from cats considered signals of 0.4-s duration presented at a 40-dB sensation level. *Middle:* Frequency-place maps for cat and human cocleas. *Bottom:* Frequency-discrimination performance at threshold ($d' = 1$), expressed as a spatial shift in the cochlear excitation pattern. The dashed line represents the width of a single cat inner hair cell at the specified cochlear site.

The most commonly employed explanation for frequency-discrimination performance involves determining the minimally detectable shift in the cochlear spatial excitation pattern. The amount of spatial shift of the traveling wave peak at the jnd can be calculated by taking the cochlear frequency-to-place map into account. Lieberman (1982) combined electrophysiological recordings with intracellular marking techniques to develop such a map for the cat, and Greenwood (1961) fit curves to available frequency-place data to arrive at maps for several species, humans among them. Lieberman's cat map and Greenwood's human map are shown in the middle panel of Figure 17.11. The maps allow us to convert Wier's (human) jnds and Elliott's (cat) jnds to coordinates in cochlear space and plot them as a function of frequency. This has been done in the lower panel of Figure 17.11. The dashed line was adapted from data published by Lieberman and Oliver (1984) and has been included for reference purposes. It represents the width of an inner hair cell at cochlear sites corresponding to the indicated frequency. The interesting points here are that (1) for frequencies below 2 kHz the amount of shift of the traveling wave at the jnd is approximately equal to (for human listeners) or greater than (for cats) the width of single inner hair cell, (2) plotting human jnd's as a spatial shift produces a graph with little relative decrease in performance at low frequencies, and (3) performance is substantially poorer at high frequencies than at low frequencies.

Goldstein and Srulovicz (1977) developed a theoretical approach to predicting frequency-discrimination performance that is based entirely on temporally encoded frequency information. In this the listener assigns frequency based on ISIs and bases perceptual decisions about frequencies below 3–4 kHz on that information. Above 4 kHz, of course, temporal determinations of acoustic frequency fail because neural discharge synchronization is lost. In that case the ear must base frequency judgements solely on spatial excitation patterns.

An important feature of the Goldstein-Srulovicz model is that the longer the ISI the listener is allowed to use, the better the performance that results. To appreciate this, consider two tones, one at 1 kHz and another at 1.01 kHz. The difference in period between these is approximately 10 μs. THis is the amount of time by which mean ISIs would differ if spikes occurred on every stimulus period. However, if the observer monitors ISIs occurring when successive spikes skip one stimulus period, then performance should improve by a factor of 2 because the difference in signal period accumulates over the two intervening periods, 20 μs in this example. Likewise, performance continues to improve as ISI order increases, i.e., 30 μs for the third-order ISIs, 40 μs for fourth-order ISIs, and so on. Obviously, the longer the ISI used in the analysis, the easier the discrimination task becomes. This approach is described in more detail in Javel and Mott (1988).

Javel et al. (1988) used standard psychophysical two-alternative forced-choice (2AFC) paradigms to investigate the ability of single auditory nerve fibers to discriminate acoustic frequencies when only temporally encoded frequency information entered the decision process. In their task a tone was presented and the times of occurrence of discharges were digitized. Then another tone of slightly higher frequency was presented and the discharge times digitized once again. Assuming that the frequency of the standard was known, the differences between the obtained and expected ISIs were summed, taking into account the number of intervening stimulus cycles in each ISI. Finally, the mean frequency was computed as the reciprocal of the average response period, and the signal interval possessing the higher mean was selected as the response to the 2AFC trial. On the basis of that answer, which was either correct or incorrect, the frequency separation was either increased, decreased, or unchanged according to standard up-down decision rules (Levitt, 1971). Fibers tracked preselected performance levels, typically 70.7% correct (a value commonly taken as threshold performance). In conformance with standard psychophysical procedures, the minimally discriminable frequency separation was computed as the average of the reversal points on the adaptive track.

Data on frequency separations producing 70.7% correct performance on the 2AFC task are shown in Figure 17.12. The filled circles represent frequency difference limens obtained from single auditory nerve fibers at the stated frequency, the solid line represents a moving window average of the neural data, and the dotted line represents the best perfomance of Elliott's, Stein, and Harrison's (1960) cats. There is a close correspondence between the two lines for frequencies below 1 kHz. Above 1 kHz neural performance declines rapidly, and difference limens are unobtainable above 2 kHz. As stated earlier, neural synchronization of cat auditory nerve fibers to pure tones also declines above 1 kHz (Figure 17.1), so a decrease in performance is not at all surprising. What is surprising is the rapidity at which performance declines; i.e., the decline occurs at frequencies well below those predicted by the Goldstein-Srulovicz model. Thus, although temporal coding accounts relatively well for freqency discrimination performance below 1 kHz, it fails at higher frequencies.

An important and troublesome aspect of temporal processing of ISIs, not shown here, is that temporal sampling predicts frequency discrimination performance to be a steeply rising function of frequency separation. That is, as the two frequencies to be discriminated move apart, decisions based on temporal sampling of ISIs rapidly achieve perfect performance. Costalupes (1988) obtained psychometric functions for frequency discrimination of a 1 kHz tone in cats. Like the human data, performance improves rather slowly (about 0.75 percent correct per hertz). The neural

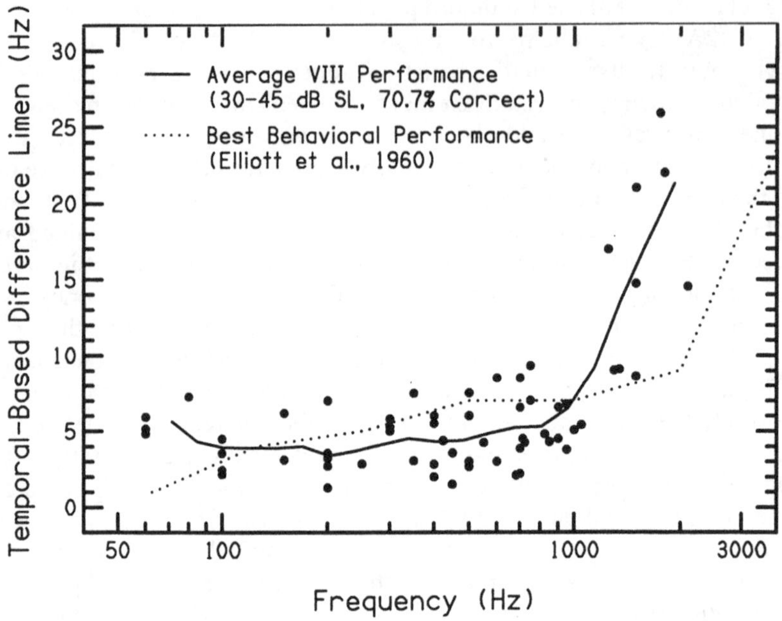

FIGURE 17.12. Pure-tone frequency discrimation performance of single auditory nerve fibers in cats. Data were obtained at 20 to 40-dB sensation level using an adaptive two-interval forced-choice procedure. The solid line represents a third-octave-width moving-window average of the neural data. The dotted line indicates the best behavioral performance obtained by Elliot, Stein, and Harrison (1960).

data, on the other hand, improve at a rate of 10–30 percent correct per hertz. Thus, although temporal frequency coding produces difference limens of reasonable magnitude at frequencies below 1 kHz, other aspects of temporal coding at the level of the auditory nerve are simply not consistent with behavioral findings.

Merging the data on pitch of complex tones and frequency discrimination, it appears that the upper-frequency limit for temporal coding is not at the 3–4 kHz upper limit for discharge synchronization in the auditory nerve. Rather, the upper limit for use by the perceptual processor appears to be under 1 kHz. This conclusion is consistent with findings in frequency discrimination experiments on listeners with cochlear implants (Shannon, 1983), who cannot easily discriminate pitch changes above 0.5–0.7 kHz. It is also consistent with observations that the upper limit for the pitch of complex tones (Ritsma, 1962) and the upper limit for the pitch of AM noise (Burns and Viemeister, 1976) are both under 1 kHz.

Temporal Encoding of Electrical Stimuli

Time Structure of the Response

An auditory nerve fiber's response to an electrical stimulus, be it sinusoidal or pulsatile, has basically the same form. The response, however, is considerably different from what is observed acoustically. Some of the differences are shown in Figure 17.13. At the top is a period histogram obtained from an auditory nerve fiber that was stimulated acoustically by a 200 Hz sinusoid. As shown earlier, the response is

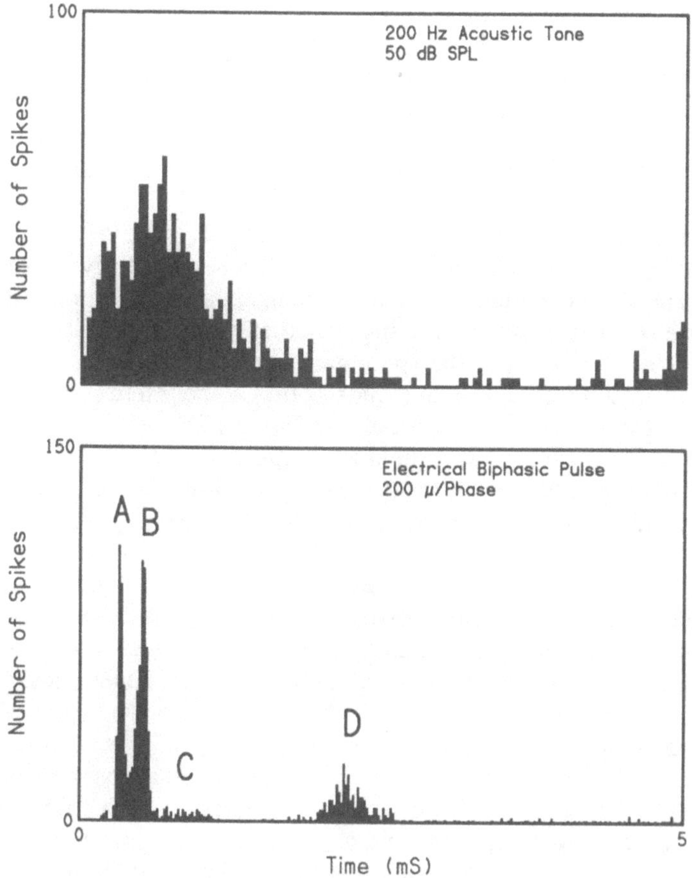

FIGURE 17.13. *Top:* Period histogram obtained by acoustically stimulating an auditory nerve fiber with a 200-Hz sinusoid. *Bottom:* Composite period histogram obtained by electrically stimulating a different fiber with a biphasic pulse train presented at a 200-Hz rate. Letters indicate times at which spikes tend to cluster.

half-wave-rectified and resembles a half cycle of the signal. In contrast, the response to an electrical stimulus, in this case a biphasic pulse, exhibits much tighter synchronization, and discharges arise at four discrete latencies. These are denoted by **A, B, C,** and **D.** The latencies, of course, reflect the time needed for the action potential to be initiated by the electrical stimulus and propagate to the more centrally located recording microelectrode.

The **D** response occurs at latencies >1.5 ms and is indistinguishable from that generated by an acoustic click. It possesses a relatively low threshold and wide dynamic range, and it is absent when the stimulated ear exhibits no acoustic sensitivity. Moxon (1971) named this the δ response and surmised that it arises from stimulation of hair cells by a traveling wave established as a result of capacitive events near the stimulating electrode. That is, the electrical signal repels or attracts the (negatively charged) basilar membrane, generating a clicklike response that propagates along the basilar membrane and is analyzed in the usual manner by the cochlea. Since the **D** response is not a result of direct stimulation of spiral ganglion cells, its relevance to cochlear implants is minimal.

The **C** response occurs at 0.8–1.2 ms, is usually relatively weak, exists prinicpally at near-threshold intensities, and is not as firmly phase-locked as the earlier occurring responses. Although the precise origin of the **C** response is unclear, its latency suggests that it arises from the vicinity of the peripheral process of the spiral ganglion cell.

The **B** response is the one most often encountered in recordings obtained from undeafened animals. It has a latency of 0.5–1.0 ms, is usually observed at near-threshold intensities, possesses a dynamic range of 1–9 dB (depending on stimulus parameters, primarily stimulation rate), and is highly synchronized to the stimulus. The overlapping of **B** and **C** response latencies suggests the possibility that the **C** response is merely a less highly synchronized, near-threshold extension of the **B** response. The temporal characteristics and input-output behavior of the **B** response are consistent with the notion that it arises from spikes initiated at the peripheral processes of spiral ganglion cells (White, Finely, and Wilson, 1987).

The **A** response possesses a latency of 0.3–0.5 ms. Using bipolar electrode pairs in undeafened animals, this response is observed predominantly at high intensities. In deafened animals it is by far the most commonly observed response and is the response observed near threshold. The **A** response is the most highly synchronized response and, at <2 dB, possesses the narrowest dynamic range. As will be shown below, the **A** response commonly appears in undeafened animals after a **B**-latency response has already been established. In this the **A** response supplants the **B** response without changing the slope of the rate-intensity function. The latency, dynamic range, and temporal dispersion of the **A** response are all consistent with its arising from the central process of the spiral ganglion cell.

The **A, B,** and **C** responses together form the α response described by Moxon (1971).

Input–Output Relationships

Figure 17.13 shows that individual components of an auditory nerve fiber's response to electrical stimulation are highly phase-locked. For pulsatile stimuli high degrees of synchronization are evident even at near-threshold intensities. Examples of period histograms obtained at several intensities from the same fiber are shown in Figure 17.14. The stimulus was a biphasic pulse train, with each phase of the pulse being 50 μs in duration. The signal was presented at a rate of 200 pulses/s in 100 ms bursts, and the pulse waveform was initially positive at the more apical stimulating electrode. Intensities indicated in the figure are in decibels re 1 μA. Thus, 40 dB implies a peak pulse amplitude of 0.1 mA, 60 dB implies 1 mA, and so on.

The period histograms in Figure 17.14 principally show a **B**-latency response at all intensities, although a few **C**-latency spikes can be seen at the lower intensities. Even at the lowest intensity, namely 46.6 dB, the few driven spikes occurred within the 0.5–1.0-ms **B**-latency window. Spikes occurring outside that window represent spontaneous activity, or discharges occurring in the absence of a stimulus. As intensity was increased, the response became stronger, the latency decreased slightly, the spikes were somewhat more tightly distributed, and the spike distribution became skewed to the right.

Input-output functions for these data are shown in Figure 17.15. The solid symbols depict the discharge rate as a function of intensity, and the open symbols depict the synchronization index. The synchronization index approaches 1.0 at all intensities. This extraordinarily high degree of phase locking is particular to the use of pulsatile electrical stimuli. Hartmann, Topp, and Klinke (1984) used sinusoidal stimuli and obtained lower values for the synchronization index at near-threshold intensities. They also documented the existence of a small dynamic range for synchronization growth. At suprathreshold intensities, values for the synchronization index in response to electrical sinusoids is roughly the same as for pulses. In both cases, however, synchronization is considerably higher than to acoustic tones at the same frequency, and it possess a much narrower dynamic range.

The rate-intensity function shown in Figure 17.15 exhibits an extraordinarily linear rate of growth. The maximum or saturation discharge rate is about 200 spikes/s, which coincides with the stimulus pulse rate. In general the saturation rate observed for electrical stimulation is the same

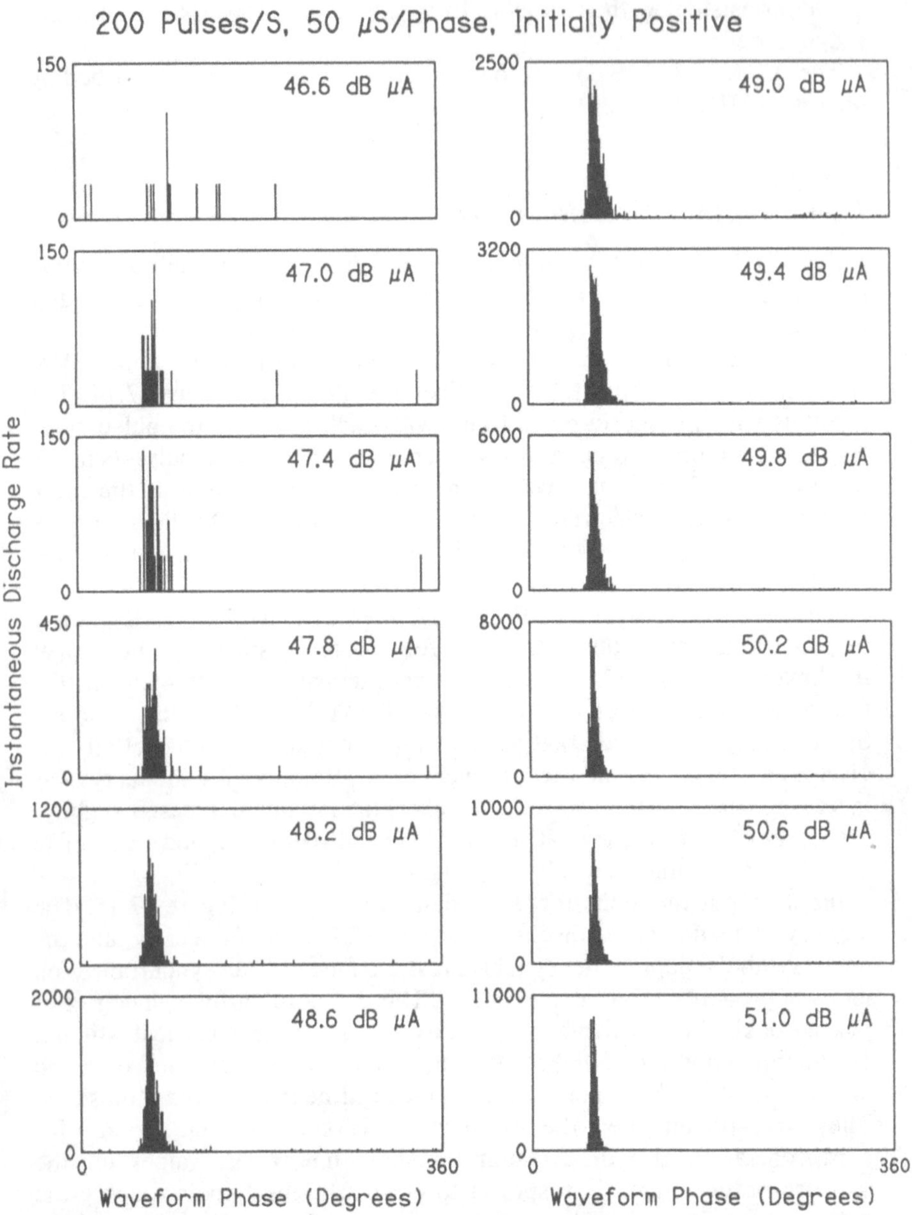

FIGURE 17.14. Period histograms obtained at several intensities from an auditory nerve fiber stimulated by a 200 Hz biphasic pulse train. Pulse width was 50 μs/phase. The response becomes greater and more highly synchronized as intensity increases.

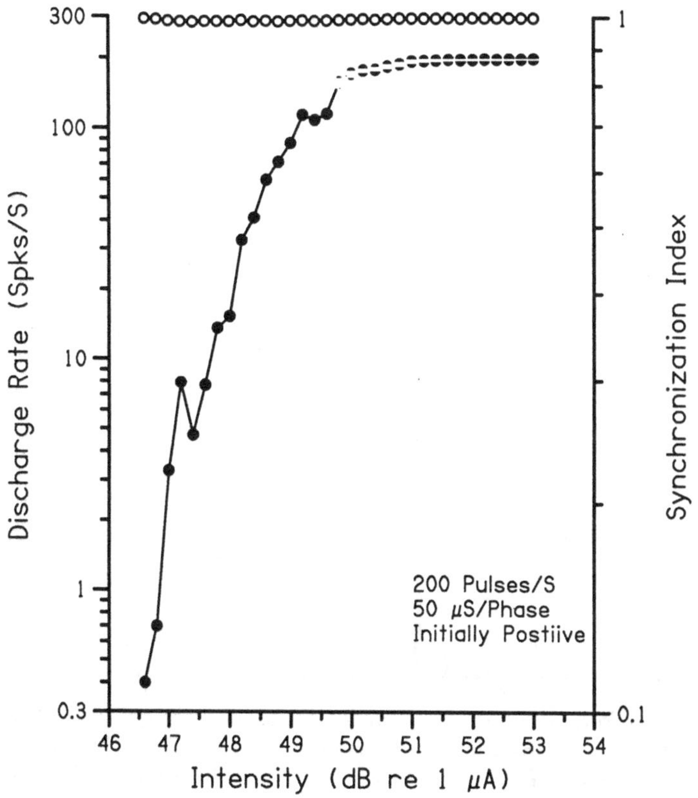

FIGURE 17.15. Rate-intensity (filled symbols) and synchronization-intensity (open symbols) functions for the data shown in Figure 17.14. Synchronization is maximal at all intensities, whereas discharge rate grows linearly over a 2 dB dynamic range and saturates at the pulse frequency.

as the stimulation rate, even for rates as high as 1000 pulses/s. Thus, maximum discharge rates obtained in response to electrical stimuli can be as much as 8 times higher than those observed acoustically.

The dynamic range of the response, or the intensity range over which discharge rate increased from 10% to 90% of the maximum, is about 2 dB in the case shown. This is a typical value for pulse rates of 200 pulses/s. As will be shown later, dynamic range is a direct function of stimulus pulse rate.

Period histograms obtained from a fiber whose response exhibited **A**-latency spikes as well as **B**-latency spikes are shown in Figure 17.16. This particular fiber possessed a relatively high threshold to electrical stimulation, suggesting that it was not located close to the stimulating electrodes. At intensities that were just suprathreshold (e.g., 63.8 dB) the

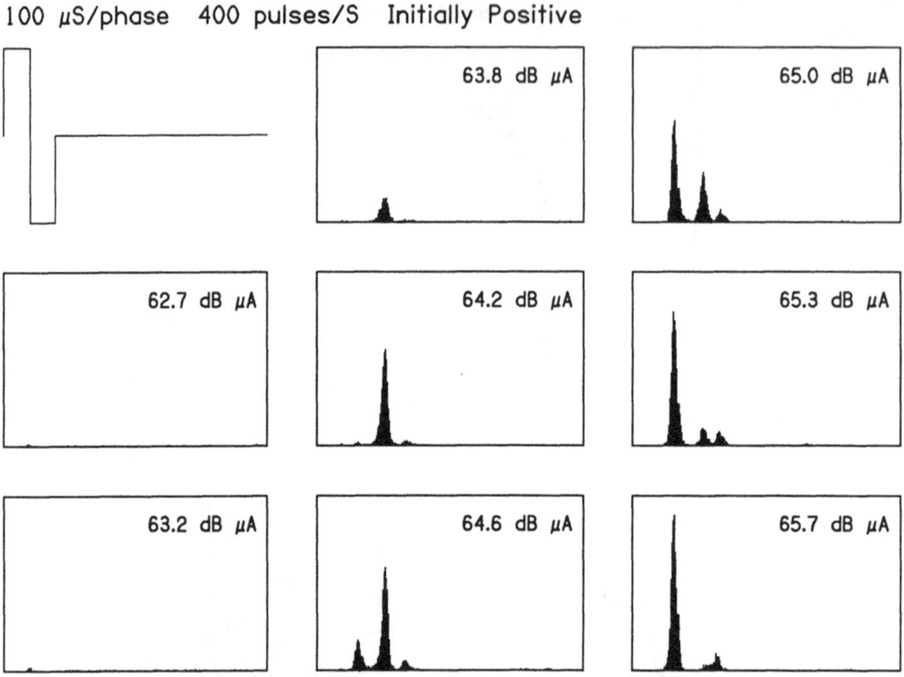

FIGURE 17.16. Period histograms obtained from an auditory nerve fiber whose response underwent a **B-A** latency transition. Near threshold the response is of the **B**-latency variety. Beginning at 64.2 dB μA the **B** response is supplanted by the **A** response.

response was in the **B**-latency range. This response became stronger at 64.2 dB, and a few **C**-latency spikes appeared. At 64.6 dB a shorter, **A**-latency response arose. The **A** response grew rapidly at higher intensities while the **B** response declined. The **C** response stayed relatively constant, however.

Input-output relationships for discharge rate, latency, and standard deviation of the reponse distribution are shown in Figure 17.17. These data were obtained from a fiber different from the one that provided the date in Figure 17.16, but the response was similar in that it underwent a **B-A** latency transition. Cosidering the rate-intensity function (upper panel) first, the **B** response (filled circles) was the one observed from threshold. With the inclusion of spontaneously occurring spikes, the **B** response dictated the shape of the overall rate-intensity function at intensities <58 dB. Just below 58 dB an **A** response appeared. This grew rapidly at higher intensities, at the expense of the **B** response. The rate of growth of the **A** response was considerably greather than that of the **B** response. At the highest intensity studied the **A** response replaced the **B**

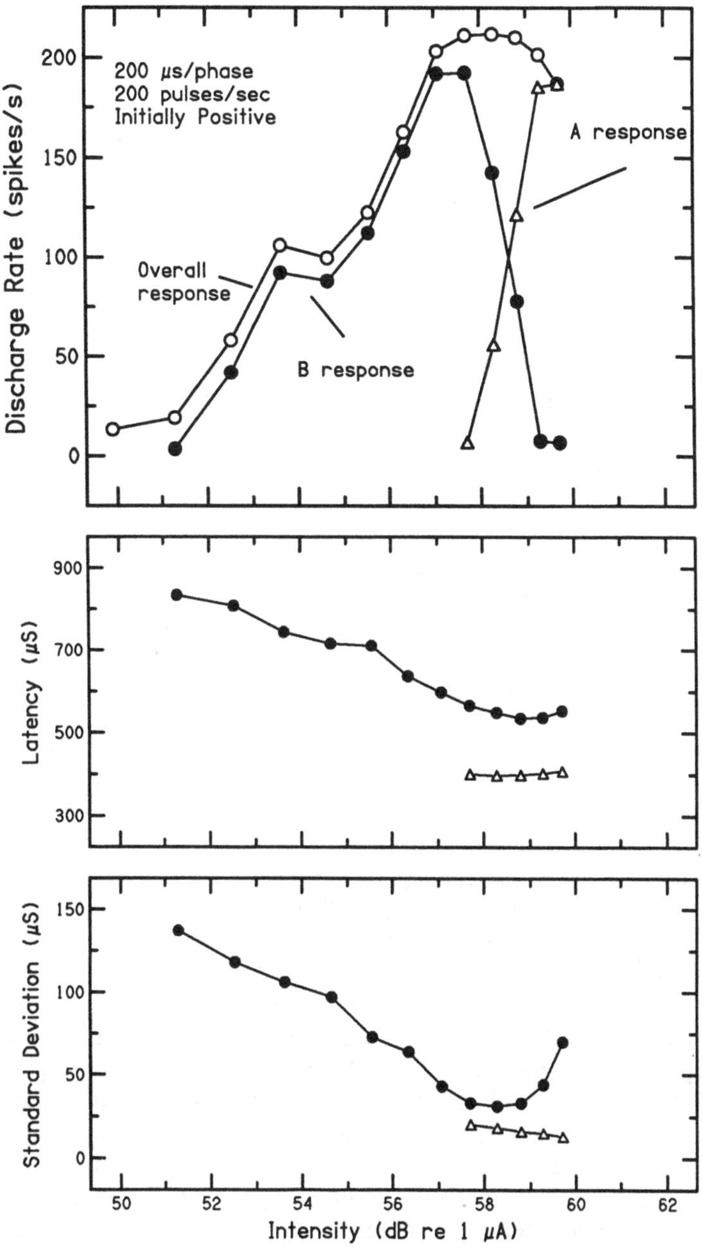

FIGURE 17.17. Rate versus intensity (*top*), latency versus intensity (*middle*), and standard deviation versus intensity functions obtained from a fiber whose response underwent a **B-A** latency transition. **A**-latency responses are indicated by triangles, **B**-latency responses are indicated by filled circles, and the overall response is indicated by open circles.

response almost completely. The overall rate-intensity function did not change slope when the **B-A** trasition occurred.

Latency-intensity functions for the **A** and **B** responses are shown in the middle panel of Figure 17.17. The **B** response underwent a 315 μs cumulative latency shift in 6 dB. Although latency shifts of this magnitude suggest that the site of action potential initiation moved centrally as intensity increased, examination of period histograms of the type shown in Figure 17.14 indicated that most of the latency shift was due to a tightening of the distribution of spike occurrences. The **A** response underwent only a minimal latency shift with increasing intensity. For electrical sinusoids the cumulative latency shift can be much greater than for biphasic pulses (Hartmann, Topp, and Klinke, 1984).

Date on the dispersion of sychronized **A**- and **B**-latency spikes are shown in the lower panel of Figure 17.17. The standard deviation of **B**-latency spikes changed considerably as intensity varied through the dynamic range, but the standard deviation of **A**-latency spikes did not.

*Time Course of **A** and **B** Responses*

Some insight into the time course of **A**- and **B**-latency responses is provided by the data shown in Figure 17.18. The figure presents dot rasters of **A** and **B** responses obtained at several intensities from an auditory nerve fiber stimulated with biphasic, initially positive pulse trains presented at a rate of 400 pulses/s in 100 ms bursts. Each dot in the display represents a spike, and individual spikes were categorized as **A** or **B** on the basis of latency following pulse onset. Spikes from the first of 50 bursts are presented as the uppermost row of dots at each intensity, with data from successive burst presented in subsequent rows.

The response shown in Figure 17.18 underwent a **B-A** transition. At near-threshold intensities (not shown) all the spikes were of the **B**- latency variety. **A**-latency spikes arose at 63.2 dB and supplanted the **B**-latency spikes at higher intensities. The interesting feature of Figure 17.18 is the location of **A**- and **B**-latency spikes at times following burst onset. When the response exhibited both **A**- and **B**-latency spikes, for example at 65.0 and 65.3 dB, the **A** spikes tended to cluster at the beginnings of trials, whereas the **B**- latency spikes tended to occur later. The amount of time the fiber spent generating only **A**-latency spikes depended on intensity, with higher intensities causing the neuron to emit **A**-latency spikes for successively longer periods of time. If the hypothesis that spike latencies reflect the distance from the initiation site to the recording microelectrode is correct, then these data suggest that the initiation site moved from the central process to the peripheral process as stimulation continued. Whether this is actually the case cannot be determined from these data, although it is conceivable that spike initiation at different points along the spiral ganglion cell, for example the peripheral and central processes, can

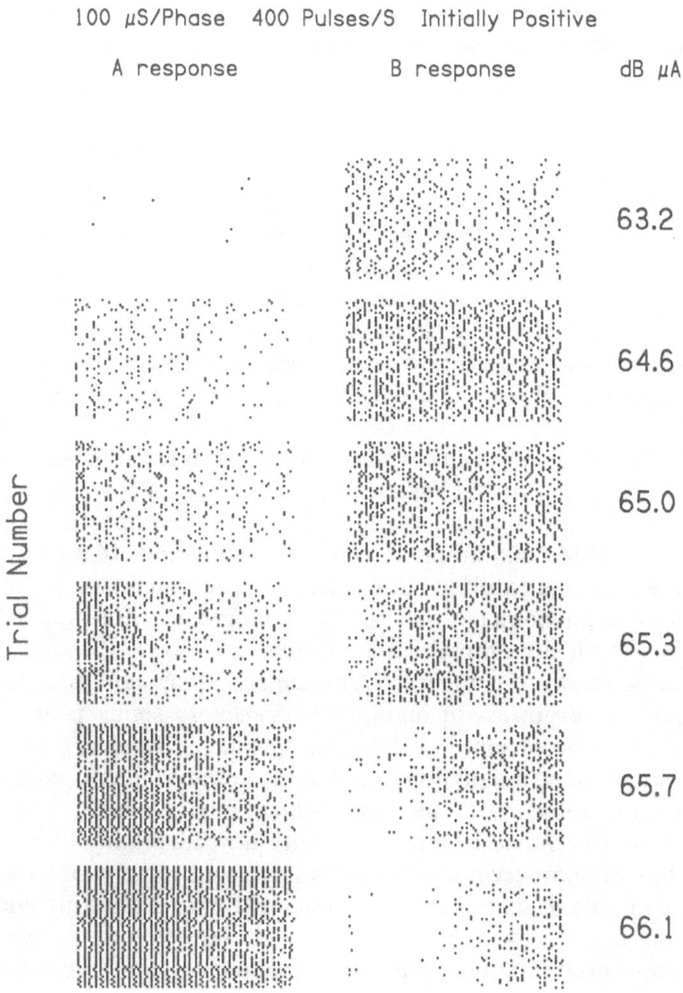

FIGURE 17.18. Dot rasters for **A**- and **B**-latency responses, obtained from an auditory nerve fiber whose response underwent a **B-A** latency transition. **A** responses tend to cluster at the beginning of the trial, and **B** responses tend to cluster at the end. The amount of time spent eliciting **A**- and **B**- latency spikes depends on intensity.

undergo different rates of polarization over time, thereby producing the effect.

In a similar vein, van den Honert and Stypulkowski (1987) showed data indicating that **B-A** latency transitions only occur when biphasic pulses are used as stimuli, and that **A** and **B** responses arise because both stimulus phases become capable of exciting the neuron. Although **B-A** latency transitions are unlikely to be important for perception, they are undoubtedly relevant to theories of electrical stimulation and to analyses of intracochlear current spread. The phenomenon clearly deserves more study.

Poststimulus-Time Histograms and Adaptation

Most electrically stimulated auditory nerve fibers exhibit time-dependent response decrements that are reminiscent of adaptation. Representative data on this are shown in Figure 17.19, which consists of a series of poststimulus-time (PST) histograms obtained at several intensities from a fiber excited by biphasic pulse trains presented at a rate of 200 pulses/s. The horizontal bar in each histogram represents the time when the pulse train was present. When the discharge rate is still growing with intensity, that is, when the rate lies within the fiber's dynamic range, the response is greatest at the beginning of the train, settling into a steady-state discharge rate after 30–40 ms. At the highest intensity, when each stimulus pulse is capable of eliciting a spike, the PST histogram assumes a rectangular shape that has no counterpart in acoustic stimulation. Many but not all fibers in our sample exhibited this behavior. The remainder displayed no adaptationlike phenomena; that is, PST histograms were predominantly rectangular at all suprathreshold intensities.

The data shown in Figure 17.19 suggest that not all adaptation observable in responses of auditory nerve fibers stems from the hair cell/auditory nerve synapse, as is usually assumed (Smith and Brachman, 1982). Rather, some adaptation arises in the spiral ganglion cell itself. An observation of some importance for cochlear implants is that only over a relatively narrow range of intensities does any adaptation like behavior exist. Thus, if short-term adaptation is important in perceptual processing, for example in determining amounts of forward masking and voice onset times and in enhancing the neural representation of plosive consonants, appropriate inputs must be supplied by the implant speech processor because the cochlea and auditory nerve will not supply adaptation at all intensities.

Distributions of Interspike Intervals

Given the observation that an auditory nerve fiber's response to pulsatile and most sinusoidal stimuli is very highly phase-locked, one would expect the distributions of time intervals between successive discharges to be equally sharply defined. That this is indeed the case is demonstrated by Figure 17.20, which depicts ISI histograms obtained from an auditory nerve fiber excited by biphasic pulse trains presented at 200 pulses/s (left column) and from a different fiber excited acoustically by a 200 Hz sinusoid (right column). Considering the acoustic results first, the existence of discharge synchronization appears as a tendency of the ISIs to

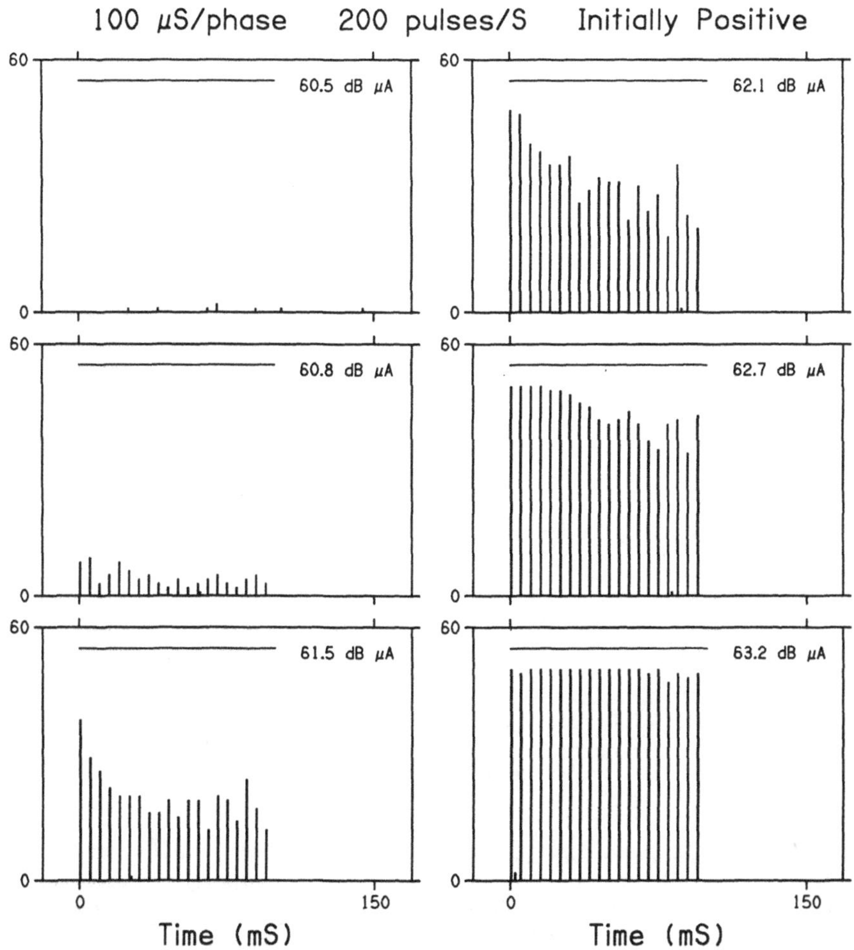

FIGURE 17.19. PST histograms obtained in response to electrical stimulation with biphasic pulse trains of 100 ms duration presented at 200 pulses/s. Horizontal lines indicate times when the pulse train was present. The response exhibits a form of adaptation when the response is submaximal. At high intensities the adaptation disappears.

cluster at integral multiples of the stimulus period. Moreover, the relative numbers of the first- and higher-order intervals (i.e., discharges occurring on successive stimulus cycles versus discharges skipping cycles) follow a characteristic exponential decay as interval order increases. The rate of decay is a simple function of discharge rate. Third, the response never becomes entrained; that is, the stimulus is incapable of eliciting a spike on every cycle. Lastly, the dispersion of ISIs in any cluster is a direct function of stimulus period.

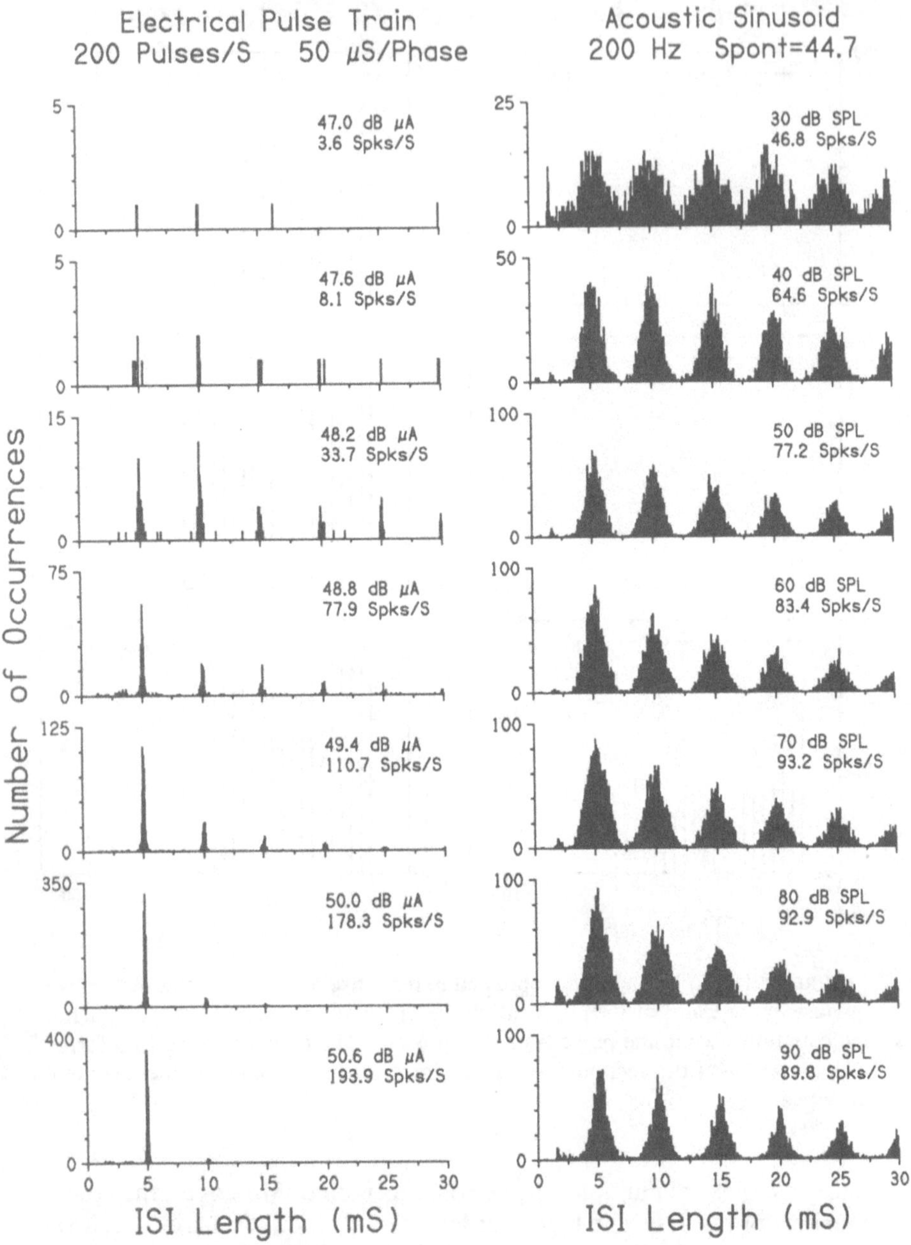

FIGURE 17.20. *Left:* ISI histograms obtained in response to biphasic electrical pulse trains presented at 200 pulses/s. The distribution of ISIs is an exponentially decaying function of ISI length when the response is submaximal. *Right:* ISI histograms obtained in response to acoustic tones at 200 Hz. Distribution of ISIs is an exponentially decaying function of ISI length at all intensities.

Consider now the response to electrical pulse trains, shown in the left column of Figure 17.20. The ISI histograms differ in several respects from their acoustic counterparts. First and most prominent, the dispersion of the peaks is considerably smaller. This is in accord with the much greater degree of synchronization of responses to waveform cycles, discussed earlier. Second, although there is some evidence of an exponential decay of ISI clusters, this exists only when the fiber responds at submaximal rates. At high intensities the response is entrained, and the exponential decay is lost entirely when a discharge occurs in response to every stimulus pulse. ISI histograms obtained in response to sinusoidal electrical stimuli behave in much the same manner (Hartmann, Topp, and Klinke, 1984).

Behavior of Input–Output Functions at Different Stimulation Rates

In Figure 17.21 are shown rate-intensity functions obtained from one fiber at several different electrical stimulus pulse rates. On the left are shown overall discharge rates plotted as a function of intensity, and on the right the same data have been replotted, now in terms of discharge probability (i.e., average number of spikes per stimulus pulse). The important features of this figure are that (1) maximum discharge rate is equal to stimulus pulse rate over a wide range of rates, (2) dynamic range is also a direct function of pulse rate, (3) slopes of rate-intensity functions are constant across pulse frequency, (4) thresholds are roughly equal across pulse rate, and (5) spike probability is an intensity- and frequency-dependent variable.

The findings that maximum discharge rates and dynamic ranges depend on stimulation rate, but thresholds and rates of response growth do not, have potentially important consequences for cochlear implant speech processing strategies. For example, the potential for driving neurons at rates well beyond those observed acoustically is clearly something to be avoided because the cell's inability to sustain high discharge rates can lead to tone decay. Issues such as this have not yet been addressed by contemporary implants.

Temporal-Response Anomalies

Figure 17.21 shows that an auditory nerve fiber responds at a constant discharge rate regardless of stimulus frequency. This statement holds as long as the driven rate is lower than or equal to stimulus frequency. Moreover, the constant rate is usually not distributed over an exponentially decreasing range of ISIs, as is the case acoustically (Figure 17.20).

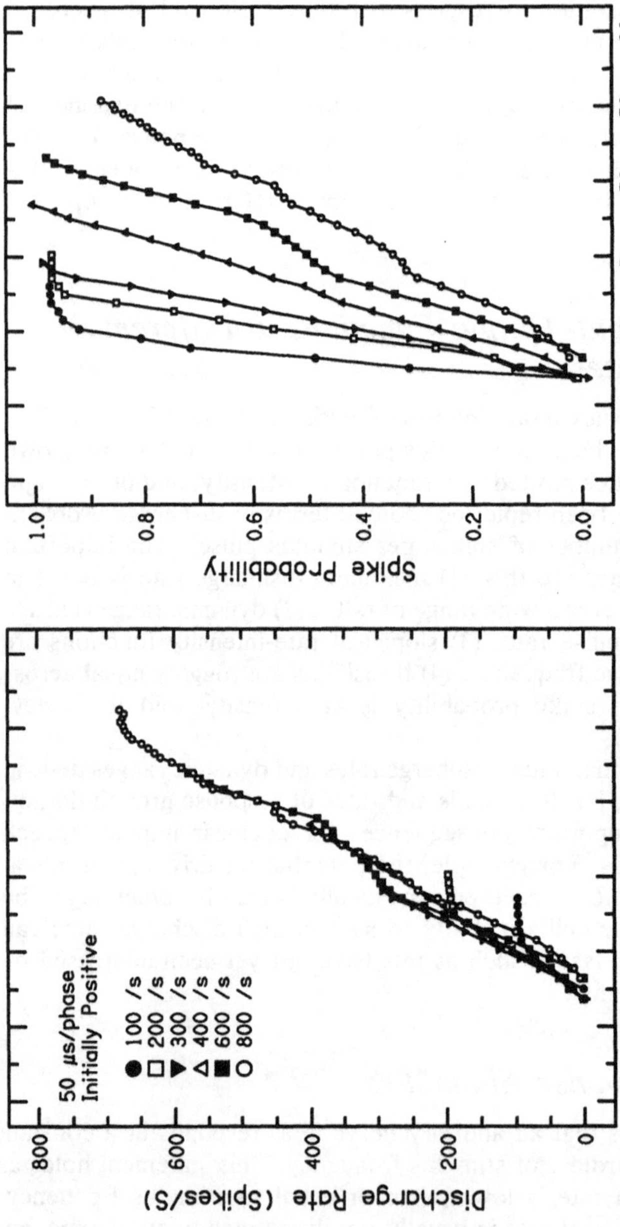

FIGURE 17.21. Input-output functions obtained from an auditory nerve fiber in response to biphasic electrical pulse trains presented at rates ranging from 100 to 800 pulses/s. *Left:* Discharge rate as a function of intensity. Dynamic range and maximum discharge rate are functions of pulse rate, and rate of growth is constant at all rates. *Right:* Same data, plotted as probability of a spike (spikes/pulse).

Rather, action potentials tend to occur regularly at times corresponding to the reciprocal of the discharge rate. Thus, at 50 spikes/s action potentials tend to occur every 20 ms, at 100 spikes/s they occur every 10 ms, and so on.

One consequence of the regularity of discharge occurrence is that spike probability can depend strongly on the temporal order of stimulus pulses. An example of this is shown in Figure 17.22, which is a PST histogram obtained in response to biphasic pulses presented at a rate of 800 pulses/s in 100 ms bursts. The overall discharge rate was 330 spikes/s. The first pulse in the train generated a high-probability (1.0) response, and the second pulse also generated a high-probability (0.82) spike. However, beginning with the third pulse and continuing for the next 40 ms, spike probability alternated between low and high, ultimately converging on a probability of approximately 0.4. Thus, the PST histogram resembles a "chopper"-type response reminiscent of those observable in cells of the ventral cochlear nucleus. The reason why the response chops is quite different, however. In the case shown the chopping occurs because the neuron discharges every 3.1 ms. At 800 pulses/s, this corresponds to one spike for every 2.5 pulses. When a spike occurs in response to a pulse, there will be a strong tendency for spikes not to occur again for another 2.5 pulses. It is for this reason that the PST histogram shows spikes alternating between high- and low-probability responses. This type of

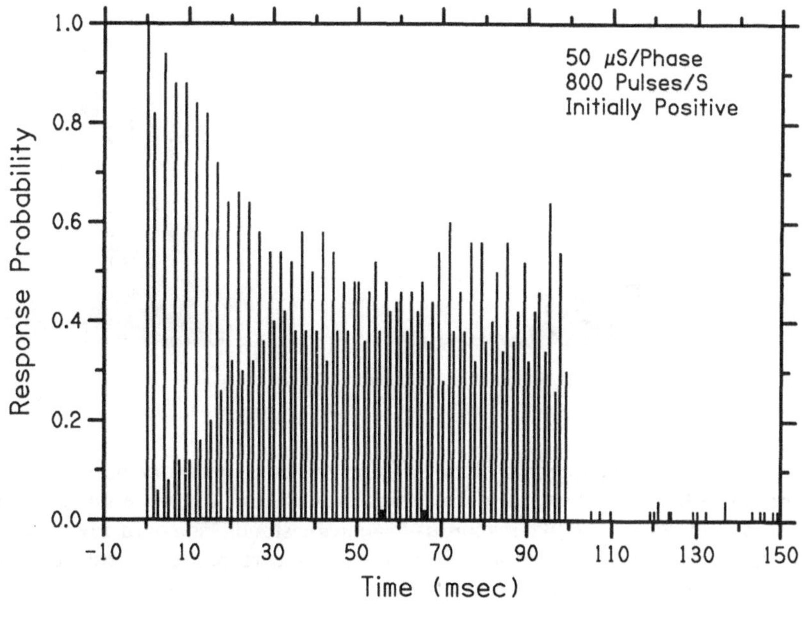

FIGURE 17.22. Example of a "chopper"-type PST histogram commonly observed when stimulation rate exceeds driven discharge rate.

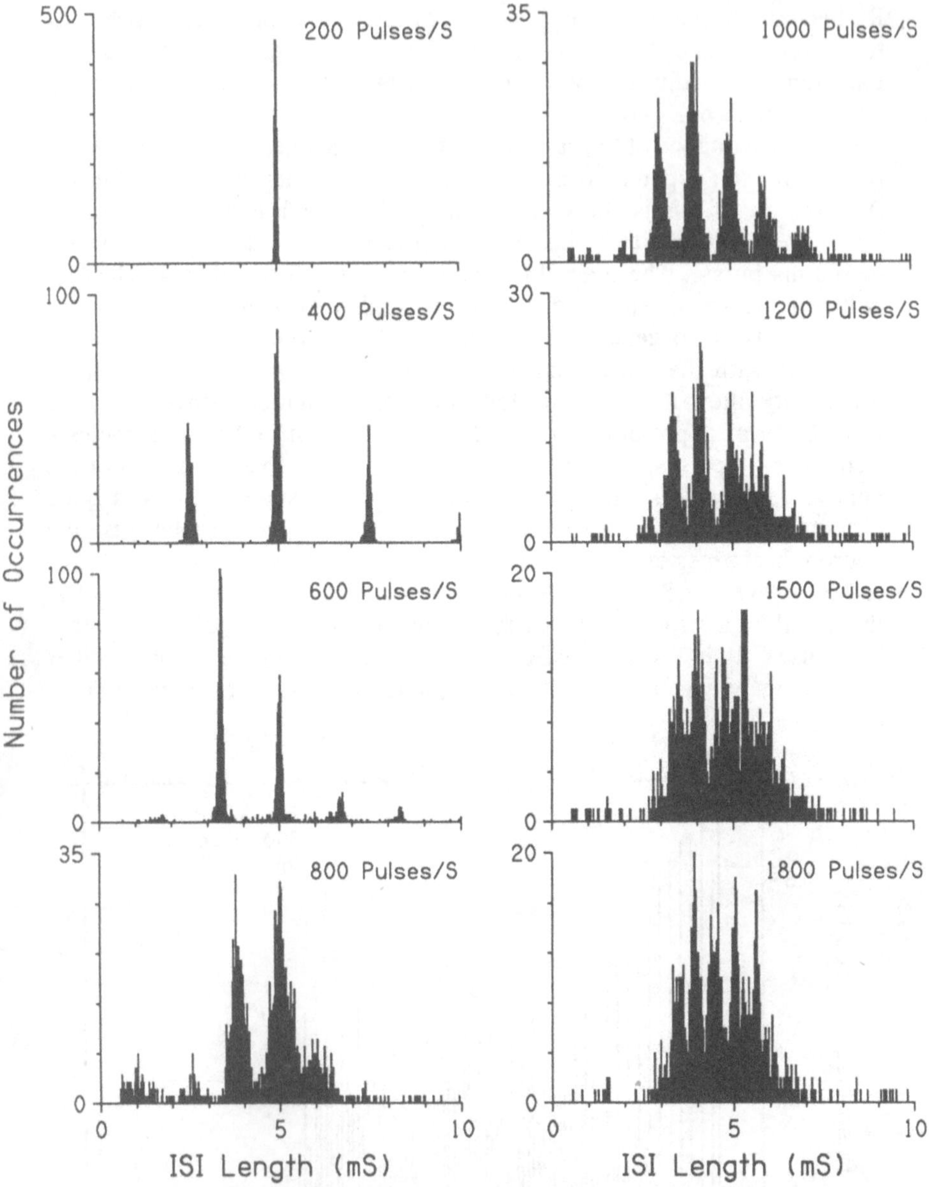

FIGURE 17.23. ISI histograms obtained from the same auditory nerve fiber in response to biphasic electrical pulse trains presented at the same intensity but different frequencies. Unlike responses to acoustic stimuli, standard deviations of ISI clusters are direct functions of pulse rate, and responses cluster at times corresponding to the reciprocal of discharge rate.

behavior is an obvious outgrowth of neural refractoriness and is very unlike that observed acoustically.

Another effect of the regularity of discharge occurrence is that ISI histograms exhibit strong tendencies for ISIs to cluster at times corresponding to the reciprocal of discharge rate, regardless of stimulation rate. This phenomenon is depicted in Figure 17.23, which shows a series of ISI histograms obtained at different pulse rates but at the same intensity. Each histogram contains data from 2 1/2 s of signal presentation. Overall discharge rates ranged from 183 to 220 spikes/s, with a mean of 196 spikes/s. Thus, spikes tended to occur every 5.1 ms. At a pulse rate of 200 pulses/s (upper left) the discharge rate is reflected as a spike on virtually every stimulus pulse, and the ISIs are grouped tightly around a single cluster at 5 ms. At 400 pulses/s, however, clusters of spikes also exist at 2.5 and 7.5 ms as well. These values, of course, are equivalent to spikes occurring every stimulus pulse and every third pulse, respectively. Moving from low pulse rates to high, one can see that in all cases ISIs tend to cluster around 5 ms. Signals presented at higher pulse rates, in which more pulses occur per unit time, generate ISI histograms with clusters at integer multiples of the pulse period, but almost exclusively for those pulses occurring approximately 3–7 ms apart. Even though pulses occurred at shorter and longer intervals than these, they are not represented in the histogram. Finally, the temporal dispersion of the ISI clusters enlarges as pulse rate increases, with the standard deviations of the clusters at rates >1 kHz approaching those values observable for acoustic stimuli (Rose et al., 1967).

The ISI histograms shown in Figure 17.22 are reminiscent of responses to harmonic complexes (Figure 17.7). The general form of the "effective" signal is such that it possesses a center frequency at the pulse rate and components spaced at frequencies equal to multiples of the discharge rate. Depending on stimulus parameters, the acoustic sensations evoked by these stimuli range from various types of frog croaks (at low discharge rates and low center frequencies) to cricket chirps (at low discharge rates and high center frequencies) to sirens (at high discharge rates and high center frequencies). In no case would they resemble speech sounds. Thus, if the brain is capable of extracting frequency information from temporal discharge cadences, it is no wonder that implantees have trouble understanding human speech: The temporal aspects of the neural responses bear little resemblance to those elicited in normal-hearing ears by speech sounds.

Discussion

Central processing of phase-locked neural activity can account for several aspects of human perceptual performance on certain auditory tasks.

Although excitation pattern models can perform equally well on the same tasks, doing so requires physiological mechanisms, such as integration over wide stretches of cochlear space and statistical independence of neural response channels, that either have not been demonstrated or are unrealistically complex. Also, excitation pattern models generally predict poorer performance at high intensities or in the presence of masking, whereas the frequency information provided by temporal codes improves with intensity and need not be degraded by masking. Despite the parsimoniousness of temporal frequency coding mechanisms, the degree to which these representations are retained at higher CNS levels and to what degree remain moot points.

Based on the limits for the existence of the pitch of complex tones and the degree to which processing of phase-locked activity accounts for frequency-discrimination performance, the upper limit for temporal frequency coding in humans appears to be <1 kHz. Available physiological data (Glass, 1984; Javel et al., 1987b) show that auditory nerve fibers in people with cochlear implants probably respond to electrical stimuli with a considerably higher degree of synchronization and entrainment than that observed in response to acoustic tones. Given the exceedingly small variance associated with synchronized neural responses to electrical stimuli, one might expect frequency discrimination performance in implanted patients to be even better than that observed acoustically in normal-hearing listeners. However, much of this improvement is offset by relative lack, particularly at high intensities, of long ISIs (which improve frequency discriminability). The fact that implant recipients generally cannot discriminate frequencies above 0.5–1 kHz (Shannon, 1983) is consistent with the acoustic single-fiber data described earlier, but it is generally inconsistent with the predictions of temporal frequency discrimination models (e.g., Goldstein and Srulovicz, 1977).

An important factor in temporal processing of phase-locked discharges is the statistical independence of discharges occurring between fibers. In the case of cochlear implants such independence is almost sure to be lacking. That is, at sufficiently high intensities, what one fiber does, they all do. There is little doubt that the CNS is a temporal processor: Most neurons in CNS nuclei discharge only when the temporal alignment of activity at two or more inputs is correct. When the alignment is not correct, no output spike occurs. An intriguing speculation in this regard is that the great redundancy of auditory nerve fiber innervation of inner hair cells may have evolved to assure that discharges arise on every cycle of an input signal (Wever, 1949). Without that redundancy neurons would not be able to discharge fast enough to provide information on every cycle. In the case of the cochlear implant the need for redundancy is partially offset by the extremely high discharge rates and synchronization indices possible in single-fiber responses. Thus, stochastic independence across fiber responses may be necessary for normal acoustic hearing but, given the high maximum discharge rates obtainable with electrical stimulation, may be unnecessary for a cochlear implant recipient.

Lastly, let us examine some possible perceptual consequences of temporal encoding of electrical stimuli. Temporal processing ability resides on a continuum that ranges from tasks requiring only gross forms of temporal processing ability (e.g., gap detection and determinations of voice onset time), through mid-level ability (e.g., pitch of complex tones and voice pitch), to fine temporal resolution (e.g., frequency discrimination and vowel formant identification). Given the precision of synchronization to electrical stimuli, the auditory nerve of a cochlear implant recipent should have no trouble providing sufficient information for any of these tasks. However, a problem arises when it comes to resolving fine temporal events, as is the case for frequency-discrimination tasks, because the upper limits of temporal resolving ability are approached, not in the auditory nerve but higher in the CNS.

Available psychophysical evidence (e.g., Shannon, 1983) suggests that most implantees perform about as well as normal-hearing listeners on gap detection tasks. Pitch, on the other hand, is a more subtle phenomenon that has not been investigated rigorously in implanted subjects. As stated earlier, frequency discrimination in implantees fails rapidly above 500 Hz, and at no frequency do absolute performance levels approach those observed acoustically. From these findings we may conclude that temporal processing ability should be retained in recipients of cochlear implants, with performance being limited only by the number and cochlear location of stimulable neurons.

Acknowledgments. This work was supported by an NINCDS grant. Coworkers involved in collecting and analyzing the data reported here were R.K. Shepherd, Y.C. Tong, and G.M. Clark of the University of Melbourne (Australia) and D.W. Smith, J.B. Mott, N.L. Rush, D.A. Clark, G. Litman, and D. Cuka of the Boys Town National Institute. Their contributions are gratefully acknowledged.

References

Arthur, R.M. (1976). Harmonic analysis of two-tone discharge patterns in cochlear nerve fibers. *Biol. Cybernet.* 22:21–31.

Brugge, J.F., Anderson, D.J., Hind, J.E., and Rose, J.E. (1969). Time structure of discharge in single auditory nerve fibers of the squirrel monkey in response to complex periodic sounds. *J. Neurophysio.* 27:287–303.

Burns, E.M., and Viemeister, N.F. (1976). Nonspectral pitch. *J. Acoust. Soc. Am.* 60:863–869.

Clopton, B.M., and Glass, I. (1984). Unit responses at cochlear nucleus to electrical stimulation through a cochlear prosthesis. *Hearing Res.* 14:1–11.

Costalupes, J.A. (1988). Frequency-difference thresholds for tone and noise stimulus combinations in the cat. In *Basic Issues in Hearing,* edited by

H. Duifhuis, J.W. Horst, and H.P. Wit (London: Academic Press), pp. 215–222.

de Boer,E. (1956). Pitch of inharmonic signals. *Nature* 178:535–536.

Delgutte, B., and Kiang, N.Y.S. (1984). Speech coding in the auditory nerve. I. Vowel-like sounds. *J. Acoust. Soc. Am.* 75:866–878.

Dye, R.H., and Hafter, E.R. (1980). Just-noticeable differences of frequency for masked tones. *J. Acoust. Soc. Am.* 67:1746–1753.

Elliott, D.N., Stein, L., and Harrison, M.J. (1960). Determination of absolute-intensity thresholds and frequency-difference thresholds in cats. *J. Acoust. Soc. Am.* 32:380–384.

Galambos, R., and Davis, H. (1943). The response of single auditory nerve fibers to acoustic stimulation. *J. Neurophysiol.* 6:39–57.

Glass, I. (1984). Phase-locked responses of cochlear nucleus units in response to electrical stimulation through a cochlear implant. *Exp. Brain Res.* 55:386–390.

Goldberg, J., and Brown, P. (1969). Response of binaural neurons of dog superior olivary complex to dichotic tonal stimuli: Some physiological mechanisms of sound localization. *J. Neurophysiol.* 32:613–636.

Goldstein, J.L. (1973). An optimum processor theory for the central formation of the pitch of complex tones. *J. Acoust. Soc. Am.* 54:1496–1516.

Goldstein, J.L., and Srulovicz, P. (1977). Auditory-nerve spike intervals as an adequate basis for aural frequency measurement. In *Psychophysics and Physiology of Hearing* edited by E.F. Evans and J.P. Wilson (New York: Academic Press), pp. 337–346.

Greenwood, D.D. (1961). Critical bandwidth and the frequency coordinates of the basilar membrane. *J. Acoust. Soc. Am.* 33:1344–1356.

Greenwood, D.D. (1988). Cochlear nonlinearity and gain control as determinants of the response of primary auditory neurons to harmonic complexes. *Hearing Res.* 32:207–254.

Hartmann, R., Topp, G., and Klinke, R. (1984). Electrical stimulations of the cat cochlea: Discharge pattern of single auditory fibers. *Adv. Audio.* 1:18–29.

Horst, J.W., Javel, E., and Farley, G.R. (1985). Extraction and enhancement of spectral structure by the cochlea. J. Acoust. Soc. Am. 78:1898–1901.

Horst, J.W., Javel, E., and Farley, G.R. (1986). Coding of spectral fine structure in the auditory nerve. I. Fourier analysis of period and interspike interval histograms. *J. Acoust. Soc. Am.* 79:398–416.

Hudspeth, A.J., and Corey, D. (1977). Sensitivity, polarity and conductance change in the response of vertebrate hair cells to controlled mechanical stimuli *Proc. Nat. Acad. Sci. (U.S.A.)* 75:2407–2411.

Javel, E. (1980). Coding of AM tones in the chinchilla auditory nerve: Implications for the pitch of complex tones. *J. Acoust. Soc. Am.* 68:133–146.

Javel, E. (1981). Suppression of auditory nerve responses. I. Temporal analysis, intensity effects and suppression contours. *J. Acoust. Soc. Am.* 69, 1735–1745.

Javel, E., Horst, J.W., and Farley, G.R. (1987a). Coding of complex tones in temporal response patterns of auditory nerve fibers. In *Auditory Processing of Complex Sounds,* edited by W.A. Yost and C.S. Watson (Hillsdale, N.J.: L. Erlbaum), pp. 237–246.

Javel, E., and Mott, J.B. (1988). Physiological and psychophysical correlates of temporal processes in hearing. *Hearing Res.* 34:275–293.

Javel, E., Mott, J.B., Rush, N.L., and Smith, D.W. (1988). Frequency discrimination: Evaluation of rate and temporal codes. In *Basic Issues in Hearing,* edited by H. Duifhuis, J.W. Horst, and H.P. Wit (London: Academic Press), pp. 224–232.

Javel, E., Tong, Y.C., Shepherd, R.K., and Clark, G.M. (1987b). Responses of cat auditory nerve fibes to biphasic electrical current pulses. *Ann. Otol. Rhinol. Laryngol.* Suppl. 128, 96:26–30.

Johnson, D.H. (1974). *The Response of Single Auditory-Nerve Fibers in the Cat to Single Tones: Synchrony and Average Discharge Rate.* Doctoral thesis, MIT, Cambridge, Mass.

Levitt, H. (1971). Transformed up-down methods in psychoacoustics. *J.Acoust. Soc. Am.* 49:467–477.

Lieberman, M.C. (1982). The cochlear frequency map for the cat: Labeling auditory-nerve fibers of known characteristic frequency. *J. Acoust. Soc. Am.* 72:1441–1449.

Lieberman, M.C., and Oliver, M.E. (1984). Morphometry of intracellularly labeled neurons of the auditory nerve: Correlations with functional properties. *J. Comp. Neurol.* 223:163–176.

Licklider, J.C.R. (1951). A duplex theory of pitch perception. *Experientia* 7:128–134.

Luce, R.D., and Green, D.M. (1974). Neural coding and psychophysical discrimination. *J. Acoust. Soc. Am.* 54:610–619.

Mathes, R.C., and Miller, R.L. (1947). Phase effects in monaural perception. *J. Acoust. Soc. Am.* 18:780–797.

Moore, B.C.J. (1973). Frequency discrimination limens for short-duration tones. *J. Acoust. Soc. Am.* 54, 610–619.

Moxon, E.L. (1971). *Neural and Mechanical Responses to Electric Stimulation of the Cat's Inner Ear.* Doctoral thesis, MIT,Cambridge, Mass.

Patterson, R.D. (1987). A pulse ribbon model of peripheral auditory processing. In *Auditory Processing of Complex Sounds,* edited by W.A. Yost and C.S. Watson (Hillsdale, N.J.:Erlbaum), pp. 167–179.

Ritsma, R.J. (1962). Existence region of the tonal residue. I. *J. Acoust. Soc. Am.* 34:1224–1229.

Rose, J.E., Brugge, J.F., Anderson, D.J., and Hind, J.E. (1967). Phase locked response to low frequency tones in single auditory nerve fibers of the squirrel monkey. *J. Neurophysiol.* 30:769–793.

Rose, J.E., Kitzes, L.M., Gibson, M.M., and Hind, J.E. (1974). Observations on phase-sensitive neurons of anteroventral cochlear nucleus of the cat: Nonlinearity of cochlear output. *J. Neurophysiol.* 37:218–253.

Russell, I.J., Richardson, G.P., and Cody, A.R. (1986). Mechanosensitivity of mammalian auditory hair cells *in vitro. Nature* 321:517–519.

Schouten, J.F. (1940). The residue, a new component in subjective sound analysis. *Proc. Koninkl. Ned. Adad. Wet.* 43:356–365.

Schouten, J.F., Ritsma, R.J., and Cardozo, B.L. (1962). Pitch of the residue. *J. Acoust. Soc. Am.* 34:1418–1424.

Shannon, R.V. (1983). Multichannel electrical stimulation of the auditory nerve in man. I. Basic psychophysics. *Hearing Res.* 11:157–189.

Siebert, W.M. (1970). Frequency discrimination in the auditory system: Place or periodicity mechanisms? *Proc. IEEE* 58:723–730.

Smith, R.L., and Brachman, M.L. (1982). Adaptation in auditory-nerve fibers: A revised model *Biol. Cybernet.* 44:107–120.
Terhardt, E., Stoll, G., and Seewann, M. (1982). Algorithm for extraction of pitch and pitch salience from complex tonal signals. *J. Acoust. Soc. Am.* 71:679–688.
van den Honert, C., and Stypulkowski, P.H. (1987). Temporal response patterns of single auditory nerve fibers elicited by periodic electrical stimuli. *Hearing Res.* 29:207–222.
Wever, E.G. (1949). *Theory of Hearing* (New York, Dover).
White, M.W., Finley, C.C., and Wilson, B.S. (1987). Electrical stimulation of the auditory nerve: Stochastic response characteristics. *IEEE/Ninth Annual Conference of the Engineering in Medicine and Biology Society,* pp. 1906–1907.
Wier, C.C., Jesteadt, W., and Green, D.M. (1977). Frequency discrimination as a function of frequency and sensation level. *J. Acoust. Soc. Am.* 61: 178–184.
Wightmann, F.L. (1973). The pattern-transformation model of pitch. *J. Acoust. Soc. Am.* 54: 407–416.
Young, E.D., and Sachs, M.B. (1979). Representation of steady-state vowels in the temporal aspects of the discharge patterns of populations of auditory-nerve fibers. *J. Acoust. Soc. Am.* 66:1381–1403.

Eric Javel: Discussion

Dr. Hartmann: These data are really intriguing. If you did the same experiment with sinusoidal electrical stimuli and looked at the interval histograms, you observe patterns interval histograms that resemble the acoustic case at low frequencies, but not at high frequencies. Therefore, a good strategy might be to use sinusoidal stimuli at low frequencies and pulsatile stimuli at high frequencies.

Dr. van den Honert: As always, Eric, I'd like to take issue with your interpretation of the **A** and **B** peaks. I submit that there are no data that the cell body necessarily lies between any two initiation sites on the nerve. We originally advanced the notion that the site of excitation could jump from the peripheral process to the proximal process, as you raise the intensity of a monophasic pulse. We did that to try to explain the discontinuous reduction in latency that we saw in the compound action potential. We have looked in approximately 2500 single fibers over 2 years and have never seen a discontinuous jump in the latency with increase in monophasic pulse intensity. When you apply a biphasic pulse, you do introduce two sites of excitation. You pass the current in one direction and polarize one part of the cell, then in the other direction and depolarize some other part of the cell, at a different distance from your recording site. Indeed you can produce excitation at two different points in time, and one can dominate as you increase the intensity, particularly if you first excite a lower threshold, more peripheral site, then a more proximal higher threshold site. Then the more peripherally excited spike won't make it to your recording electrode. There's a straight forward experiment that demonstrates that. Separate the pulses in time, and as you do, the two peaks go with the pulses. So, I agree that in the case of the biphasic pulse, there are certainly two sites of initiation, and you can get collisions and interactions between the two. But I submit there is no evidence that the cell body necessarily lies between the two.

I would also like to second Rainer's point that with sinusoidal stimulation it is possible to obtain interval histograms at frequencies up to 1kHz that look very much like the acoustically elicited ones. It's peculiar to the sinusoids and not true of any other waveform. Admittedly, you can only do it over a narrow range of intensities. But that just indicates that we need amplitude compression.

Dr. Geisler: I'd just like to comment on the acoustical responses of the auditory nerve fibers. One can account for the nonlinear behavior such as you displayed quite easily. A linear filter bank followed by an automatic gain control device does very well in matching auditory nerve responses over a wide range of stimuli. So that doesn't require a great deal of extra processing.

Dr. Javel: No. You are right. But when one is operating within these very narrow dynamic ranges, as is the case in electrical stimulation, the automatic gain control is going to be difficult to implement.

Dr. Geisler: Yes, but then it's all the more important. You have the same problem in hearing aids with people with very limited dynamic range in the acoustical world. You really have to work hard with the automatic gain control to squeeze the wide dynamic range of normal acoustic signals into the narrow range that the patients perceive.

Dr. Javel: The point is, the possibility is there and it should be investigated.

Dr. Miller: At the highest frequency stimulus you used, 1800 Hz, was there still a temporal structure that was centered at 200 Hz, or at a 5 ms interval?

Dr. Javel: That's right. The histogram resembled what one would see in response to an amplitude modulated tone.

Dr. Miller: What's your explanation for that one?

Dr. Javel: It is related to refractoriness, and it is interesting that it's so regular. The dispersion of those intervals is not nearly what one sees acoustically at 1800 Hz.

Dr. Dent: Concerning your synchrony at 200 Hz: At Stanford, when trying to implement the deconvolution scheme in a multichannel speech processor, we hoped to use pulsatile stimuli, since that gives you better control over the injection of charge. And if you are going to inject charge on multiple channels simultaneously, you want them to be canceling simultaneously. However, we wanted to recreate, if possible, the analog patterns that we saw in the nerve with acoustic stimulation. We chose an amplitude-modulated pulse scheme, which we hypothesized would give a response like that to an amplitude-modulated tone. And we've had good results with one patient so far with this processor. We've implemented it now portably in real time. It turns out in 1983, Charley Parkins in New York Symposium proposed exactly that scheme: amplitude-modulated pulses for generating a representation on the nerve which more resembles the acoustic case.

Dr. Pfingst: I wonder, Eric, if you, and maybe Rainer Hartmann, could comment: There seems to be a difference in the data that you two have shown with regard to the effects of level on synchrony. As I recall, Rainer's data show that there is an increase in synchrony from low levels to high levels, over a few decibels at least. You are indicating that the response is perfectly synchronized at threshold.

Dr. Javel: There are two differences, I think. First, there is a difference between analog stimulation and pulsatile stimulation. Second, my guess is that what Rainer is doing is including all spikes, even spontaneously occurring spikes, in his analysis. In my analyses I window-out the spontaneously occurring spikes.

Dr. Rabinowitz: How do you decide what is a spontaneous spike and what's a driven spike?

Dr. Javel: By using a time window and starting at the highest intensities, where all the spikes are occurring at the same point in time. Working backward toward threshold, window limits are set that include only the driven spikes. I might add that windowing is rarely necessary because many fibers don't exhibit spontaneous activity.

18
Theories of Speech Perception as Guides to Neural Mechanisms

JAMES D. MILLER

Introduction

In this paper a brief overview of the processes of speech perception will be given. The goal is to place in the record of this conference a summary of a rather general view of the process of speech perception that seems to be consistent with current linguistic theory. From this perspective, thumbnail sketches of three classes of theories will be presented that deal with the acoustic-to-linguistic transformation that is performed by the human listener. Finally, it will be proposed that these three theories suggest rather different neural mechanisms, at least at the higher levels of the nervous system.

Speech Understanding

The Structure of Speech

Speech is conceived as being composed of linguistic segments usually referred to as consonants and vowels. These segments are the phonetic elements or phonemes of a language. All of the syllables and words of a language are composed of a relatively small number of phonemes. In the case of English the inventory of phonemes consists of about 25 consonants and 15 vowels, for a total of about 40 elements. However, phonemes are often pronounced in slightly different ways depending on surrounding context. When these finer phonetic distinctions are included, the number of distinguishable speech sounds or allophones of English may rise to as high as 50 or 60.

Larger linguistic units are formed when phonemes are combined into morphological entities called morphemes. A morpheme is a minimal sequence of phonemes that has its own meaning or grammatical function. A word is made of one or more morphemes. For example, the word "walked" is make up of the verb morpheme "walk" and the past tense morpheme "ed." According to this view morphemes are stored in the lexicon, and words are formed by appropriate combinations of morphemes.

Speech Production

A description of how an utterance is planned and executed helps to define the sensory, perception, and linguistic problems faced by the listener as he seeks to recover, from the acoustic information reaching his ear, the talker's intended meaning.

The process of production of an utterance can be modeled as a step-by-step procedure. Much of this process is controlled by rules or functions that are part of a grammar that is internalized in each user of a language. Furthermore, this grammar can be subdivided into recognizable components that come into play at various points in the production process.

Consider the steps that occur once the message is conceived. The syntactic component of the grammar generates a syntactic tree with a structure appropriate to the intended message. Then the morphological component of the grammar combines the relevant morphemes into words and inserts them into the proper nodes of the syntactic tree. The syntactic tree may or may not undergo transformations, such as transformation into passive voice. Next, the rules of a phonological component of the grammar apply, converting any not-acceptable sequence of phonemes into acceptable ones as well as determining the allophones to be used. Then, the so-called phonetic implementation rules convert sound sequences into sequences of motor commands to the relevant articulators such as the tongue and lips. Speech is finally generated by forcing air through the appropriately shaped vocal tract, and the acoustic wave radiates from the lips and travels to the hearer's ear.

Consider the example of the message: "The cat chased the mouse." After the message is conceived, the syntactic component of the internalized grammar generates a syntactic tree. This tree specifies that the subject of the sentence be made up of an article and a noun. The predicate is subdivided into a verb and an object, and the object is subdivided into an article and a noun. The morphological component of the grammar then assigns words to the end branches of the tree as strings of phonemes. Finally, the phonological component of the grammar generates the string of allophones to be produced. In this case, certain phonemes are dropped or altered in the natural utterance. These changes are ubiquitous and describable and are called phonological rules. Finally, of course, an acoustic waveform that is informative of the allophonic string is generated.

A theory of speech perception must explain how a listener extracts allophones and phonemes from the acoustic waveform; how he groups the phonemes into morphemes and words; how he determines the syntactic structure of the utterance; and finally how he determines the speaker's intended meaning.

In this paper the focus shall be on theories of the process whereby the acoustic wave is converted to a sequence of allophonic units.

Extensive discussions of models of the cognitive processes whereby allophonic or spectral information is used for word recognition and lexical access can be found elsewhere (Church, 1987; Frauenfelder and Tyler, 1987; Marslen-Wilson, 1987; Pisoni and Luce 1987). The higher-level processes whereby the listener decodes the talker's syntax and semantics to arrive at his intended meaning are reviewed in textbooks on psycholinguistics.

Theories of Phonetic Perception

Motor Theories

The *motor theory of phonetic recognition* posits that a special module of the human perceptual system examines the acoustic patterns of speech and determines the abstract speech motor commands that would be required to produce that particular array of informative acoustic elements. Once the abstract commands have been determined, the corresponding phonetic code can be activated. The system is thought to run automatically without significant input from other parts of the linguistic-cognitive system of the brain. Arguments for the theory include the presumed efficiency of a specialized coordinated system for speech production and speech perception (Liberman, 1982; Liberman and Mattingly, 1989). Also, numerous seemingly inexplicable relations between acoustic patterns and phonetic perceptions seem to be potentially understandable in terms of the motor theory. And, finally, a variety of experiments that indicate that human infants and untutored adults are aware of correspondences between articulation and speech sounds also provide apparent support for the motor theory.

Feature Theories

In feature theories, as in all other theories, the auditory system is thought to convert the acoustic waveform into a series of short-term spectra. These spectra are then examined for auditory-acoustic features that may be signaled by spectral shapes, by formant locations, by the locations of the troughs in the spectra, by durations, by rates of spectral change, or by rates of rise of amplitudes. Pisoni and Sawusch (1975) have described feature theories in general terms. The auditory system is assumed to analyze the incoming waveform for a variety of auditory-acoustic features such as those mentioned above. In a second stage, the auditory-acoustic features are mapped onto phonetic features. Phonetic features are classificatory in nature and are based on linguistic analysis of phonological rules, speech production, and historical shifts in languages. In a third stage, the phonetic features are analyzed to specify an allophone. The output of the device is a sequence of allophones, which must then be submitted to a lexical access system to determine the sequence of words. Of course, higher levels of syntactic and sematic analysis are needed to determine the meaning of the utterance.

Major proponents of feature theory have been Gunnar Fant and Kenneth Stevens. Examples of their work can be found in Fant (1973) and Stevens and Blumstein (1981). A cognitive model of speech perception that incorporates aspects of feature theory has been presented by Massero and Ogdin (1980). An interesting use of the connectionist neural net approach to speech perception that seems to converge on featurelike descriptors can be found in Elman and Zipser (1987).

Pattern-Matching Theories

One approach to pattern matching has been suggested by Klatt (1979). His idea was that templates that corresponded to amplitude (decibels) by frequency by time patterns could be developed for each demi-syllable of American English. He estimated that several thousand such templates would characterize speech and that by using such templates one could recognize words and/or phonetic sequences by appropriate processing.

Recently, Miller (1984, 1987, 1989) has proposed a theory of phonetic perception in which pattern matching is achieved through the concept of target zones. In this theory, it is hypothesized that the input waveform in converted by the auditory system into a sequence of spectral patterns. It is further hypothesized that these patterns can be represented in a three-dimensional space, with the position in the space being influenced not only by the spectral patterns of the incoming speech but also by their loudnesses and changes in loudnesses. In this way, the input waveform is converted into a path through the hypothesized space, which is referred to as an auditory-perceptual space (APS). A sequence of allophones is then generated by activation of successive target zones corresponding to each allophone of the language. Two major classes of target zones are envisaged in this theory. One type is called the simple target zone. It involves the recognition of location in the APS. In this case the target zone represents a continuous subspace of the APS. A simple target zone is activated when the "path" generated by the speech input enters it and when the variables controlling segmentation cross a threshold value. Variables controlling segmentation are believed to be several. One is the velocity of movement along the path, or the rate of spectral change. Another is related to the degree of curvature in the path, as segmentation is often associated with changes in the direction of spectral change. Another is whether the path is exhibiting a local extreme in position in APS. Peaks and valleys in pitch and intensity are also variables believed to participate in the segmentation process.

A second type of target zone is the complex target zone. It involves the recognition of a pattern of movement through the APS, and thus corresponds to patterns of spectral change. In this case a class of movements are required not just to activate the target zone but also to define the identity of the associated allophone. For example, the diphthong [AY], which occurs in the word height, appears to be defined by a nucleus of [AA] and a spectral glide from an [AA]-like pattern to an [IH]-like pattern. Preliminary evidence suggests that more complicated movement patterns characterize allophones such as [J] in yet.

Neural Mechanisms

Auditory-Sensory Mechanisms

All theories of speech perception require that the auditory system perform certain analyses. These include short-term spectral analyses that result in relatively smoothed spectral envelopes so that the pattern of spectral peaks and valleys can be used for speech recognition, mechanisms for identifying the perodicity and low pitch of periodic speech signals, and mechanisms for extracting aperiodic speech signals and separately characterizing their spectral envelopes. Preliminary experimental studies have been reported wherein the speech stimuli are used to stimulate anesthetized animals and responses are recorded from the eighth nerve or the cochlear nucleus (Carney and Geisler, 1986; Delgutte, 1986, 1987; Delgutte and Kiang, 1984; Deng and Geisler, 1987; Sachs and Young, 1979).

Along with the continuation of work of the kind just cited, work is needed to clarify the linear and nonlinear auditory mechanisms that allow the listener (1) to separate the desired speech signal from other nonspeech signals in the auditory scene (Darwin, 1984; Darwin and Sutherland, 1984), (2) to separate the desired speech signal from other background speech sounds, and (3) given that the desired speech signal has been isolated from the background, to separate and analyze separately its components.

All of this implies a very high resolution analysis in both time and frequency. For according to the current data, detailed harmonic analysis is required for scene analysis and pitch recognition, as well as for the separation and analysis of burst-friction components, that is, generated at supraglottal loci in the vocal tract from glottal-source components (generated at the glottis). For example, the relatively weak bursts of stop consonants may be superimposed on a low-frequency voice bar and immediately followed by a high-amplitude vowel. The auditory system seems to be able to separate the burst from the voice bar and the following vowel and analyze its characteristics. Another example is provided by the voiced fricatives. These often have only a brief period of simultaneous voicing and friction noise and are bounded by a high-amplitude vowel sound and a low-amplitude friction sound. The analyses of voiced stops and fricatives challenge our current engineering methods of spectral analysis. To discover neural mechanisms used in such analysis not only would add to neuroscience but might also improve our understanding of signal processing generally.

Approaches to the Neural Bases of Phonetic Perception

Background

As stated in the previous section, it appears that auditory analysis requires that the desired speech signal is extracted from the background auditory scene, that it has been successfully separated into supraglottal and glottal components, and that each of these has been analyzed to determine its phonetically relevant spectral characteristics, including its low pitch. The perceptual system must then use these auditory variables to generate a set of phonetic codes.

Each of the theories described previously in the Theories of Phonetic Perception section II of this chapter would encourage different strategies of scientific search for the neural mechanisms that generate the phonetic codes. Adherents of a motor theory would search for special regions of the higher motor centers that might be involved in such perception. Feature theorists might look for anatomical and physiological correlates of significant auditory and/or phonetic features. Pattern-matching or target-zone theorists might search for the anatomical and physiological correlates of the hypothesized target zones. Feature theorists and target-zone theorists would probably expect the more auditory of their concepts to be located in auditory areas or auditory-association areas of the brain. The correlates of the more phonetic of their concepts may be expected to be located in either higher sensory or motor centers. A summary of available knowledge can be found (Lass et al., 1982).

Approaches to these issues can be made in a variety of ways. Experiments with animals provide several avenues of approach. Animals can be studied to determine how they process their own communication signals. This has been extremely successful in the case of birds and bats (Konishi, 1985; Suga, 1988a, 1988b). Trained and untrained animals can also be studied to see how they process the communication sounds of other species. Indeed, studies of how animals perceive and discriminate human speech sound have been extremely successful in elucidating which variables are powerful across species and which may represent specialized species-specific signals. Given a background of perceptual data, animals provide excellent opportunities of elucidating the anatomical and physiological bases for such perception. The human listener has provided a vast amount of perceptual data. New methods promise to enable us to use the human listener as an important source of knowledge of the anatomical and physiological bases of speech perception.

Approaches to Physiological and Anatomical Bases of Phonetic Perception

The neural organization and patterns of neural activity of both animal and human subjects can be studied in a variety of ways, and many of these have only recently emerged as viable techniques.

For example, some indications of chronic levels of activity can be found by staining for cytochrome oxidase (Wong-Riley, 1979; Wong-Riley et al., 1978; Wong-Riley et al., 1981). In the visual system various cortical layers and areas have been shown to have characteristic patterns of distribution of this enzyme (Horton, 1984; Tootell, Hamilton, and Silverman, 1985; Tootell et al., 1988). Furthermore, these patterns can be related to functions of the tissue (Livingstone and Hubell, 1984; Silverman et al., 1989) and can be shown to be altered by long-term removal of afferent stimulation (Wong-Riley, 1980; Wong-Riley and Carroll, 1984; Wong-Riley and Riley, 1983). Human work by Horton and Hedley-Whyte (1984) and by Martin S. Silverman (unpublished) indicates that the method of staining for cytochrome oxidase can be usefully applied to the human brain postmortem. Thus, it may be possible to see informative patterns of the concentration of cytochrome oxidase in the animal and human brains that may relate to the processing of communication signals such as speech.

Stimulus-driven activity can be studied in a variety of ways. One technique that also can be used to survey anatomical loci of response to stimuli involves the use of radioactivity-labeled 2-deoxyglucose (Sokoloff et al., 1977). With such techniques, different patterns of activation might be found for relevant and irrelevant communication signals whether these are "natural," as in the case of birds responding to a specific song, or trained, as in the case of animals responding to human speech sounds. Of course, similar mapping should be undertaken by recording from neural clusters in awake trained and untrained animals. Such measures would be extremely useful in relating the discrimination and categorization of speechlike stimuli to central neural mechanisms.

Of course, the mapping techniques of electrical recording from neural clusters in awake trained and untrained animals should be extremely useful in relating the discrimination and perception of speechlike stimuli to central neural mechanisms (Suga, 1988a, 1988b). In another approach, Ojemann (1983) continues to demonstrate the scientific usefulness of electrical stimulation of the surface of the human brain at the time of surgery. Also, in the case of human subjects, a variety of other options are becoming available. For example, the previously cited work of Horton and Hedley-Whyte and of Silverman indicates that the technique of staining for cytochrome oxidase can be usefully applied to the human brain postmortem.

Additionally, a whole variety of noninvasive procedures are becoming available, and many of these may be usefully applied to the human subject. Judith Lauter of the University of Arizona has developed a lecture entitled "Windows on the Brain" that describes and summarizes the advantages and disadvantages of these techniques.

For our purposes, I will simply list them. (1) The magnetic resonance imaging provides an anatomical description similar to that of dissection of postmortem specimens (Brant-Zawadzki and Norman, 1987). (2) Position emission tomography (PET) provides information of stimulus-driven physiological activity at a similar level of resolution (Lauter et al., 1985; Lauter, Herscovitch, and Raichle, 1988; Raichle, 1987). (3) New approaches to computer processing of evoked potentials can provide information on individual differences and differences between the ears (Berlin, Hood, and Allen, 1984; Lauter and Loomis, 1986, 1988). (4) Quantitative BEG techniques—variously known as qEEG, Beam, or EAP—use computer processing to perform spectral analyses of the EEGs from multiple electrodes to provide rather detailed mapping of the electrical activity of the brain (Duffy, Burchifiel, and Lombardo, 1979; Gevins and Schaffer, 1980; Glass, 1984; John, 1977; Lauter, 1988). (5) The method magneto encephalography—SQUID—offers very high spatial resolution, about 1 mm, of generators in the brain. By this technique it may be possible to localize phonetic modules, feature detectors, or target zones in the human brain (Bak et al., 1981; Eiberling et al., 1982; Reite, Zimmerman, and Zimmerman, 1982; Romani et al., 1982). Finally, magnetic resonance spectrography (MRS) is now beginning to be used in conjunction with MRI to localize chemical activity in the brain (Cohen, 1987). Finally, I would like to mention an obvious, but important, innovation that is emerging in my own laboratory at CID. Without high-speed computers and high-volume disk storage, we can now, through synthesis, generate and store hundreds of syllables that systematically cover the space of all possible stimuli of various classes. These can then be randomized and presented so that "maps" of similar responses can be made. Of course, the responses may be either behavioral or physiological.

It is not hard to imagine similar physiological experiments that might define the receptive fields of neurons or perhaps "receptive area maps" similar to those described by Merzenich's group in the somatosensory area.

Concluding Comments

The material presented above sketches the opportunities to uncover neuroanatomical bases of phonetic perception. Clearly, an understanding of the details of the auditory analysis of the speech waveform will aid in the design of prosthetic devices. Techniques for use in experimental animals and people which reveal the physiological effects of cochlear stimulation in the higher centers would, of course, be invaluable for the evaluation of various strategies for the electrical stimulation of the cochlea.

References

Bak, C., Kofoed, B., Lebech, J., Saermark, K., and Elberling, C. (1981). Auditory evoked magnetic fields from the human brain. Source localization in a single-dipole approximation. *Phys. Lett.* 82A:57–60.

Berlin, C.I., Hood, L.J., and Allen, P. (1984). Assymetries in evoked potentials. In *Hearing Science,* edited by C.I. Berlin (San Diego: College-Hill), pp. 461–478.

Brant-Zawadski, M., and Norman, D. (eds.). (1987). *Magentic Resonance Imaging of the Central Nervous System* (New York: Raven Press).

Carney, L.H., and Geisler, C.D. (1986). A temporal analysis of auditory-nerve fiber responses to spoken stop consonant-vowel syllables. *J. Acoust. Soc. Am.* 79:1896–1914.

Church, K.W. (1987). *Phonological Parsing in Speech Recognition* (Boston: Kluwer Academic Publisher).

Cohen, S.M. (ed.). (1987). Physiological NMR spectroscopy: From isolated cells to man. *Ann. N.Y. Acad. Sci.* 508:1–537.

Darwin, C.J. (1984). Perceiving vowels in the presence of another sound: Constraints on formant perception. *J. Acoust. Soc. Am.* 76:1636–1647.

Darwin, C.J., and Sutherland, N.S. (1984). Grouping frequency components of vowels: When is a harmonic not a harmonic? *QJ Exp Psychol.* 36A:193–208.

Delgutte, B. (1986). Analysis of French stop consonants with a model of the peripheral auditory system. In *Invariance and Variability of Speech Processes,* edited by J.S. Perkell and D.H. Klatt (Hillsdale, N.J.: Erlbaum), pp. 163–177.

Delgutte, B. (1987). Peripheral auditory processing of speech information: Implications from a physiological study of intensity discrimination. In *The Psychophysics of Speech Perception,* edited by M.E.H. Schouten (Dordrecht: Nijhof), pp. 333–353.

Delgutte, B., and Kiang, N.Y.S. (1984) Speech coding in the auditory-nerve: V. Vowels in background noise. *J. Acoust. Soc. Am.* 75:908–918.

Deng, L., and Geisler, C.D. (1987). A composite auditory model for processing speech sounds. *J. Acoust. Soc. Am.* 82:2001–2012.

Duffy, F.H., Burchifiel, J.L., and Lombroso, C.T. (1979). Brain electrical activity mapping (BEAM): A method for extending the clinical utility of EEG and evoked potential data. *Ann. Neurol.* 5:309–321.

Elberling, C., Bak, C., Kofoed, B., Lebech, J., and Saermark, K. (1982). Auditory magnetic fields from the human cerebral cortex: Location and strength of an equivalent current dipole. *Acta Neurol. Scand.* 65:553–569.

Elman, J.L., and Zipser, D. (1987). Learning the hidden structure of speech. ICS Report 8701. La Jolla, Calif.: University of California, p. 18.

Fant, G.M. (ed.). (1973). *Speech Sounds and Features* (Cambridge, Mass.: MIT Press), p. 227.

Frauenfelder, U.H., and Tyler, L.K. (1987). The process of spoken word recognition: An introduction. *Cognition* 25:1–20.

Gevins, A.V., and Schaffer, R.E. (1980). A critical review of electroencephalographic (EEG) correlates of higher cortical functions. *CRC Crit. Rev. Bioeng.* 4:113–164.

Glass, A. (1984). Round table on hemispheric specialization and lateral asymmetries in the EEG: Introduction. *Biol. Psychol.* 19:151–157.

Horton, J.C. (1984). Cytochrome oxidase patches: A new cytoarchitectonic feature of monkey visual cortex. *Phil. Trans. Roy. Soc. Lond.* B301:199–253.

Horton, J.C., and Hedley-Whyte, E.T. (1984). Mapping of cytochrome oxidase patches and ocular dominance columns in human visual cortex. *Phil. Trans. Roy. Soc. Lond.* B304:255–272.

John, E.R. (1977). Neurometrics: Clinical applications of quantitative electrophysiology. In *Functional Neuroscience* (Hillsdale, N.J.: Erlbaum), vol. 2.

Klatt, D.H. (1979). Speech perception: A model of acoustic-phonetic analysis and lexical access. *J. Phonetics* 1:279–312.

Konishi, M. (1985). Birdsong: From behavior to neuron. *Ann. Rev. Nerosci.* 8:125–170.

Lass, N.J., McReynolds, L.V., Northern, J.L., and Yoder, D.E. (eds). (1982). *Speech, Language and Hearing*. vol. I, *Normal Processes,* Chaps. 1, 4, and 11.

Lauter, J.L. (1988). Functional-activation asymmetries in normal humans studied with quantitative EEG (qEEG): First tests in the CNS Project. Presented to the Acoustical Society of America, Honolulu.

Lauter, J.L., Herscovitch, P., and Raichle, M.E. (1988). Human auditory physiology studies with positron emission tomography. In *Auditory Pathway,* edited by J. Syka and R.B. Masterton (New York: Plenum), pp. 313–317.

Lauter, J.L., Herscovitch, P., Formby, C., and Raichle, M.E. (1985). Tonotopic organization in human auditory cortex revealed by positron emission tomography. *Hearing Res.* 20:199–205.

Lauter, J.L., and Loomis, R.L. (1986). Individual differences in auditory electric responses: Comparisons of between-subject and within-subject variability. I. Absolute latencies of brainstem vertex-positive peaks. *Scand. Audiol.* 15:167–172.

Lauter, J.L., and Loomis, R.L. (1988). Individual differences in auditory electric responses: Comparisons of between-subject and within-subject variability. II. Amplitudes of brainstem vertix-positive peaks. *Scand. Audiol.* 17:88–92.

Liberman, A.M. (1982). On finding that speech is special. *Am. J. Psychol.* 37:148–167.

Liberman, A.M., and Mattingly, I.G. (1989). A specialization for speech perception. *Science* 243:489–494.

Livingstone, M.S., and Hubell, D.H. (1984). Anatomy and physiology of a color system in the primate visual cortex. *J. Neurosci.* 4:309–356.

Marslen-Wilson, W.D. (1987). Functional parallelism in spoken word-recognition. *Cognition* 25:71–102.

Massero, D.W., and Ogden, G.C. (1980). Speech perception: A framework for research and theory. In *Speech and Language: Advances in Basic Research and Practice,* edited by N.J. Lass (New York: Academic Press).

Miller, J.D. (1984). Auditory processing of the acoustic patterns of speech. *Arch. Otol.* 110:154–159.

Miller, J.D. (1987). Auditory-perceptual processing of speech waveforms. In *Auditory Processing of Complex Sounds,* edited by W.A. Yost and C.S. Watson (Hillsdale, N.J.: Erlbaum), pp. 257–266.

Miller, J.D. (1989). Auditory-perceptual interpretation of the vowel. *J. Acoust. Soc. Am.,* in press.

Ojemann, G.A. (1983). Brain organization for language from the perspective of electrical stimulation mapping. *Behav. Brain Sci.* 2:189–230.

Pisoni, D.B., and Sawusch, J.R. (1975). Some stages of processing in speech perception. In *Structure and Process in Speech Perception,* edited by A. Cohen and S.G. Nootabaum (New York: Springer-Verlag), pp. 16–35.

Raichle, M.E. (1987). Circulatory and metabolic correlates of brain function in normal humans. In *Handbook of Physiology. The Nervous System V. Higher Functions of the Brain,* Part 2, edited by F. Plum (Maryland: American Physiological Society), pp. 643–674.

Reite, M., Zimmerman, J.T., and Zimmerman, J.E. (1982). MEG and EEG auditory responses to tone, click and white noise stimuli. *Electroenceph. Clin. Neurophysiol.* 53:643–651.

Romani, G.L., Williamson, S.J., Kaufman, L., and Brenner, D. (1982). Characterization of the human auditory cortex by the neuromagnetic method. *Exp. Brain Res.* 47:381–393.

Sachs, M.B., and Young, E.D. (1979). Encoding of steady-state vowels in the auditory nerve: Representation in terms of discharge rate. *J. Acoust. Soc. Am.* 66:470–479.

Silverman, M.S., Grosof, D.H., De Valois, R.L., and Elfar, S.D. (1989). Spatial frequency organization in primate striate cortex. *Proc. Natl. Acad. Sci.* 86:711–715.

Sokoloff, L., Reivich, M., Kennedy, C., Des Rosiers, M.H., Patlak, C.S., Pettigre, K.D., Sakurada, O., and Shinohara, M. (1977). The (14C) deoxyglucose method for the measurement of local cerebral glucose utilization: Theory, procedure, and normal values in the conscious and anesthesized albino rat. *J. Neurochem.* 28:897–916.

Stevens, K.N., and Blumstein, S.E. (1981). The search for invariant acoustic correlates of phonetic features. In *Perspectives on the Study of Speech,* edited by P.D. Eimas and J.L. Miller (Hillsdale, N.J.: Erlbaum), pp. 1–38.

Studdert-Kennedy, M., Liberman, A.M., and Harris, K.S. (1970). Motor theory of speech perception: A reply to Lane's critical review. *Psychol. Rev.* 77:234–239.

Suga, N. (1988a). What does single unit analysis in the auditory cortex tell us about information processing in the auditory system? In *Neurobiology of Neocrotex,* edited by T. Rakic and W. Singer (Berlin: Wiley, S. Bernhard Dahlem Konferenzen, pp. 331–349.

Suga, N. (1988b). Neuroethology, audition and speech. In *Auditory Function,* edited by G.M. Edelman, W.E. Gall, and W.M. Cowan (New York: Wiley), pp. 679–720.

Tootell, R.B.H., Hamilton, S.L., and Silverman, M.S. (1985). Topography of cytochrome oxidase activity in owl monkey cortex. *J. Neurosci.* 5:2786–2800.

Tootell, R.B.H., Silverman, M.S., Hamilton, S.L., De Valois, R.L., and Switkes, E. (1988). Functional anatomy of macaque striate cortex. III. Color. *J. Neurosci.* 8:1569–1593.

Wong-Riley, M. (1979). Changes in the visual system of monocularly sutured or enucleated cats demonstrable with cytochrome oxidase histochemistry. *Brain Res.* 171:11–28.

Wong-Riley, M. (1980). Histochemical changes in cytochrome oxidase of cortical barrels after vibrissal removal in neonatal and adult mice. *Proc. Natl. Acad. Sci.* 77:2333–2337.

Wong-Riley, M., and Carroll, E.W. (1984). Effect of impulse blockage on cytochrome oxidase activity in monkey visual system. *Nature* 307:262.

Wong-Riley, M., and Riley, D.A. (1983). The effect of impulse blockage on cytochrome oxidase activity in the cat visual system. *Brain Res.* 261:185–193.

Wong-Riley, M., Walsh, S.M., Leake-Jones, P.A., and Merzenich, M.M. (1981). Maintenance of neuronal activity by electrical stimulation of unilaterally deafened cats demonstrable with cytochrome oxidase technique. *Ann. Otol.* 90:30–32.

Wong-Riley, M., et al. (1978). Changes in endogenous enzymatic reactivity to DAB induced by neuronal inactivity. *Brain Res.* 141:185–192.

James D. Miller: Discussion

Question: The target zone is complicated. What is involved in defining those target zones?

Dr. James Miller: One of the big problems in theories of speech perception has been the fact that a particular expression of any allophone depends a great deal on the allophones preceding it and following it. Once you take the point of view that these target zones are large, a great deal of that problem goes away. You can make an "ooh" that's almost identical to an "ih," an "ooh" that's almost identical to a "W," or an "ooh" that's almost identical to an "ah." And they are all classified as "ooh" as long as they are inside this target zone. So if you are coming from one zone and going to another, you might just dip into the "ooh" target zone briefly. Presumably a great deal of the co-articulation effects can be accounted for by these very large target zones. But I don't believe that all of them can.

Dr. Shannon: Are these data produced by responses to different speakers or just one speaker?

Dr. James Miller: These are based on a database that we have collected at CID, and extracted from the literature. So the original Pearson and Barney measures are included. There are a variety of speakers, speaking rates, sexes, ages, but they all produce spoken syllables. The data are not responses to running speech.

Dr. Rabinowitz: What do the three dimensions exactly represent?

Dr. James Miller: Well, in the original three dimensions, X is the logarithmic distance between the second and third formant, Z is the logarithmic distance between the first and second formant, and Y is the logarithmic distance between the low-frequency reference and the first formant.

19 Fundamental Limitations on Sensory Encoding of Electrical Stimulation

GREGORY H. WAKEFIELD

Introduction

In the design of an auditory prosthesis, certain criteria have been established, either implicitly or explicitly, with respect to the desired performance of the device. Although the precise specifications may be argued, the auditory prosthesis is intended, in general, to restore the full range of normal auditory function to deafened individuals. Measures of the success to which this restoration is accomplished also differ in their specifics, but in general these measures consider speech communication as primary among the many auditory functions. All currently implanted auditory protheses have been shown to provide some improvement in speech communication, although there appears to be considerable variability in the extent of such improvement. No implanted auditory prosthesis has been demonstrated to restore auditory function to normal levels.

As our discipline begins to develop the second generation of auditory prostheses, it is important to determine the source of this fundamental failure to completely restore auditory function by any of the first-generation systems. If we can show that the residual function of the auditory nerve following sensorineural loss at the auditory periphery is sufficient to support auditory function, then the failure clearly lies in the technology of the prosthesis. However, to the extent to which the residual function limits sensory transmission, no efforts, no matter how great, to design a better peripheral device will achieve the goal of complete restoration.

In the following, we discuss several approaches to understanding the transmission of information through the peripheral auditory system and outline the structure of one approach in detail. It is our belief that these approaches may help quantify the impact of sensorineural loss on auditory function and may lend insight into the design of a better prothesis. Much of this paper constitutes "work in progress," either what we are doing in our laboratory or what we believe the fruits of other laboratories will produce in the next 2 years. This paper is a preliminary reaction to the question of fundamental limits in sensory coding for the auditory prosthesis; as such, the title could be rewritten either as "Why are there 30,000 fibers in the auditory nerve?" or, from a more practical perspective, "Is the cochlear prosthesis the Holy Grail of hearing science?"

Sources of Information Loss in the Auditory Periphery

As sound is transduced at the auditory periphery, it is possible for information about the acoustic signal to become degraded. Such degradation, in turn, limits the amount of information conveyed by the signal to the auditory system. There are several points in the transduction process which are candidates for information loss: the transformation of the acoustic wave into basilar membrane motion, the spatial sampling of the basilar membrane motion by a finite set of sensors (hair cells), and the temporal sampling of basilar membrane motion by the point-process generator at the spiral ganglion.

Each of the transduction steps for normal acoustic stimulation is paralleled by similiar transformations in the electrically driven auditory system. Thus, transduction from acoustic waves to basilar membrane motion is replaced by a transduction of acoustic waves to a current field that is generated by driving an electrode implanted in the cochlea. The spatial composition of this current field is sampled by a finite set of sensors, but in this case hair cells are replaced by dendritic and axonal processes and the geometry differs substantially from that of the acoustic system. Finally, the temporal sampling differs from that in the acoustically driven cochlea by virtue of the fact that an "electrical synapse" replaces the dynamics of the hair cell membrane and chemical synapse in the organ of Corti.

Given these two different transduction systems, we can ask to what extent and in what form information is preserved between the acoustic input and neural output. The former question reflects the issue of capacity, i.e., the extent to which information is not lost through transduction, whereas the latter question focuses primarily on whether the representation of acoustic information is in a form that can be utilized by the central auditory system.

To address the question of sensory capacity, it is necessary to determine the information transmitted through each transduction step for each system and then to compare the aggregate performance of each system. Although many of the tools exist for such analysis, to our knowledge no one has combined these tools and the relevant experimental data and applied them to the present problem despite the success analysis for other sensory systems (Williams, William, and Fuller, 1984).

The Proximal Stimulus Field

The transformation of the acoustic (or electrical) stimulus to the proximal stimulus has been characterized through basilar membrane modeling (Allen and Sondhi, 1979) or through current field modeling (Eddington, 1988; Finley, Wilson, and White, Chapter 5, this volume; Spelman, Chapter 4, this volume). In the former case, the models require highly nonlinear components in order to accurately portray membrane dynamics, particularly at low stimulus levels. The presence of these nonlinear components complicates the information-theoretical analysis, but does not present an insurmountable barrier. In the latter case, the models are most often linear but are very sensitive to boundary and initial conditions, such as the transmission properties of the surrounding media and the geometry of the stimulating sites along the electrode.

Spatial Sampling

Each model provides a representation of the proximal stimulus either as the state of the basilar membrane or as that of the current field. Given this representation, it is possible to consider the effects that sampling in time and space has on information transmission. In general, sampling a continuous waveform at discrete points in time or space represents a severe loss of information since it is not possible to recover the continuous signal from its sampled points. The so-called sampling theorem (Roberts and Mullis, 1987) states conditions under which the continuous waveform can be recovered from its sampled points. These conditions require that the continuous waveform is bandlimited and that the sampling frequency is at least twice the highest frequency of the original continuous signal. If the samples are not sufficiently dense, then the original signal cannot be reconstructed exactly from the sampled points and false components (aliasing) are introduced into the reconstruction.

Whenever a sensing system utilizes a set of discrete sensors to transmit information about the original signal, sampling is involved, and therein lies the potential for a loss of information to occur. In the human auditory system, hair cells can be interpreted as the discrete sensing elements whose placement may lead to information loss due to undersampling the state of the basilar membrane. Spatial sampling in the normal acoustically driven auditory system has not been studied as extensively as it has in the visual system. In the latter case, it has been argued that the retinal mosaic within the fovea is sufficiently dense to prevent aliasing of the retinal image. However, in the off-foveal region, the sampling density decreases and therefore aliasing (information loss) occurs (Yellot, 1983).

The analysis of spatial sampling in the auditory system would proceed as in the visual system by considering as a worst case the sharpest pattern along the basilar membrane and determining whether the spacing among hair cells is sufficiently dense to prevent aliasing. This analysis may also shed some light on the general effects that hair cell loss and the pattern of hair cell loss have on auditory processing in the impaired auditory system. Extension of these results to the case of electrical stimulation would utilize the finite-element analysis suggested by Finley, Wilson, and White (Chapter 5, this volume) and assumptions about the distribution and number of nerve fibers within the field.

Temporal Sampling

In comparison with the spatial sampling properties of the auditory periphery, a substantial amount of research has focused on the temporal sampling induced by the point-process generator in the acoustically driven auditory system. This approach was first considered by Siebert (1968) with respect to characterizing behavioral intensity and frequency differences limens as reflecting the fundamental limits imposed by information loss through auditory transduction. Since Siebert's work, more refined point-process models have been used to account for the limits in behavioral sensitivity to various acoustic variables (Colburn, 1973; Goldstein and Srulovicz, 1977; Viemeister, 1988; Wakefield and Nelson, 1985). These models have been further refined through neurophysiological estimates of the driving and recovery functions of the point-process generator (Johnson, 1974; Johnson and Swami, 1983; Miller, 1985). From a different perspective, Beutler has generalized sampling theory for random sampling (Beutler and Leneman, 1966); and Bar-David (1969), among others, has considered the general problem of communication over a point-process channel.

In contrast to normal auditory function, these point-process models have not been used for modeling impaired or electrically driven auditory function even though these stochastic models present the best theoretical tool for addressing the relative importance of hair cell/synapse transduction over the "electrical" synapse introduced by the current field in transmitting information. These tools are currently being refined in our laboratory for such analysis.

More generally, the transmission of information through the point-process generator presents the most difficult analysis of the three steps in auditory transduction. The analysis is most readily approached using estimation theory, in which it is clear that ensemble averaging over conditionally independent point processes is an important criterion for recovering the driving function of the point-process generator. In lieu of such averaging, the deadtime introduced by the recovery period leads to complete loss of information about the driving stimulus. Although these effects can be related qualitatively to an information-theoretical analysis, quantitative relationships have proved difficult to establish beyond very general principles (Bremaud, 1981; McFadden, 1965).

Answers to questions of the previous three subsections will provide insight into the relative importance of each component to the transmission of information in audition. The relevance of this analysis to the question of whether we are searching for a Holy Grail in our design of a cochlear prosthesis lies in the fact that this approach can reveal quantitatively the relative importance of nerve survival and the pattern of such survival to the capacity of the auditory system for transmitting acoustic information. Though difficult, this approach may provide an upper bound on the performance of a cochlear prosthesis based on clinical measures of nerve survival, electrode design, and stimulator design.

Fidelity Criteria

Of the three transduction steps, the final step involves stochastic sampling of the driving stimulus at the auditory nerve fiber, which, by its nature, represents a loss of information for acoustic transmission. Whether this loss is significant depends, on the one hand, on the extent to which the preceding transduction steps preserve information and, on the other, on the extent to which the central auditory system utilized the encoded acoustic information. Broadly speaking, this latter question addresses the issue of fidelity in information transmission. For noisy (or lossy) channels, information theory provides a means for relating the transmission rate to the information loss through the twin notions of a fidelity criterion and a rate-distortion function. We conclude our discussion with an introduction to the issue of fidelity and its use in the design of a cochlear prosthesis.

One of the principle results in information theory is that for a large class of channels there exists a trade-off in the rate at which information can be transmitted through the channel and the distortion (or information loss) that is introduced by the channel such that distortion and rate are inversely related for the rate-distortion function that characterizes the channel. The relevance of this principle to auditory processing is that degradations in any of the steps of peripheral transduction will degrade the channel and will therefore lead to an increase in the distortion of the transduced signal. The extent to which this distortion becomes a limiting factor in information transmission depends on the degree to which information transmitted beyond the auditory periphery is preserved.

Whereas information theory explicitly defines information for an ensemble of random signals, it leaves open the definition of the distortion function, or alternatively, the fidelity criterion, with which the quality of the received signal is judged. The issue of a fidelity criterion is directly relevant to understanding auditory perception as well as the losses that occur when the system is damaged. Particularly in the case of the design of an auditory prosthesis, it is useful to understand the criteria by which received signals are judged to be similar.

Despite its importance, relatively little is known about the fidelity criterion that is determined by auditory processing. In general, psychophysical experiments on detection and discrimination provide some bounds on stimulus variations that are mapped into relatively small regions of the perceptual space. That is, if S_1 and S_2 are acoustic stimuli which are discriminated only 75% of the time, then it is consistent to assume that the fidelity, or distance, $d(S_1, S_2)$ between these two stimuli in some "perceptual" space is also relatively small when compared with the distance between stimuli that are discriminated 100% of the time. On the other hand, it is more difficult to determine the fidelity or distance metric used to characterize the similarity of suprathreshold stimuli. Historically, scaling studies have mapped the relationships between the physical and psychological dimensions of sound with some success. However, it is not clear how the scaling of loudness, pitch, timbre, or prosody relate to the fidelity of a signal and its "reproduction" or resynthesis, such as in telephony, hearing aids, or cochlear prosthetics. In such cases, it has proved more fruitful to predict speech intelligibility through the design of measurement devices based directly on empirically derived measures of speech intelligibility, e.g., the speech articulation index or the speech transmission index (Steeneken and Houtgast, 1980).

The design goal of restoring normal auditory function by an auditory prosthesis can be translated within the present context as one of designing a prosthesis such that the patient is unaware of any difference between the original acoustic percepts and those elicited electrically. In such a case, the fidelity of the prosthetic system would be high indeed. A less lofty (and more realistic) goal would be to design the auditory prosthesis such that meaningful discriminations between signals are preserved and all other discriminations are destroyed. In this case, the fidelity (as measured in terms of discriminability) of the prosthetic system would equal that of the acoustic system although the two systems could generate markedly different percepts. In other words, the auditory prosthesis should preserve, at a minimum, the relative distances among stimuli that should be discriminated and guarantee that acoustic stimuli which are not discriminated normally remain so.

To help characterize the scope of the fidelity problem and of stimulus encoding for the auditory prosthesis, we introduce the concept of an equivalence class. In our context, an equivalence class will always be associated with a given signal and a transformation that relates all of the signals within the equivalence class to that given signal. For example, the *discrimination equivalence class* (DEQ) for a given stimulus $x(t)$ is that set of signals that cannot be discriminated from $x(t)$ by an observer. Then, the goal of stimulus encoding for a sensory prosthesis is to preserve, at a minimum, the DEQs for that sensory system. If the DEQs are not preserved, then no matter how the psychological stimulus space scales, the information transmitted will be poorer than that for the normal auditory system. We believe that this notion of equivalence class is useful for understanding audition, particularly with respect to the design of a sensory prosthesis. Its advantages lie in that discrimination equivalence classes can be characterized by objective psychophysical procedures since they are based on the discriminability of the stimulus set rather than its suprathreshold properties. The concept also provides a measure of the minimum performance that an encoding scheme should achieve and therefore is useful as a first test of a new prosthesis design. We close with two examples of equivalence classes and a discussion of their implications for signal transmission/enhancement systems.

Equivalence Classes for Single Auditory Neurons

In our example, we consider the definition of a DEQ for a single neuron in the auditory nerve for acoustic and for electrical stimulation. As in Johnson and Swami (1983) and Miller (1985), we assume that the discharge record of the auditory nerve in response to a stimulus is a self-excited point process in which the excitation function $e(t)$ can be separated into the product of a stimulus-dependent driving function $d(t)$ and a response-dependent recovery function $r(t)$. Furthermore, we assume that there is no cumulative effect of discharge on neural response; that is, the recovery function is a monotonically increasing function of time from the last spike occurrence.

The factored form of the excitation function allows us to ignore refractory effects (the recovery function) for deriving the equivalence class, since these depend only on the renewal properties of the nerve. Instead, we claim that the equivalence class for a neuron is that set of acoustic stimuli which yield the same driving function. Under acoustic stimulation, Johnson (1974) among others, has demonstrated that the driving function is an invertible nonlinear transformation of the envelope of the acoustic waveform, defined at the best frequency of the auditory nerve fiber. Thus, the equivalence class for an acoustic stimlus $x(t)$is

$$DEQ\{x(t)\} = \{y(t) \mid \; |\tilde{y}(t)|^2 = |\tilde{x}(t)|^2; f\}$$

where $\tilde{y}(t)$ and $\tilde{x}(t)$ are the low-pass equivalent complex signals defined with respect to a common narrowband filter center frequency f. If the common narrowband filter has a perfectly flat passband at the center frequency f, it can be shown that the equivalence class for an acoustic stimulus with a bandwidth substantially smaller that the flat passband includes all possible shifts in carrier frequency such that the narrowband signal remains within the flat passband of the filter; otherwise, if the acoustic stimulus is broadband with respect to the narrowband filter and sufficiently rich in spectral content, then the equivalence class is reduced primarily to those signals varying only in group delay.

On the other hand, the response of the auditory nerve to electrical stimulation can modeled, to a first approximation, as an integrate-and-dump mechanism. Thus, $y(t) \in DEQ\{x(t)\}$ if $\forall i = 1, N - 1$,

$$\int_{t_i}^{t_{i+1}} y(t)dt = \int_{t_i}^{t_{i+1}} x(t)dt$$

where $\{t_i\}$ are the occurrence times at which the integral of $x(t)$ exceeds the firing threshold g_{thresh} for the nerve fiber and $\forall i = 1, N - 1$,

$$\int_{t_i}^{s} y(t)dt < g_{\text{thresh}}, \forall s < t_{i+1}$$

The equivalence class for this form of stimulation is much different from that for acoustic stimuluation. Rewriting $y(t) = x(t) + d(t)$, then the conditions for equivalence require that

$$\int_{t_i}^{t_{i+1}} d(t)dt = 0$$

and

$$\int_{t_i}^{s} d(t)dt < g_{\text{thresh}} - \int_{t_i}^{s} x(t)dt$$

Since there is no restriction on whether the driving signal is positive, the equivalence class for the electrically driven fiber is difficult to predict on the basis of signal spectrum or temporal waveform shape. Indeed, this class of signals need share little similarity, either spectrally or temporally, in order to belong to the same equivalence class. It is this irregular mapping of signals to one set that characterizes the DEQ for the auditory nerve in electrical stimulation and poses problems for any consistent encoding of stimulus information through this form of stimulation.

We claim that the DEQ for the electrically driven auditory nerve is too broad to be useful for stimulus encoding directly and suggest that some form of preconditioning, or limiting, of the class of possible signals presented to the VIIIth nerve is necessary in order to obtain a predictable, and interpretable, relationship between the input signal and its neural representation. Clearly, one possible class of signals is that of pulsatile waveforms in which the waveform peak is sufficient to cross the fiber threshold following the integrator mechanism. Such a class of signals also has the added advantage that the time of occurrence is relatively easy to determine from the occurrence of the neural discharge. This suggests that speech encoders should be designed on the basis of pulse position modulation (PPM), for codes up to the discrimination limits of the central auditory system, and that the relevant psychophysical experiments in implanted patients concern the discrimination of PPM codes.

Equivalence Classes for a Population of Auditory Neurons

The above analysis for the single auditory neuron presents the limiting case for an auditory system that "listens" through one single channel or neural element. We commonly assume that the population of auditory neurons presents a greater source of information for auditory encoding than does the single channel. However, the strength of this assumption rests on the basis that the population behavior is not completely predicted from the individual neural behavior. Under acoustic stimulation in the normal auditory system, this assumption is reasonable from the standpoint of tonotopic organization (not all neurons innervate the same frequency region, and therefore, not all neurons encode the same envelope) and relatively weak conditional dependence of the driven activity of neurons innervating the same frequency region. The latter conditioning prevents the loss of information that otherwise occurs when neural discharge is inhibited by the response-dependent recovery function.

In contrast, the electrically driven auditory system appears to be far less differentiated spatially than the acoustic system, thereby reducing the degree to which stimulus differentiation increases the effective capacity of the system, and also appears to exhibit strong conditional dependence of driven activity, thereby reducing the precision by which the driving function can be estimated from the discharge activity across the population of fibers. Our present efforts are focused at quantifying this loss of information at the level of the population of auditory nerve fibers.

Conclusions

We have outlined several fundamental sources for information loss in the normal and electrically driven auditory system and have provided an example of one approach for analyzing encoding strategies for prosthetic stimulation. Our motivation for this research lies in our general concern that the goals of a cochler prosthesis be clearly defined within the capabilities of an impaired, electrically driven system. The strength of an information-theoretical approach lies in the fact that information transmission represents a basic measure of system performance since it completely characterizes the statistics of the transmitted signal; the performance of any subsequent processing of this transmitted signal must be determined by the transmission statistics. The weakness of this information-theoretical approach lies in the difficulty of the analysis. A weaker estimation-theoretical approach was outlined using the concept of an equivalence class. This approach provides greater tractability at the expense of stronger assumptions concerning the form of the decision rules for the auditory system. We propose that discrimination measures, and the limits of psychophysical discrimination, are more conservative criteria upon which to build one's analysis and design of signal encoders for an auditory prosthesis, since they require far less theoretical justification than broader suprathreshold scaling measures.

Acknowledgments. This work was supported by funds provided by the Vice President's Office of Research and Development of the University of Michigan. The author thanks Drs. David Neuhoff, Ben Clopton, and Bryan Pfingst for the many *gedanken* experiments performed and Mr. Brent Edwards for his useful questions and succinct answers.

References

Allen, J.B., and Sondhi, M.M. (1979). Cochlear macromechanics: Time domain solutions, *J. Acoust. Soc. Am.* 66:123–132.

Bar-David, I. (1969). Communication under the poisson regime, *IEEE Trans. Info. Theory* 15:31–37.

Beutler, F., and Leneman, O. (1966). Random sampling of random processes: Stationary point processes, *Inform. Control* 9:324–346.

Bremaud, P. (1981). *Point Processes and Queues: Martingale Dynamics* (Springer-Verlag: Berlin).

Colburn, H.S. (1973). Theory of binaural interaction based on auditory nerve data. I. General strategy and preliminary results on interaural discrimination. *J. Acoust. Soc. Am.* 54:1458–1470.

Eddington, D. (1988). A three dimensional, electro-anatomical model of the implanted cochlea. Presentation at the Models of the Electrically Stimulated Cochlea Symposium, October 3 and 4, 1988, Ann Arbor, MI.

Goldstein, J., and Srulovicz, L. (1977). Auditory-nerve spike intervals as an adequate basis for aural frequency measurement. In *Psychophysics and Physiology of Hearing,* edited by E.F. Evans and J.P. Wilson (New York: Academic Press).

Johnson, D. (1974). *The Response of Single Auditory-Nerve Fibers in the Cat to Single Tones: Synchrony and Average Discharge Rate.* Ph.D. Dissertation, Department of Electrical Engineering and Computer Science, MIT, Cambridge, Mass.

Johnson, D., and Swami, A. (1983). The transmission of signals by auditory nerve fiber discharge factors, *J. Acoust. Soc. Am.* 74: 493–501.

McFadden, J.A. (1965). The entrophy of a point process, *J. Soc. Indust. Appl. Math.* 13:988–994.

Miller, M. (1985). Algorithms for removing recovery-related distortion from auditory nerve discharge patterns, *J. Acoust. Soc. Am.* 77:1452–1464.

Roberts, R., and Mullis, C. (1987). *Digital Signal Processing* (Reading, Mass.: Addison-Wesley).

Siebert, W. (1968). Stimulus transformations in the peripheral auditory system. In

Recognizing Patterns, edited by P.A. Kohlers and M. Eden (Cambridge, Mass.: MIT Press), pp. 104–133.

Steeneken, H.J., and Houtgast, T. (1980). A physical method for measuring speech-transmission quality, *J. Acoust. Soc. Am.* 67:318–326.

Viemeister, N. (1988). Intensity coding and the dynamic range problem, *Hearing Res.* 34:267–274.

Wakefield, G. and Nelson, D. (1985). Extension of a temporal model of frequency discrimination: Intensity effects in normal and hearing-impaired listeners, *J. Acoust. Soc. Am.* 77:613–619.

Williams, W.J., and Fuller, M. (1984). A continuous information approach to the analysis of cutancous receptors, *Biol. Cybern.* 47:13–16.

Yellott, J. (1983). Spectral consequences of photoreceptor sampling in the rhesus retina, *Science* 221:382–385.

Greg H. Wakefield:Discussion

Dr. Smoorenburg: It seems to me that an important aspect of the electrostimulation is that the equivalent class will increase.

Dr. Wakefield: No, I think I did make the equivalence class increase—the size of a given equivalence class will undoubtedly increase. And that is very objectionable in my opinion.

Dr. Smoorenburg: Not just the size, across dimensions.

Dr. Wakefield: Yes. That's what I meant by the bad equivalence class property of this electrical stimulation following the integrate and dump operation. So I think we're in agreement there.

Dr. Smoorenburg: I think I've tried to point out in my paper that that's an essential aspect of electrostimulation, and that we have to focus on reduced central space and work back from that.

Dr. Wakefield: The long and the short of it is that I think I would disagree in the following sense: that if, in fact, we can drive small populations of fibers with these pulse codes, that in some sense we are going to be preserving the same type of equivalence class as the standard auditory system. I don't want to deal with the perceptual argument. I'm just taking a very stimulus-oriented approach. Let's assume that we'll preserve those equivalence classes and hope, obviously, that my observer can use those.

Question: There is a central nervous system above the auditory nerve, and it puts constraints on what can be realized from input delivered from the nerve. It's not that the central nervous system does not generate highly adapted constants; it does, but it operates within those constraints, and the anatomical and connectional constraints necessarily require a treatment within those limitations.

Dr. Wakefield: I've no disagreement with that. In fact, it's why I cited two examples showing that a pulse code is invertible. With invertibility there is no loss of information; we then simply have to choose which of the operators to use as a model. Zero crossings won't work, although theoretically they can, because bandwidths are wrong. As you're saying, the central nervous system cannot work with those types of cues. Something like an encoding envelope around a given carrier frequency will work.

Dr. Merzenich: From another point of view, it might be exactly because equivalence classes are larger that the system can be driven to generate new constructs as quickly and efficiently as it does with the corrupted information it receives.

Question: This is an extension of the central nervous system question. I just wonder if the information to your approach can incorporate, or needs to incorporate, this axis from its entry into the central nervous system. The pathway is a minimum of eight parallel pathways, each of which encodes differently the information that it receives from the auditory nerve, each of which does a different transform, so your encoder-decoder boxes are a series of pairs of matched encoder-decoders. You have an issue then of synthesis or resynthesis.

Dr. Wakefield: Yes, you're right, and I'm again making a hard assumption here that there is at least some level of adaptation in the system that, once we present a clean, well-defined equivalence class of signals to the central nervous system, we can ask the system to begin to adapt and learn the new code. My argument is that up until now a lot of the coding schemes, in fact, don't do that, and the failure of these codes to work doesn't necessarily reflect whether you're stimulating it with a pulse or stimulating it with other waveforms; the failure of those codes lies in the fact that they have poor equivalence classes, in the sense that they are not easily learned by the auditory system.

20 Psychophysical and Speech Perceptual Studies on Cochlear Implant Patients

Y.C. TONG, H.H. LIM, AND G.M. CLARK

Introduction

One of the most important findings in cochlear implant research has been the orderly variation in perceptual characteristics produced by intracochlear electrodes in accordance with the tonotopic organization of the cochlea. The electrical signal dimension of electrode position has therefore been used extensively for presenting speech information to cochlear implant patients. This paper describes further psychophysical and speech perceptual results on the perceptual characteristics produced by intracochlear electrodes.

Hardware for Bipolar Stimulation

The psychophysical and speech perceptual studies were conducted on patients implanted with the Nucleus multichannel cochlear implant device. During the implant surgery (Clark, Pyman, and Bailey, 1979), an array of 22 electrodes, spaced 0.75 mm apart, was inserted through the round window into the scala tympani for a distance of up to 25 mm. The residual auditory nerve fibers were activated by charge-balanced biphasic current pulses. The implanted electrodes are numbered from 1 to 22 in the apical-to-basal direction. Bipolar stimulation, produced by passing an electric current between two electrodes, was used. The spatial extent of each bipolar electrode pair is defined as the distance between its apical and basal members. An electrode pair is numbered according to its basal electrode member. For example, electrode pair EP-12 activated with a spatial extent of 2.25 mm has electrodes 12 and 9 as its basal and apical electrode members, respectively, while EP-14-10 denotes electrical stimulation using two temporally nonoverlapping electrode pairs, EP-14 and EP-10, activated in quick succession in a stimulus period.

Forward-Masking Patterns at Different Stimulus Current Levels

This study (Lim, Tong, and Clark, 1988) investigated the forward-masking patterns produced by a bipolar electrode pair at different stimulus current levels. This study has been conducted on one of our patients (FK). The duration of the masker was 300 ms, while the duration of the probe was 18 ms. The pulse rate for both masker and probe was 166 pps. The last pulse of the masker pulse train led the first pulse of the probe pulse train by 6 ms. The masker electrode pair (EP-12) was fixed in the middle of the electrode array. The threshold electric current for each probe electrode pair activated in isolation was first estimated using a four-interval forced-choice procedure. The increase in threshold current for each probe electrode pair along the electrode array in the presence of the masker was then estimated. This increase in threshold current will be referred to as the amount of forward masking.

Figure 20.1 shows the forward-masking patterns of a masker electrode pair (EP-12) at four stimulus current levels. The amount of masking is shown on the ordinate. The electrode-pair number for the probe, ranging

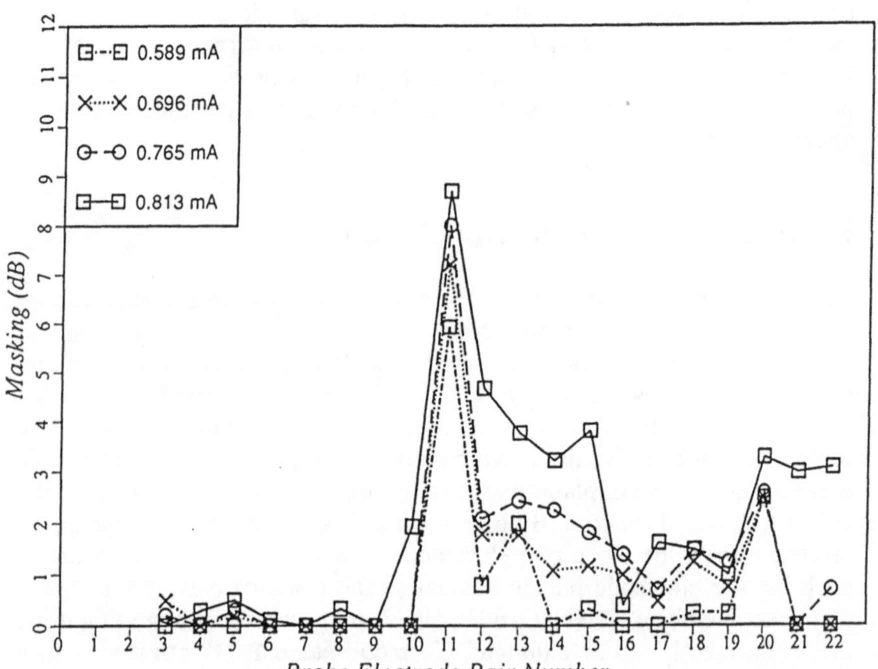

FIGURE 20.1. Forward-masking patterns of electrode pair EP-12 at four stimulus current levels.

from 3 to 22 in the apical-to-basal direction, is shown on the abscissa. The four stimulus currents used are shown in the inset. These masking patterns show that the amount of masking at each probe electrode pair increased with masker current level. The neural activity at each probe location therefore increased with stimulus current, and the overall loudness of the hearing sensation produced by the maskers also increased. The location of the maximum and the general shape of the masking pattern, however, did not change significantly with masker current level. These results indicate that the location of the maximum and the general shape of the neural excitation distribution along the cochlea for a fixed masker electrode pair do not change significantly with stimulus current level, and that the pitch and timbre produced by a fixed electrode pair should not, therefore, change significantly with current or loudness.

Identification of Electrode Positions at Different Current Levels

To further investigate the effects of stimulus current on the perceptual characteristics produced by intracochlear electrodes, an absolute identification study (Tong et al., 1988b) has been conducted on one of our patients (RS). Twenty-one stimuli, consisting of seven electrode positions at three different loudness (or stimulus current) levels, were used in a single interval task. The seven electrode positions were electrode pairs 6 to 18 in the apical-to-basal direction, and were assigned response numbers from 1 to 7 in order of increasing electrode-pair number. Each electrode pair was presented at three different loudness (or stimulus current) levels: 33%, 66%, and 100% of comfortable loudness. Note that only one response number was assigned to each electrode pair. For example, the three stimuli of different loudnesses on electrode pair 6 were assigned response number 1, and the patient was instructed to nominate "1" as the response if he thought that one of these three stimuli on electrode pair 6 had been presented. Data analysis was performed on the combined confusion matrix constructed by pooling the responses for the twenty-one stimuli, and on three individual confusion matrices constructed by including only the responses for the seven stimuli at each individual loudness level.

Figure 20.2 shows the combined confusion matrix for patient RS. Each row represents the response pattern for the three stimuli of different loudnesses on the same electrode pair. The black dot on top of each pattern represents the center of gravity of the response pattern, while the dotted line represents the center of gravity for a response pattern that is symmetrical about the response number assigned to the electrode pair in question. For example, in the case of the response pattern for electrode pair 6, the black dot was located on the right of the dotted line because of

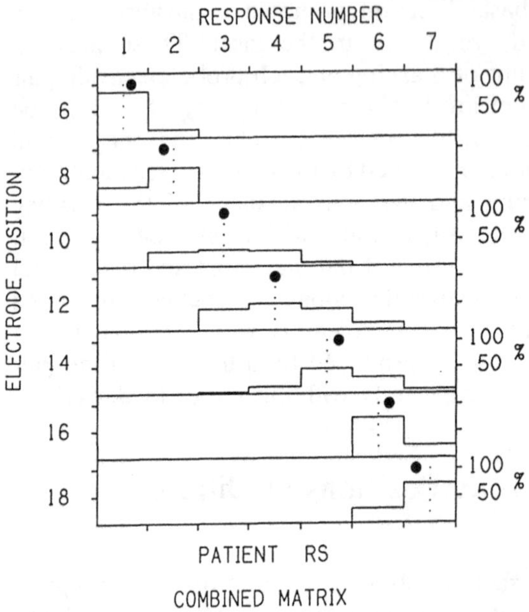

FIGURE 20.2. Combined confusion matrix for the identification of electrode positions at different current levels.

the incorrect responses given in the response number 2 category. The location of the black dot with respect to the dotted line gives an indication of the deviation of the patient's response from the designated response number. This deviation or bias could be toward a lower or higher response number corresponding to a bias of response toward an apical or basal electrode pair, respectively. Figure 20.3 shows the amount of deviation versus response number for the four confusion matrices: the combined matrix and the three individual matrices at the three different loudness levels. The deviations changed from predominantly positive for the 33% comfortable loudness matrix, close to zero for the 66% matrix, and predominantly negative for the comfortable loudness matrix. The deviations for the combined matrix were also close to zero and were similar to those of the 66% matrix. Using the 66% matrix as a reference, the predominantly positive deviations for the 33% matrix indicate a bias toward a higher response number or an apparent increase in pitch and sharpness when the electrical stimuli were soft. The predominantly negative deviations for the matrix at comfortable loudness indicate a bias toward a lower response number or an apparent decrease in pitch and sharpness. Note that the variations in pitch and sharpness with loudness were not large in that the deviations in Figure 20.3 are within the range of ± 1. It is also worth noting that this decrease in pitch and sharpness with loudness for electrical stimulation is in the same direction as the decrease in pitch with loudness for acoustic tones below 1 kHz (Stevens, 1935).

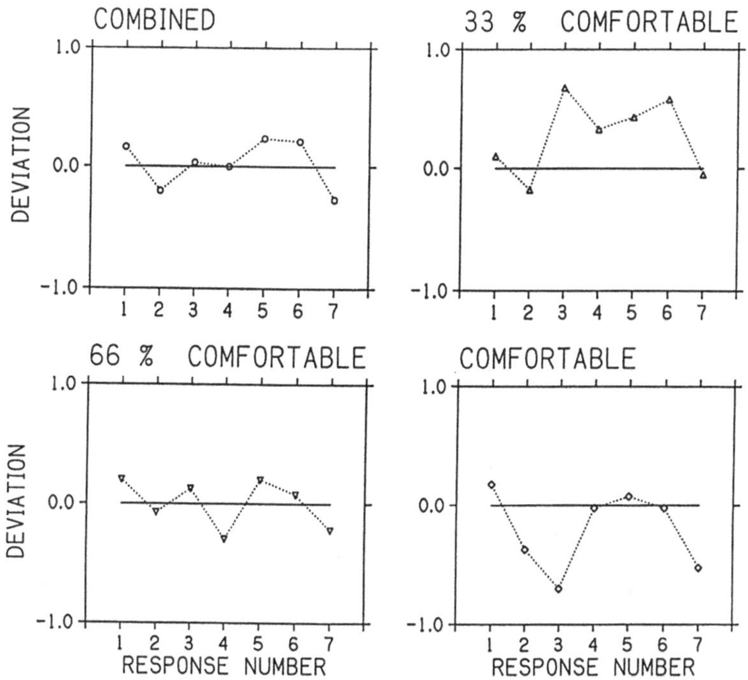

FIGURE 20.3. The amount of deviation versus response number for the combined matrix and the three individual matrices at three different loudness levels.

Returning to Figure 20.2 the diagonal pattern of the combined confusion matrix indicates reasonably good identification performance for the 21 stimuli. A quantitative measure of identification performance is to calculate, on the basis of the confusion matrix, the sensitivity index d' representing the perceptual distance between two successive electrode positions. These d' measures are shown in cumulative form in Figure 20.4 for the combined matrix and the three individual matrices. In Figure 20.4, better identification performance is indicated by steeper cumulative curves. The results in Figure 20.4 indicate that identification performance for electrode position was similar for the different loudnesses.

Forward-Masking Patterns Produced by Two Bipolar Electrode Pairs Activated in Quick Succession

This study (Lim, Tong, and Clark, 1988) investigated the forward-masking pattern produced by two bipolar electrode pairs activated in quick succession within a stimulus period. This study has been conducted on patient FK. The stimulus configuration for this study is almost

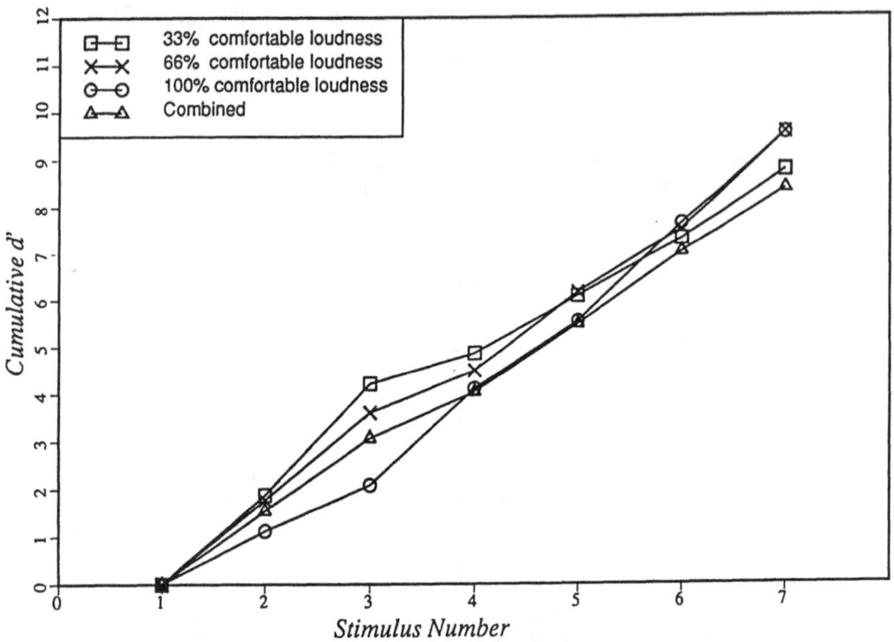

FIGURE 20.4. Cumulative d' curves for the combined matrix and the three individual matrices.

identical to that described in the previous Forward Masking study section with the exception that two masker electrode pairs were used. The two masker electrode pairs were activated in quick succession within a stimulus period of 6 ms. Within a stimulus period, the biphasic pulse on the more basal masker (electrode pair 16) leads the pulse on the more apical masker (electrode pair 8) by 0.8 ms. There was no temporal overlap between the pulses on the two maskers.

Figure 20.5 shows three forward-masking patterns for one of our patients: the basal masker (EP-16) and the apical masker (EP-8) in isolation and the two maskers activated in quick succession in a stimulus period. The forward-masking pattern for each masker activated in isolation shows a single dominant peak in the vicinity of the masker electrode pair in question. The forward-masking pattern for the two maskers activated in quick succession in a stimulus period shows two peaks in the vicinity of the two masker electrode pairs.

These masking patterns suggest that the interaction between two electrode pairs activated in quick succession was small, and the individual perceptual characteristics of the two electrode pairs were preserved.

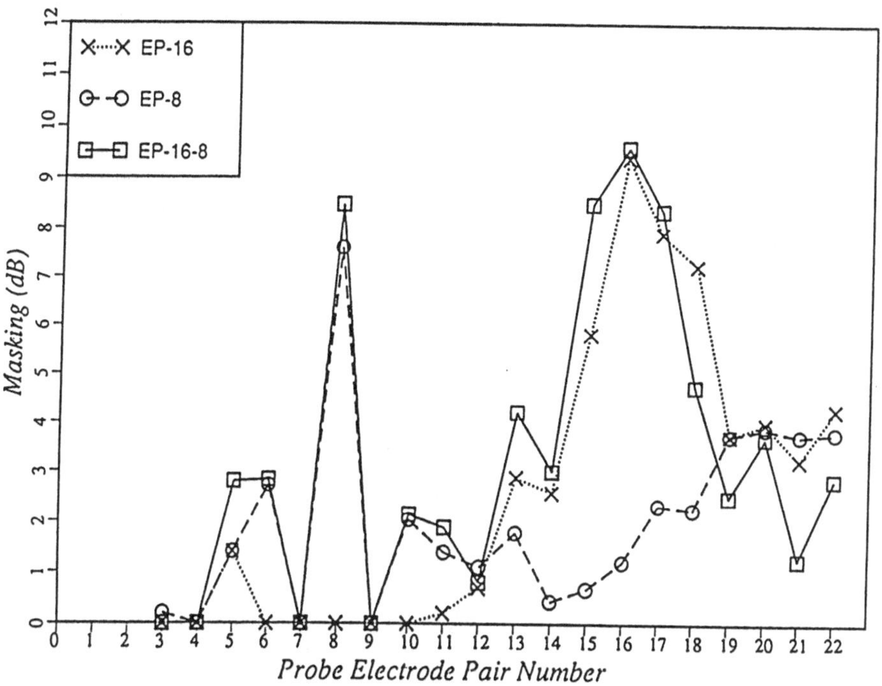

FIGURE 20.5. Forward-masking patterns for the basal masker (EP-16) and the apical masker (EP-8) in isolation and the two maskers (EP-16-8) activated in quick succession in a stimulus period.

Synthetic Vowel Study

To further investigate the interaction between two electrode pairs activated in quick succession and the usefulness of this stimulus configuration in terms of speech processor design for cochlear implant patients, a synthetic vowel study (Tong, Lim, and Clark, 1988a) was conducted. Eleven electric pulse trains were constructed on the basis of eleven natural vowels in Australian English. The pulse trains were at a fixed repetition rate of 125 rep/s. Within each stimulus period, two electrode pairs were activated in quick succession. The location of the first electrode pair in the stimulus period was selected according to the second formant frequency of the natural vowel, and the second pair according to the first formant frequency. The electrode assignments for the 11 pulse trains are shown in Figure 20.6. The electrode pair encoding second formant frequency information is represented on the abscissa, and the electrode pair encoding first formant frequency information is represented

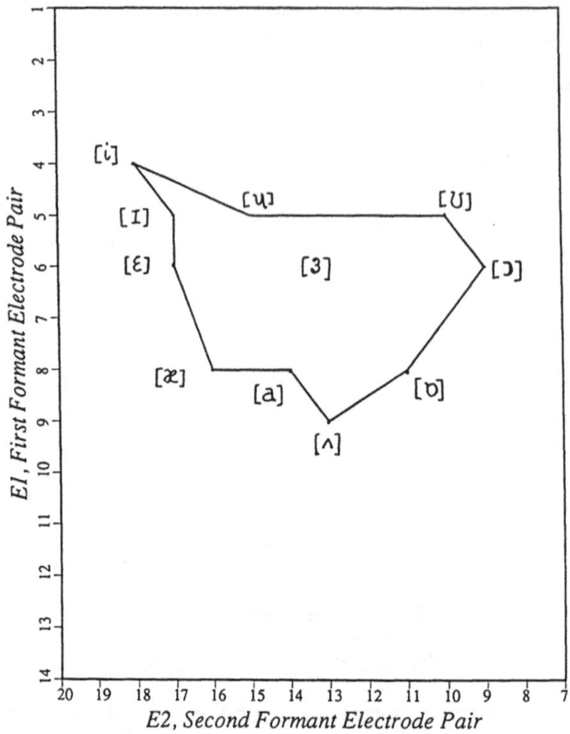

FIGURE 20.6. Electrode assignments for the 11 synthetic vowels.

on the ordinate. The electrode assignment for each pulse train is specified by the coordinates of the phonetic symbol of the corresponding natural vowel. For example, the pulse train corresponding to the natural vowel /I/ was specified by electrode pairs 17 and 5, respectively.

The 11 pulse trains or synthetic vowels were presented in random order in a single interval task. The response pattern was recorded in a confusion matrix, which was further analyzed using information transmission analysis. Table 20.1 shows the synthetic vowel results for two patients. The overall percentage scores for the two patients were approximately 75%. There was a significant amount of information transmitted about the duration of the vowels and the second formant and the first formant of the vowels. Note that the information transmitted about these three features is partially redundant. This is illustrated by computing (F1)′, which is the amount of information transmitted about the first formant when its redundancy with the second formant and duration has been accounted for. The values of 0.36 and 0.45 for (F1)′ indicate that even after accounting for redundancy, a significant amount of information was transmitted about the first formant. These results confirm that the

TABLE 20.1. Percentage correct and information transmission scores for the synthetic vowel study.

		Information transmitted (bits)			
Patient	% Correct	Dur.	F2	F1	(F1)′
MO	76	0.94	1.28	0.65	0.36
LL	73	0.98	1.22	0.64	0.45

interaction between two electrode pairs activated in quick succession is small, and that this stimulus configuration is useful for speech coding for cochlear implant patients.

The Effects of Temporal Order on Perceptual Characteristics

The psychophysical and speech perceptual studies so far described suggest that by activating a number of electrode pairs in a stimulus period, a corresponding number of spectral components of the speech signal can be conveyed to cochlear implant patients. The question then is, What are the effects of the temporal order of the different electrode pairs (in the stimulus period) on perceptual characteristics? We have conducted a number of psychophysical studies (Tong et al., 1988b) to investigate the differences in perceptual characteristics between different temporal orders.

One of the studies was to ask the patients to discriminate between a pulse train of fixed temporal order and another pulse train in which the temporal order was randomized from period to period. The stimulus configuration for this study is shown in Figure 20.7. The repetition rate of the pulse trains was 100 rep/s. Four electrode pairs, nominally numbered from 1 to 4, were activated in a stimulus period. The bottom half shows a pulse train with a fixed temporal order in each period, while the top half shows a pulse train with its temporal order of the four electrode pairs changed randomly from period to period. Note that the same four electrode pairs were used in the two pulse trains.

Discrimination studies using 2IFC and 4IFC procedures showed that the pulse train of the randomized temporal order was easily discriminated from that of the fixed temporal order. The major difference between these two pulse trains was that the randomized pulse train sounded fussy and scratchy, while the pulse train of the fixed temporal order sounded (relatively) smooth. The results of this study indicate that the temporal order of the electrode pairs in a stimulus period does have significant effects on perceptual characteristics and that it may be possible to use

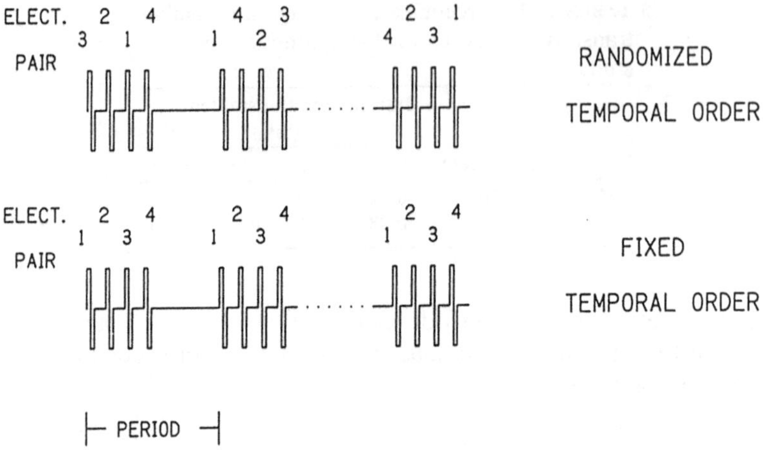

FIGURE 20.7. Stimulus configuration for the psychophysical studies using pulse trains of randomized temporal order and fixed temporal order.

these randomized pulse trains to convey information about unvoiced consonants or noiselike signals to cochlear implant patients.

To further investigate the possibility of using randomized pulse trains for conveying information about unvoiced consonants and noiselike signals, two identification studies were conducted. The stimulus specifications and response numbers for the two studies are shown in Table 20.2. The stimuli for the first study shown in the top half of Table 20.2 were seven pulse trains of randomized temporal order. Four electrode pairs were activated in a stimulus period for each pulse train. The electrode pairs varied progressively in the apical-to-basal direction for the seven pulse trains, which were assigned response numbers from 1 to 7. The electrode pairs for each pulse train spanned over seven banded electrodes on the electrode array, and there were considerable overlaps in terms of electrode position among the seven pulse trains. In a single interval task, the seven stimulus pulse trains were presented in random order and the patient was instructed to identify each stimulus presentation as one of the pulse trains and to respond by nominating the appropriate response number.

The seven stimuli for the second study shown in the bottom half of Table 20.2 were seven pulse trains, with a single electrode pair activated in each stimulus period. The electrode pairs varied in the apical-to-basal direction for the seven pulse trains, which were assigned response numbers from 1 to 7. Note that the spacing in terms of electrode position between two successive stimuli in the second study is the same as that in the first study. The performance measured in the second study using a

TABLE 20.2. Stimulus specifications for two identification studies investigating the perceptual characteristics of pulse trains of randomized temporal order.

	Study 1	
Electrode pairs	Temporal order	Response number
6-8-10-12	Randomized	1
7-9-11-13	Randomized	2
8-10-12-14	Randomized	3
9-11-13-15	Randomized	4
10-12-14-16	Randomized	5
11-13-15-17	Randomized	6
12-14-16-18	Randomized	7
	Study 2	
10	—	1
11	—	2
12	—	3
13	—	4
14	—	5
15	—	6
16	—	7

single electrode pair in each stimulus can therefore be used as a reference for the first study.

Two confusion matrices were constructed from the results of the two studies, respectively. Measures of d' as described before were calculated for the two matrices. The d' results are shown in cumulative form in Figure 20.8 for one of our patients (RS). The open squares are cumulative d' measures for the seven pulse trains of randomized temporal order, while the crosses are for the seven pulse trains with a single electrode pair in each stimulus period. These two curves show that identification performance was almost identical for the two sets of pulse trains. When the patient was asked to describe the hearing sensations produced by the seven pulse trains of randomized temporal order, he reported that despite the scratchy and fussy sensation, he was able to rank these randomized pulse trains from dull to sharp in accordance with the tonotopic organization of the cochlea.

Summary

The results of a forward-masking study indicate that a spatially localized neural excitation pattern can be produced by bipolar electrical stimulation in the human cochlea. The location of the maximum and the general shape of this pattern does not change significantly with electric current level.

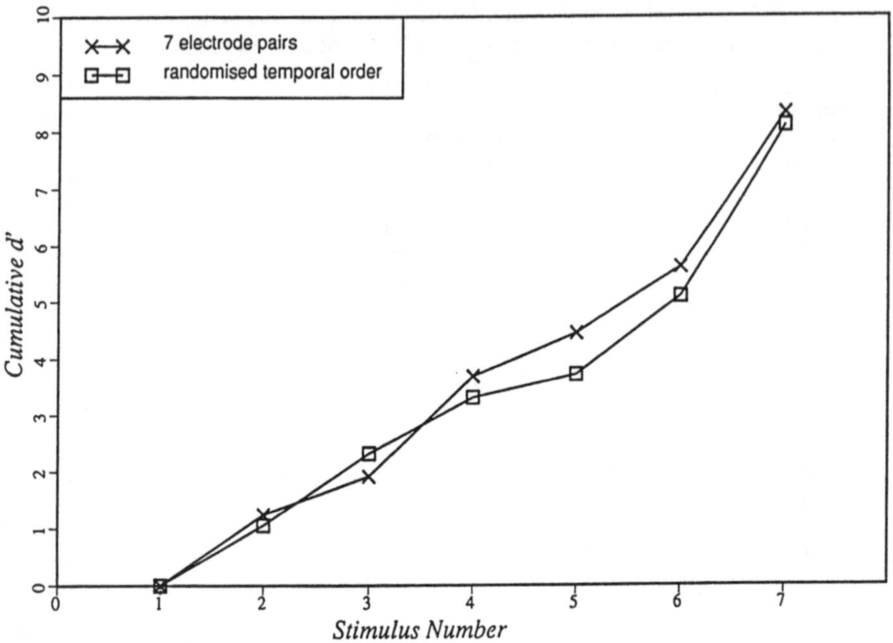

FIGURE 20.8. Cumulative d' curves for seven pulse trains of randomized temporal order and seven pulse trains with a single electrode pair in each period.

These results suggest that, despite the increase in loudness with current level, the pitch and timbre of the hearing sensation should not change significantly with electric current level. This lack of significant change in pitch and timbre with current was confirmed by a further psychophysical study which measured a patient's ability to identify different electrode positions at different current levels.

The results of a second forward-masking study indicate that the interaction between two electrode pairs activated in quick succession in a stimulus period is small, and the individual perceptual characteristics of the two electrode pairs are preserved. The results of a speech perceptual study using synthetic vowels indicate that useful information about the first two formants of speech can be conveyed to cochlear implant patients by activating two electrode pairs in quick succession in a stimulus period. These results suggest that by activating a number of electrode pairs in quick succession in a stimulus period, information about a corresponding number of spectral components of speech can be conveyed to cochlear implant patients.

Discrimination and identification studies were conducted to investigate the effects of the temporal order of the different electrode pairs in a stimulus period on perceptual characteristics. Pulse trains in which the temporal order was randomized from period to period were easily discriminated from those of a fixed temporal order, and produced scratchy and fussy hearing sensations. However, despite these fussy and scratchy characteristics, patients were able to identify these pulse trains of randomized temporal order in accordance with the tonotopic organization of the cochlea. These results suggest that the perceptual effects of temporal order do not significantly affect the identification of the overall electrode position of a pulse train, and that pulse trains of randomized temporal order could be useful in conveying information about unvoiced consonants and noiselike signals to cochlear implant patients.

The results described above also indicate that the tonotopic variation in perceptual characteristics produced by individual intracochlear electrode pairs is very robust. The tonotopic variation is retained at different stimulus current levels and in the presence of other nonsimultaneous electrode pairs; it is also not significantly affected by the temporal order of nonsimultaneously activated electrode pairs in a stimulus period. Further psychophysical and speech perceptual studies are being carried out on a larger number of patients to establish the generality of these results.

References

Clark, G.M., Pyman, B.C., and Bailey, Q.R. (1979). The surgery for multiple-electrode cochlear implantation, *J. Laryngol. Otol.* 93:215–223.

Lim, H.H., Tong, Y.C., and Clark, G.M. (1988). Forward masking patterns produced by intracochlear electrical stimulation of one and two electrode pairs in the human cochlea, *J. Acoust. Soc. Am.* (submitted for publication).

Stevens, S.S. (1935). The relation of pitch to intensity, *J. Acoust. Soc. Am.* 6:150–154.

Tong, Y.C., Lim, H.H., and Clark, G.M. (1988a). Synthetic vowel studies on cochlear implant patients, *J. Acoust. Soc. Am.* (in press).

Tong, Y.C., et al. (1988b). *Speech Processors for Auditory Prostheses.* Eleventh quarterly progress report, NIH Contract N01-NS-5-2388.

Y.C. Tong: Discussion

Dr. Dent: I just wanted to put your *d′* results in context. You showed a cumulative *d′* of 9 or 10. Was that your average or your best patient? The best we've ever gotten with a Stanford electrode, or with deconvolution on our patients, is 4 or 5, and that was on a pitch-ranking experiment, which is presumably less difficult than an absolute identification experiment. In addition, the step to vowel identification is surprising.

Apparently you reported the output bits of information (because you had some numbers that were greater than 1), and what we need to know is how that relates to the input bits.

Dr. Tong: The number of bits in our results refers to the amount of information transmitted. It is difficult to go from the d' results to the synthetic vowel results because of interaction between the perceived speech features.

Dr. Dent: Well, it's just the point that Bob Helfert tried to make, which was that our results look more impressive if we don't say what the relative amount of information was that was transmitted. So if you only have 1.5 bits in $F2$ and you transmitted 1.25, that looks very good. However, if you had 2 bits or more in $F2$ and transmitted 1.25 the it is not as effective.

Dr. Tong: About 1.5 bits: three categories.

Dr. Dent: The other question was about your masking patterns. Did you have any sense that they would corroborate what Don Eddington found? I noticed the patterns went to the left not to the right.

Dr. Tong: Our results are for bipolar stimulation, while Don Eddington's results are for monopolar stimulation. For monopolar stimulation, the earth is the basal region; there is, therefore, a large spread of current toward the base. For bipolar stimulation, the current distribution should be more restricted. However, when an electric current is passed between two electrodes in the cochlea, it is very difficult to predict the current path. There is definitely some evidence of a basal spread of current for our bipolar electrodes. However, to interpret the results properly, we must use a mathematical model with the right geometry.

Dr. Rabinowitz: I would like to follow up on that. There was noticeable noise in the masking pattern for the apical electrode. The masking first went down and then came up quite substantially.

Dr. Tong: The irregular masking pattern at the apical end could be the result of the proximity of the apical electrodes to the neural elements. For bipolar stimulation, using two apical electrodes that are close to the neural elements, the current distribution may consist of two peaks instead of one. The masking pattern is, therefore, likely to be irregular.

Dr. Wilson: In our studies with patients implanted with the UCSF electrode array, we see nice tonotopic rankings, similar to the one that you described, with small covariations between loudness and pitch, in the same direction that you described. That is, increases in loudness can produce small decreases in perceived pitch. In other patients we see strong covariation between loudness and pitch in the opposite direction. That is, when you increase stimulus intensity, you get huge increases in perceived pitch. One or two of these patients also have anomalous tonotopic rankings and high channel interactions and other presumptive signs of poor nerve survival. So it may be that in your series you were especially fortunate to get patients that are blessed with good nerve survival.

Dr. Tong: Or maybe it's the characteristics of the electrode array.

Dr. Wilson: There is some difference there.

Dr. Soli: Use of the *d′* measure implicity assumes that you are working with a unidimensional percept and that the spatial ordering of the electrodes corresponds to some kind of inner dimensional percept. What I would suggest is that you might want to look at the dimensionality of these percepts using something like multidimensional scaling. When we've done that with our patients, we've seen that the percepts corresponding to different places of stimulation are not unidimensional. We see that they may be two-dimensional. Your schematized confusions data suggest that perhaps some of the same things might be happening with your patients as well.

Dr. Tong: Well, if the two dimensions are used together as correlated information, then it doesn't really matter, but you can use multidimensional scaling and so on to look at it.

Dr. Smoorenburg: When you presented the vowel data it wasn't quite clear to me whether the F1-F2 coding was just the Nucleus type of stimulation where you pick out two electrodes or whether it was the full pattern that you were giving.

Dr. Tong: It was a Nucleus device. Just two electrodes, one corresponding to F1 and one corresponding to F2.

Dr. Smoorenburg: Suppose you would present the full spatial pattern. Did you try that?

Dr. Tong: We tried up to three formants, and it seemed to work in that significant information was transmitted for F1 to F3. We haven't tried a full spectrum, not in the synthetic setting.

21 Representations of Speech Features with Cochlear Implants

BLAKE S. WILSON, CHARLES C. FINLEY, AND DEWEY T. LAWSON

Introduction

The development and application of cochlear prostheses have improved the quality of life for many deaf individuals. Much work remains to be done, however, in order to achieve high levels of speech recognition in a majority of patients. In particular, we do not fully understand how different speech processor and implanted electrode designs affect the perception of speech and other sounds. Also, we have only fragmentary and primitive knowledge of how various differences among patients affect their outcomes.

The principal characteristics of five different cochlear implant systems are presented in Table 21.1. These characteristics include the type of electrode used, the number of stimulation channels, and the method for processing speech inputs. As is evident from the table, a tremendous diversity exists in current approaches to prosthesis design. Further details on the systems listed in Table 21.1 can be found in recent reviews (Gantz, 1987; Millar et al., 1984; Moore, 1985; Parkins, 1986; Pfingst, 1986) and in primary sources (Clark et al., 1987; Danley and Fretz, 1982; Eddington, 1983; Hochmair and Hochmair-Desoyer, 1985; Merzenich, 1985).

A remarkable finding from evaluations of the disparate approaches to prosthesis design is that several of these approaches can produce high levels of speech perception in some patients. Unfortunately, the converse is also true in that poor levels of performance are found for other patients using the same approaches.

These facts are illustrated in Table 21.2, which compares the average values and standard deviations of speech recognition scores for the three multichannel systems listed in Table 21.1. All the data presented in Table 21.2 were obtained from studies in which single presentations of recorded material were used. The data reported for the Nucleus device are those for the new "FO/F1/F2" processing strategy. Note that the standard deviations are large for all measures and devices. This variability reflects the observation that, for any of the listed devices, excellent performance

TABLE 21.1. Cochlear implant systems.

Device	Electrode(s)	Stimulus channels/ stimulus sites	Processing strategy
3M/House	Monopolar	1 / 1	Amplitude modulation of 16-kHz carrier
3M/Vienna	Longitudinal bipolar or extracochlear	1 / 1	Compressed analog with frequency equalization
Nucleus	Longitudinal bipolar	2 / 21	Feature extraction (F0, F1, and F2), pulsatile stimulation
Symbion	Monopolar	4 / 4	Compressed analog with filtering
Storz	Radial bipolar	4 / 4	Compressed analog with filtering

is found for some patients, while poor performance is found for others. Finally, it is worth noting that experience with an implant can have a profound effect on the scores for these (and other) tests. With the Storz device, for example, both the NU6 word and CID sentence scores show significant increase ($p < .02$ for the NU6 test and $p < .01$ for the CID test) from the 3-month to the 12-month studies.

Much of this heterogeneity of outcomes may be attributed to variation among patients. The importance of learning effects associated with experience has just been mentioned. Other potentially important variables include differences among patients in the survival of neural elements in the implanted ear, integrity of the central auditory pathways, and cognitive and language skills. The likely influence of patient variables on outcome obviously complicates comparisons aimed at identifying the best types of electrode and speech processor designs for cochlear prostheses. Indeed, such comparisons are not meaningful when small populations of

TABLE 21.2. Average percent correct scores for recognition of NU6 words and CID sentences with multichannel cochlear prostheses.*

Device	NU6	CID	N	Months postimplant	Citation
Nucleus	6.5 (6.4)	20.7 (19.5)	53/49†	3	Brimacombe et al., 1988
Symbion	8.5 (10.9)		11	>7	Gantz, 1987
Storz	7.6 (8.2)	21.0 (16.5)	14	3	Wilson et al., 1988d
	20.2 (15.0)	45.9 (26.8)	12	12	Wilson et al., 1988d

* The standard deviations of these scores are given in parentheses.
† N = 53 for the NU6 test, and N = 49 for the CID test.

subjects are used for the evaluation of each system or when test procedures used at the various laboratories involved in the evaluation of individual systems are different.

Recognition of the problem just described helped to initiate two major studies in which relatively large populations of patients implanted with different devices are being tested in a uniform and consistent manner. One of these studies is a cooperative effort among VA medical centers, and the other study is being conducted at the University of Iowa (Gantz et al., 1988). Results from these studies should be of great value in establishing expected levels of performance for contemporary cochlear prostheses.

A complementary method for the comparison of prosthesis systems is to evaluate different processing strategies and electrode coupling configurations in tests with the same implant patient. A key advantage of such tests is that controls are provided for patient variables. Thus, for a given patient with a fixed pattern of nerve survival and fixed levels of cognitive skill, etc., the performance levels of different prosthesis systems can be compared directly.

In recent studies conducted in collaboration with investigators at the University of California at San Francisco (UCSF) and at Duke University Medical Center, our team compared a variety of speech processing stragegies in tests with patients implanted with the UCSF/Storz electrode array (Wilson et al., 1988a; Wilson et al., 1988b, 1988c; Wilson et al., 1988d). Some of the largest differences in performance among processing strategies were found in comparisons between the compressed analog (CA) processor of the present UCSF/Storz prosthesis and a type of "interleaved pulses" (IP) processor which delivers pulses in sequence to the different channels in the implanted electrode array. To show how the design of the processor can affect the outcome for individual patients, we will restrict ourselves here to descriptions of tests to evaluate and compare the performance of these two processors. The emphasis will be on the results obtained in tests of consonant and vowel identification. In addition, results for the open-set tests of the Minimal Auditory Capabilities (MAC) battery (Owens et al., 1985) will be mentioned. Results for the full MAC battery and other tests of speech perception are presented elsewhere (Wilson et al. 1988b, 1988c; Wilson et al., 1988d).

Methods

Processing Strategies

In the clinical UCSF/Storz device, alternate pairs of the 16 available electrodes are stimulated simultaneously with the CA outputs of a four-channel speech processor. The basic functions of this processor are to compress the wide dynamic range of input speech signals into the narrow dynamic range available for electrical stimulation of the cochlea and then to filter the compressed signal into individual frequency bands for presentation to each pair of stimulated electrodes. Typical waveforms of the CA processor are shown in Figure 21.1. The top trace in each panel is the input signal, which in this case is the word "bought." The other waveforms in each panel are the filtered output signals for four channels of intracochlear stimulation. The bottom left panel shows an expanded display of waveforms during the initial part of the vowel in "bought," and

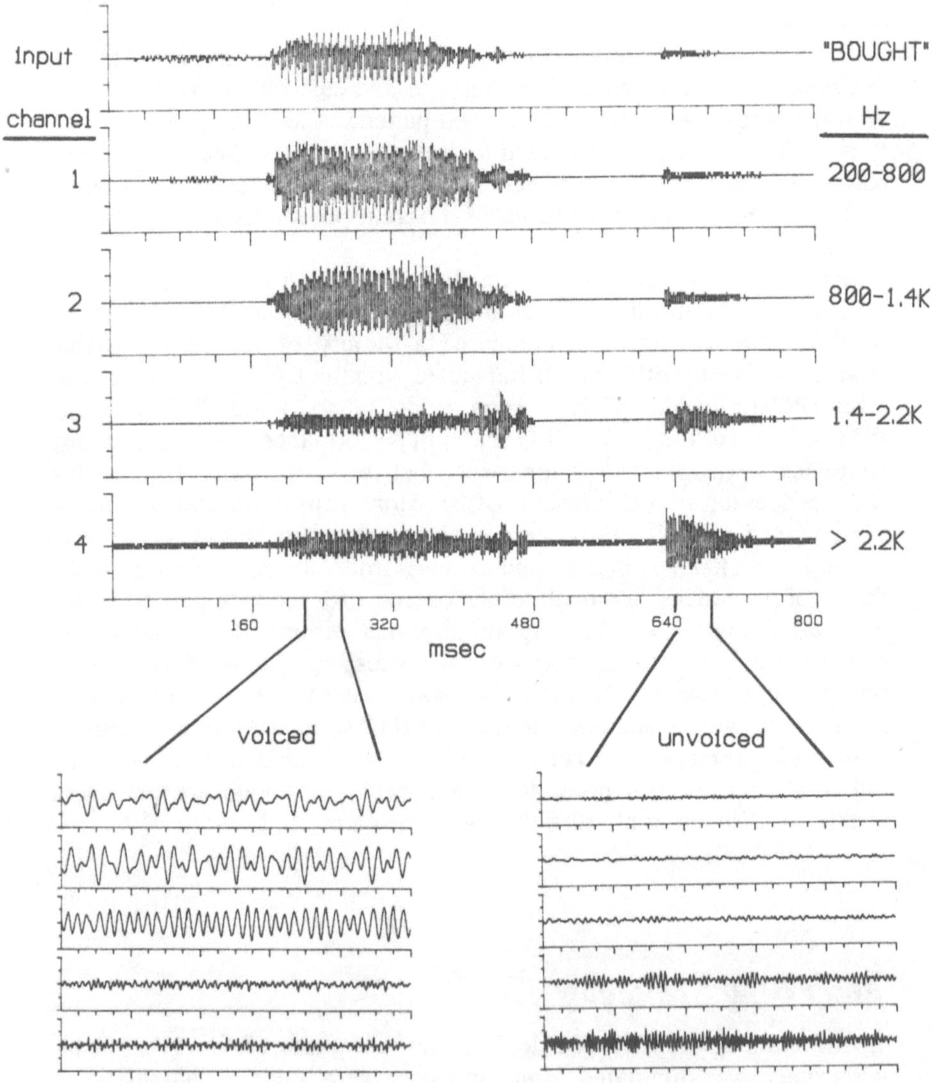

FIGURE 21.1. Waveforms of a CA processor.

the bottom right panel shows an expanded display of waveforms during the final /t/. The lower panels in Figure 21.1 thus exemplify differences in waveforms for voiced and unvoiced intervals of speech.

In the voiced interval the relatively large outputs of channels 1 and 2 reflect the low-frequency formant content of the vowel, and in the unvoiced interval the relatively large outputs of channels 3 and 4 reflect the high-frequency noise content of the /t/. In addition, the clear periodicity in the waveforms of channels 1 and 2 reflects the fundamental and first formant frequencies of the vowel during the voiced interval, and the lack of periodicity in the output of any channel reflects the noiselike quality of the /t/ during the unvoiced interval. As has been described elsewhere (Schindler and Kessler, 1987; Schindler et al., 1987; Schindler et al., 1986; Wilson et al., 1988d), this representation of speech features can support high levels of open-set recognition for many (but not all) of the patients implanted with the UCSF/Storz prosthesis.

A concern associated with the use of multichannel CA processors is that of channel interactions (White, Merzenich, and Gardi, 1984). Simultaneous stimulation of two or more channels with continuous waveforms results in summation of the electrical fields from the individual bipolar pairs of electrodes. This summation can exacerbate interactions among channels, especially for patients who require high stimulation levels. Summation of stimuli from multiple channels also depends on the phase relationships among the waveforms. Because these relationships are not controlled in a multichannel CA processor, representation of the speech spectrum may be further distorted by continuously changing patterns of channel interaction. A reduction of channel interactions might increase the salience of channel-related cues for implant patients.

The problem of channel interactions is addressed in the IP processor of Figure 21.2 through the use of nonsimultaneous stimuli. There is no temporal overlap between stimulus pulses, so that direct summation of electrical fields produced by different electrode channels is avoided. The energy in each frequency band of the input signal is coded as the amplitude of the pulses delivered to the corresponding stimulus channel. Distinctions between voiced and unvoiced segments of speech are represented by the timing of cycles of stimulation across the electrode array. In this particular processor stimulation cycles are timed to occur in synchrony with the detected fundamental frequency for voiced speech sounds and at the maximum rate (with one stimulation cycle immediately following its predecessor) for unvoiced speech sounds. The timing of stimulation cycles for voiced and unvoiced intervals can be seen in the lower panels of Figure 21.2.

Comparison of Figures 21.1 and 21.2 shows large differences in the stimuli presented for the CA and IP processing strategies. One might expect that the CA processing strategy would provide the greatest benefits to patients who could appreciate details in the stimulus wave-

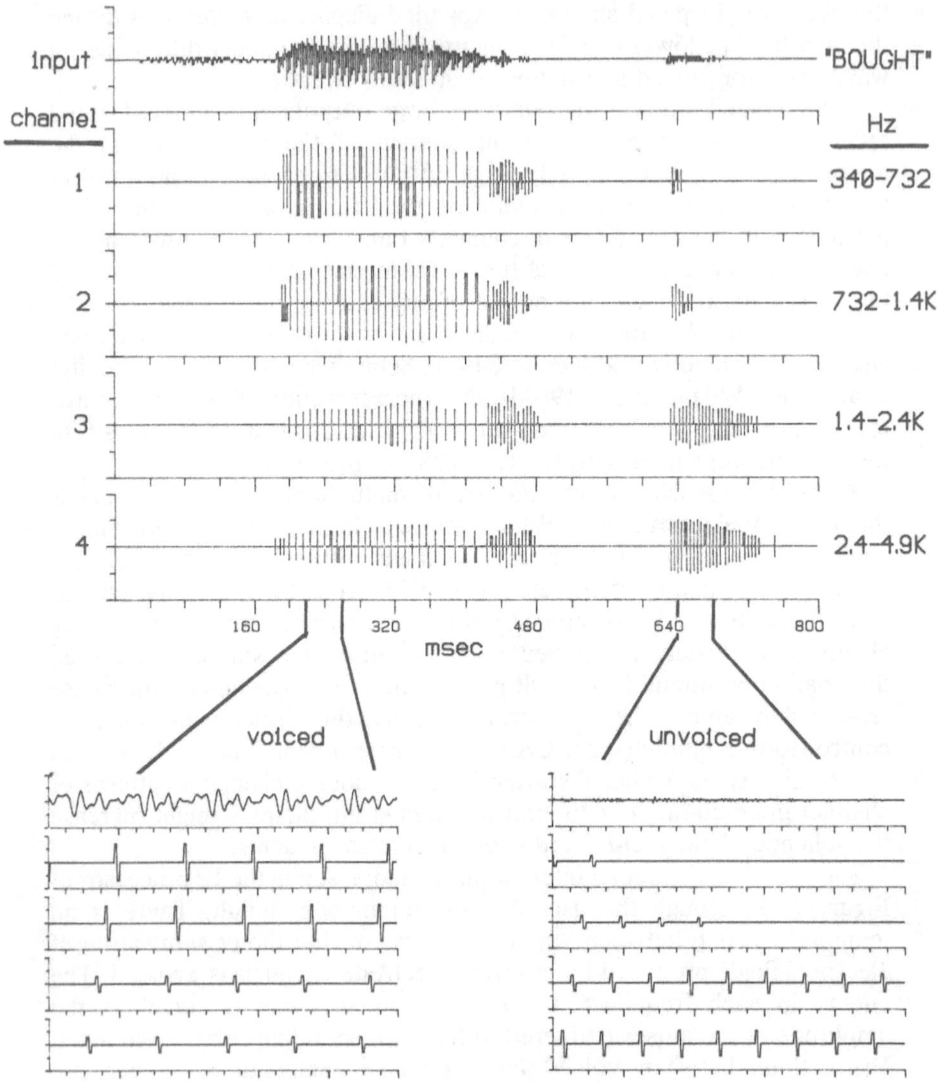

FIGURE 21.2. Waveforms of an IP processor.

forms (see above) and who have low thresholds of stimulation. In contrast, the IP processing strategy might be expected to provide superior performance for less fortunate patients who cannot make use of such details in CA stimulus waveforms and who have high thresholds of stimulation. We note that high thresholds of stimulation and high levels of measured channel interactions with simultaneous stimuli are both regarded as signs of poor nerve survival in the implanted ear (Gardi, 1985;

Merzenich et al., 1978; Pfingst and Sutton, 1983; White, Merzenich, and Gardi, 1984). Thus, application of an IP processor may confer special benefits for patients with poor nerve survival.

Subjects

Six patients implanted with the UCSF/Storz cochlear prosthesis (Loeb et al., 1983; Merzenich, 1985; Schindler et al., 1986; Wilson et al., 1988d) participated as subjects in this study. Tests with the CA processor were conducted with each patient's clinical device, and tests with the IP processor were conducted either with computer simulations (Wilson and Finley, 1985) or with a real-time, microprocessor-based instrument (Finley, Wilson, and Lawson, 1987).

It is important to note that certain attributes of these subjects favored the CA processor in comparisons of the CA and IP strategies. First, all six subjects entered the study with substantial experience using the CA processor. The average experience with this processor approximated 1 year of daily use. In contrast, experience with the IP processor was limited to that obtained in a 6-day period of testing with a variety of processors with each subject. As mentioned in the Introduction (and discussed in detail elsewhere—see Dowell et al., 1987; Tyler et al., 1986; and Wilson et al., 1988d), such a disparity in experience might strongly favor the CA processor.

An additional factor weighing against the IP processor was the use of the four-channel, UCSF/Storz transcutaneous transmission system (TTS). The principal limitations of that system for IP processors were (*a*) inadequate levels of voltage compliance for stimulation with short-duration pulses, (*b*) the small number of channels, and (*c*) lack of current control in the stimulus waveforms. Half of the subjects were further limited to fewer than four channels due to a mode of device failure (Schindler et al., 1986). Because optimized fittings of IP processors require at least six channels of stimulation and short-duration pulses (Wilson et al., 1988a; Wilson et al., 1988b), compromises had to be made in the fitting of IP processors for the subjects of this study.

The parameters selected for the IP processors used by each of the six subjects are presented in Table 21.3. The best fulfillments of the fitting criteria for IP processors (Wilson et al., 1988b) were obtained for subjects HE and MC2. Each had the use of all four stimulation channels, and the average pulse width across channels was 0.5 ms/phase or less for these two subjects.

In contrast, relatively poor sets of parameters had to be used for the remaining subjects. Subjects MC1 and JM had only three usable channels and subject RC only two. In addition, long pulse durations (1.0 ms) had to be used for subjects JM and ET.

TABLE 21.3. Parameters of IP processors.*

Subject	Channels	Pulse widths/phase (ms)	Pulse sep. (ms)	Cycle time (ms)
MC1	3	0.5	0.5	4.5
HE	4	0.5	0.5	6.0
JM	3	1.0	0.1	6.3
RC	2	0.5	0.1	2.2
ET	4	1.0	0.1	6.4
		1.0		
		0.5		
		0.5		
MC2	4	0.3	0.5	5.2
		0.7		
		0.3		
		0.3		

* All six processors used symmetrical biphasic pulses with positive phase leading and with the channels stimulated in base-to-apex order. Stimulation cycles were presented at the fundamental frequency for voiced intervals and at maximum rate (period equal to cycle time) during unvoiced intervals.

Tests

Most of the results reported in this paper are from tests of consonant and vowel identification. The consonants were presented in an /aCa/ context and the vowels in a /bVt/ context. Two consonant tests were used. The first was the one developed at the University of Iowa for measurement of audiovisual consonant perception (Tyler, Preece, and Lowder, 1983). A videotape of an adult male speaker provided the visual component of each presentation. The audio track of the tape provided an input to the UCSF/Storz processor or the real-time IP processor via direct connection. The consonants were /p, b, m, f, v, ʃ, dʑ, s, z, t, d, n, g, k/. Each consonant was presented five times in a randomized list of stimulus presentations. After each presentation, the subject responded by pointing to one choice in a table of the 14 response options. No feedback on correct or incorrect responses was provided. Finally, the order of testing for the different conditions was designed to confer any benefits of learning on the CA processor. The order was first to test the IP processor plus vision, then vision alone, and then the CA processor plus vision.

A matrix of stimuli and responses was compiled for each subject and condition. The matrices were then summed across subjects for each of the conditions. These summed matrices provided the inputs to the analyses described in the Results section of this paper. The raw summed matrices may be found in Appendix 21.1.

The second consonant test was one suggested by Earl Schubert (1985) to assess the ability to distinguish the nonlabial consonants with the greatest frequencies of occurrence in spoken English. These consonants include /ð, s, z, t, d, n, k, l/ and are difficult or impossible to distinguish with speech-reading alone (particularly /s, z, t, d, n/). Schubert reasoned that a pragmatic approach to processor design and evaluation would be to concentrate on these eight important (but largely invisible) consonants. The primary purpose of the vowel test was to measure the ability to discriminate relatively large differences among the selected vowels in the frequencies of the first and second formants. The vowels included /i, I, ɔ, o, u/.

Single exemplars of the tokens in the last two tests (hereafter called the RTI tests) were recorded and digitized from representative utterances of an adult male speaker. The digitized tokens were used as inputs to the UCSF/Storz processor (after appropriate digital-to-analog conversion) or the computer simulation of the IP processor. A single block of trials included three presentations of each of the consonants or five presentations each of the vowels in random order. Multiple repetitions of a token were available at regular intervals during each presentation. At the beginning of each presentation a display of response options was shown on a computer terminal used by the subject. The subject responded by touching a key on the terminal. Usually a response was entered after the first or second repetition. At the end of a block, the subject was given the overall percent correct score and an indication of the principal confusions made during the test. With few exceptions, no feedback was given during a block. In the exceptional cases (12 out of 137 blocks), feedback was provided across conditions so that no processor would receive an advantage over another.

The conditions for both RTI tests included vision only, CA processor plus vision, IP processor plus vision, CA processor only, and IP processor only. For the conditions with a visual component, speech-reading information was provided by miming the tokens in synchrony with the stimulus repetitions. The same person (DTL) mimed the tokens for all subjects.

Blocks of trials were repeated as time permitted during the 6 days of testing with each subject. Because many other tests were being conducted during this same period (Wilson et al., 1988b, 1988c; Wilson, et al., 1988d), the total number of trials for the RTI tests was not uniform across subjects and conditions. The actual totals are presented in Table 21.4. For the great majority of subjects and conditions, the number of trials with each token for the consonant test was 6 or more, and the number for the vowel test was 10 or more.

As with the Iowa test, matrices of stimuli and responses were compiled for all subjects and conditions. Each RTI matrix was normalized to show the fraction of responses in each cell, and the normalized matrices were then summed across subjects for each of the conditions. The estimates of matrix responses calculated in this way reflect balanced contributions

TABLE 21.4. Number of presentations of each token in the RTI tests for the indicated subjects.

		Condition*				
Test	Subject	V	CA+V	IP+V	CA	IP
Consonant	MC1	3	9	15	9	18
	HE	6	6	9	3	9
	JM	9	9	6	9	6
	RC	6	6	9	6	12
	ET	3	6	6	9	6
	MC2	6	3	6	3	6
Vowel	MC1	10	15	10	15	10
	HE	10	10	30	15	15
	JM	15	10	5	10	5
	RC	10	10	10	10	10
	ET	5	10	5	10	5
	MC2	10	10	10	10	10

* Abbreviations are V for vision, CA+V for compressed analog plus vision, IP+V for interleaved pulses plus vision, CA for compressed analog only, and IP for interleaved pulses only.

from all subjects for each condition while still using all of the available data. The final matrices for the RTI tests may be found in Appendix 21.1.

In addition to the tests of consonant and vowel identification, the CA and IP processors were further evaluated with an extensive series of speech perception tests. These additional tests included all subtests of the MAC battery (Owens et al., 1985), the Diagnostic Discrimination Test (DDT) of consonant confusions (Grether, 1970), and connected discourse tracking with and without the prosthesis (De Felippo and Scott, 1978; Owens and Raggio, 1987). The results from the subtests of the MAC battery designed to measure open-set recognition will be discussed in this paper. Results from the full MAC battery, along with the results from the other tests, are presented elsewhere (Wilson et al., 1988b, 1988c; Wilson et al., 1988d).

Results

Percent Correct Scores

The means and standard deviations of overall percent correct scores for the tests of consonant and vowel identification are presented in Table 21.5. To compare results among the conditions for each test, a randomized-blocks analysis of variance (ANOVA) was conducted with the subjects as blocks and the conditions as the second factor. For the Iowa consonant test a significant effect of conditions was found [$F(2,10) = 20.56$; $p < .001$]. Post hoc comparison of the means using the

TABLE 21.5. Means and standard deviations (SD) of consonant and vowel identification scores in percent correct.

	Iowa consonants		RTI consonants		RTI vowels	
Condition*	Mean	SD	Mean	SD	Mean	SD
Vision only	33.3	5.3	42.0	8.3	83.4	8.7
CA + vision	54.5	16.6	69.6	13.6	94.0	2.5
CA only			51.8	12.6	86.0	5.1
IP + vision	64.0	6.7	79.7	13.0	87.3	9.9
IP only			65.8	14.6	83.3	10.8

* Abbreviations are CA for compressed analog processor and IP for interleaved pulses processor.

Tukey multiple comparisons procedure showed that the means for both processor-plus-vision conditions are significantly higher than the mean for the vision-only condition ($p < .01$, both processors). However, the difference between means for the processor-plus-vision conditions is not significant ($p > .05$).

A significant effect of conditions was also found for the RTI consonant test [$F(4,20) = 22.23$; $p < .001$]. Post hoc comparison of the means, with the Tukey procedure, can be summarized as follows:

1. The means for the processor-plus-vision conditions are significantly higher than the mean for the vision-only condition ($p < .01$, both processors).
2. The difference between means for the processor-plus-vision conditions is not significant.
3. The mean for the IP-only condition is significantly higher than the mean for the CA-only condition ($p < .05$).
4. The means for both processor-plus-vision conditions are significantly higher than the means for the processor-only conditions ($p < .01$ for the CA processor and $p < .05$ for the IP processor).
5. The mean for the IP-only condition is significantly higher than the mean for the vision-only condition ($p < .01$).
6. None of the differences among means for the remaining combinations of conditions is significant.

Finally, no significant differences among conditions were found for the RTI vowel test [$F(4,20) = 2.81$; $p > .05$]. We note that scores are quite high for all conditions of this test. Possibly, true differences among conditions may have been masked by ceiling effects, and if so, a more difficult test might demonstrate such differences.

Information Transmission Analysis

Although overall percent correct scores can serve as a rough indication of processor performance, they provide little or no insight into the strengths and weaknesses of specific strategies. That is, the *pattern* of confusions (and correct responses) in a consonant or vowel identification test can provide much more detailed information on processor performance than the overall percent correct score.

To evaluate the patterns of confusions for the conditions of this study, the combined matrix for the responses of all subjects for each condition (see Appendix 21.1) was used as an input to the information transmission (IT) analysis described by Miller and Nicely (1955). In this analysis the "relative transinformation" is calculated for selected articulatory or acoustic features of the phonemes in the identification tests. The relative transinformation score for each feature, expressed here as percent information transfer, indicates how well that feature was transmitted to the subjects. The consonant features selected for the present study were voicing (voice), nasality (nasal), place of articulation (place), duration (durat), frication (fric), envelope cues (envel), and visual cues (viseme). The vowel features were first formant frequency (F1), second formant frequency (F2), duration (durat), and visual cues (viseme). Assignments of these features for the phonemes in the Iowa and RTI tests may be found in Appendix 21.2.

The results from IT analysis of the Iowa consonant matrices are presented in Figure 21.3. The open bars show IT scores for the vision-only condition, the bars with diagonal lines show the scores for the CA-processor-plus-vision condition, and the solid bars show the scores for the IP-processor-plus-vision condition. Note that the viseme and place features are transmitted equally well for all three conditions. The high score for place in the vision-only condition is indicative of the high

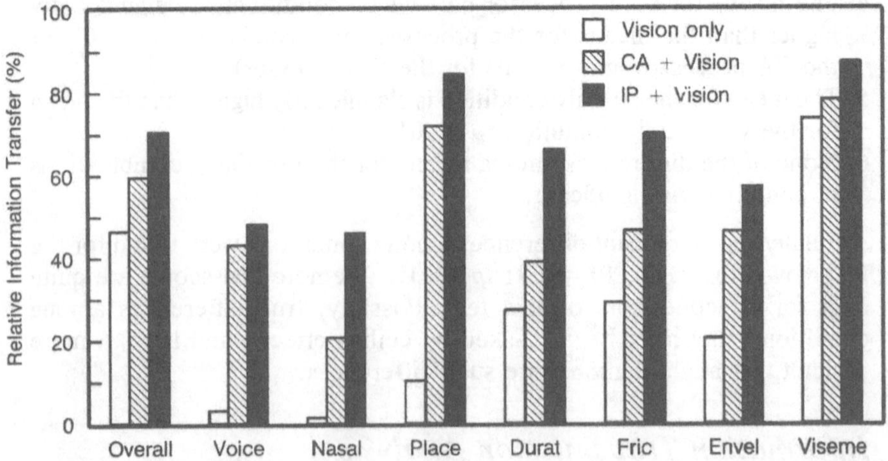

FIGURE 21.3. Relative information transfer of speech features for the Iowa consonant test.

redundancy between assignments for the place and viseme features. That is, a front (bilabial and labiodental) place of articulation usually can be distinguished from other places of articulation through speech-reading alone (Owens and Blazek, 1985), and this ability is reflected in the choices for the viseme groupings. Thus, if subjects can distinguish the groups /p,b,m,f,v/, /ʃ, dʒ/, and /d,s,z,t,d,n,g,k/ through speechreading, then the scores for both viseme and place will be high.

Other features that exhibit some redundancy with the viseme groupings are duration and frication. The relatively high scores for these features with vision alone reflect this overlap. On the other hand, the scores for voicing, nasality, and envelope are all low for the vision-only condition. These features are invisible on the lips and have little or no redundancy with the viseme groupings.

The scores for both processor-plus-vision conditions demonstrate increases over the scores for the vision-only condition. Especially large increases are found for the features of voicing, duration, and envelope. In addition, the scores for overall information transfer are higher for the processor-plus-vision conditions.

Comparison of the scores obtained with the two processors indicates superiority of the IP processor for all features except place and viseme, where the scores are about the same. Scores for the IP processor are much higher for the features of voicing, nasality, and envelope. Inasmuch as these are the very features that have little or no redundancy with the viseme groupings, the IP processor might be expected to provide a highly effective supplement to speech-reading.

The general finding of superior performance with the IP processor is also evident in the results from IT analysis of the RTI consonant matrices. Results for the vision-only and processor-plus-vision conditions are presented in Figure 21.4, and results for the processor-only conditions are presented in Figure 21.5. In Figure 21.4 the open, diagonally lined and solid bars again show IT scores for vision only, CA processor plus vision, and IP processor plus vision, respectively. In Figure 21.5 the stippled bars show IT scores for the CA processor only, and the vertically lined bars show the scores for the IP processor only.

For the conditions with a visual component (Figure 21.4), high scores again are obtained for the viseme feature. Because the consonants in the RTI test all have a nonlabial place of articulation, however, high scores for the viseme feature merely show that the groups /s,z,t,d,n/, /k,l/, and /ð/ can be distinguished. /ð/ and /l/ usually are visible through tongue protrusion and tongue flap, respectively, even though they have nonlabial places of articulation. Perception of these cues for /ð/ and /l/ can produce relatively high viseme scores for the consonants in the RTI test.

Another effect of the choice of consonants for the RTI test is to hold place of articulation essentially constant. All consonants except /k/ have a mid place of articulation (Singh and Black, 1966). Thus, the only

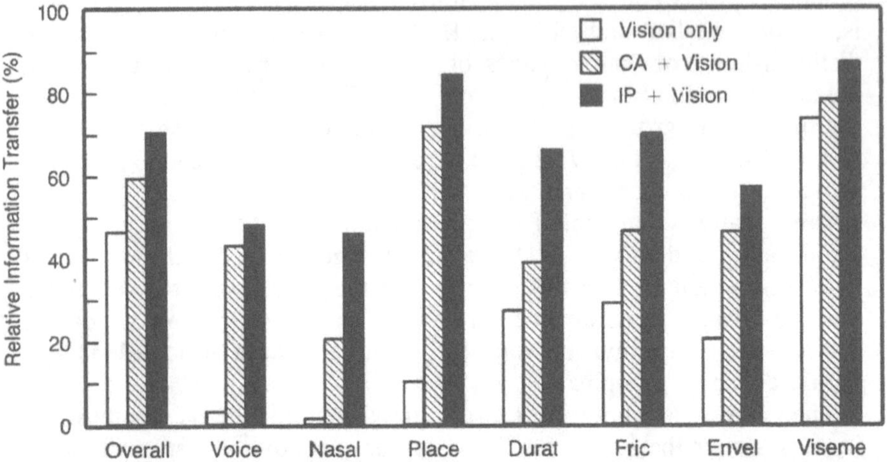

FIGURE 21.4. Relative information transfer of speech features for the vision-only and vision-plus-processor conditions of the RTI consonant test.

distinction that has to be made to produce high place scores is the one between /k/ (back place of articulation) and the remaining consonants. The low place score for the vision-only condition in Figure 21.4 reflects the fact that the place and viseme features are not redundant for the particular consonants of the RTI test. The scores for all other features (voicing, nasality, duration, frication, and envelope) are generally consistent with the scores for the vision-only condition of the Iowa test.

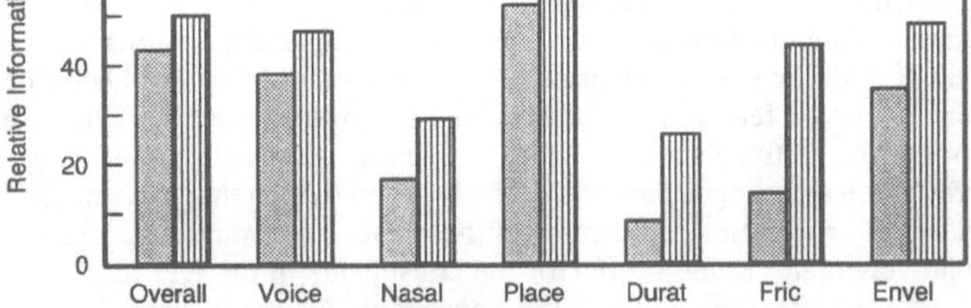

FIGURE 21.5. Relative information transfer of speech features for the processor-only conditions of the RTI consonant test.

Comparison of results across conditions again shows increases over the vision-only scores when either processor is used with speech-reading. The largest increases are found for the features of voicing, nasality, place, and envelope. The increases for voicing and envelope are quite similar to those found for the Iowa test. The increases for nasality and place, however, are not seen (place) or not as large (nasality) in the Iowa results. The difference in the increases for place can be attributed to the particular choice of consonants in the RTI test, as outlined above. The difference in the increases for nasality is one of degree in that increases are found for both tests, but the relative increase for the CA processor plus vision over vision only is not as large for the Iowa test compared with the increase for the RTI test. This difference between tests again might be a consequence of the different choices of consonants: the only nasal in the RTI test is /n/, while the Iowa test contains /n/ and /m/. The single distinction of /n/ from the remaining consonants may allow higher scores for the nasal feature in the RTI test.

As with the Iowa test, large increases are found in feature transmission scores when the IP processor is used instead of the CA processor for the vision-plus-processor conditions. The IP processor produces at least some increase in the score for every studied feature, and substantial increases are demonstrated for the features of nasality, duration, and frication. The same pattern of increases is evident in the scores for the Iowa test; however, the relative increases for the voicing and envelope features are greater with the Iowa test, while the relative increases for the duration and frication features are greater with the RTI test. These differences probably can be attributed to the differences in the consonant sets and to test variability. In all, the patterns of results from the Iowa and RTI tests are remarkably consistent. Both patterns demonstrate substantial gains over vision alone when either processor is used in conjunction with speech-reading, and both patterns shown superiority of the IP processor. In addition, the particular differences in feature scores found between conditions for one of the tests usually are found for the other test as well.

The results from the RTI test for the processor-only conditions (Figure 21.5) mirror those reviewed above for the processor-plus-vision conditions (Figure 21.4). Specifically, the IP processor again produces an increase in the score for every studied feature, and substantial increases are found for the features of nasality, duration, and frication. Moreover, for all features the ratios of the scores for the CA-processor-plus-vision and IP-processor-plus-vision conditions (Figure 21.4) closely approximate the ratios for the CA-processor-only and IP-processor-only conditions (Figure 21.5). These findings suggest that the IP processor provides additional cues which are utilized by the subjects in both the hearing-only and hearing-plus-vision conditions.

In contrast to the results from the Iowa and RTI consonant tests, the IT scores from the RTI vowel test indicate superiority of the CA processor. These scores for the vowel test are presented in Figure 21.6, where the coding of the bars for the various conditions is identical to the coding used in Figures 21.3 to 21.5. Comparison of the IT scores between processors shows that the CA processor produces higher or equivalent scores for every feature. For the processor-plus-vision conditions higher scores are obtained for overall transmission, F1, and duration; and for the processor-only conditions higher scores are obtained for these features and F2. In the cases where equivalent scores are found (F2 and viseme features, processor-plus-vision conditions), ceiling effects may have masked true differences between the processors. A more difficult test (with, for example, more vowels and less redundancy between assignments for the F2 and viseme features) would provide a more sensitive detector of any difference between processors. In any event, the present results show that the CA processor is superior at least for the transmission of F1 and duration information.

The most general observations from the IT data reviewed above are that (*a*) the IP processor produces higher or essentially equivalent scores for every studied feature of the phonemes in the Iowa and RTI consonant tests and (*b*) the opposite is found for every studied feature of the phonemes in the RTI vowel test. To evaluate the significance of these observations, a blocked ANOVA was conducted for each test with the features as blocks and the processor-plus-vision and processor-only conditions as the second factor. Because the objective was to compare the contributions of the two processors, the viseme feature was not included in the analysis. The ANOVA results supported the general

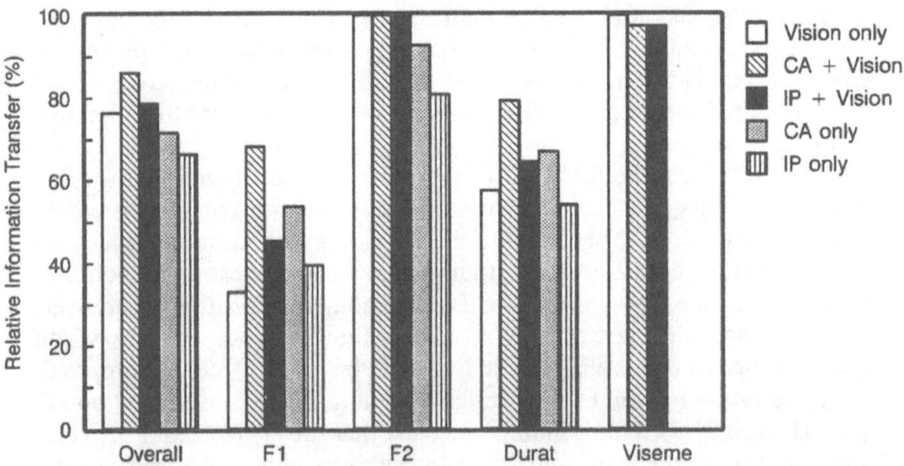

FIGURE 21.6. Relative information transfer of speech features for the RTI vowel test.

observations for each of the three tests. In particular, significant effects of conditions were found for all three tests [for the Iowa consonant test $F(1,6) = 18.19$ and $p < .01$; for the RTI consonant test $F(2,18) = 19.92$ and $p < .001$; and for the RTI vowel test $F(3,9) = 18.33$ and $p < .001$]. The significant effect for the Iowa test demonstrated superior performance of the IP processor ($p < .01$). Post hoc comparison of the means for the four conditions of the RTI consonant test (using the Tukey procedure) also demonstrated superiority of the IP processor (for the processor-plus-vision conditions $p < .01$, and for the processor-only conditions $p < .05$). Finally, post hoc comparison of the means for the RTI vowel test demonstrated superiority of the CA processor (for both sets of processor conditions, with and without vision, $p < .05$).

Sequential Information Analysis

As noted above, interpretation of the results from IT analysis is complicated by the presence of redundancies in feature assignments for the phonemes in the identification test. Because some features are highly redundant with others (e.g., viseme and place for the Iowa consonant test), IT analysis cannot determine the extent to which each separate feature is used by the subjects in making their judgments. To address this problem of IT analysis, Wang and Bilger (1973) developed a procedure designed to remove the effects of redundancies among features. In this procedure, called sequential information analysis (SINFA), the unconditional IT scores are first calculated for all features, as in the standard procedure for IT analysis. Then the feature with the highest score for percent information transfer is identified and held constant for subsequent iterations of IT analysis. In the subsequent iterations any redundancies between the previously identified feature and the remaining features are removed by holding the identified feature constant. At the conclusion of each iteration the remaining feature with the highest information transmission score is identified and added to those being held constant for all subsequent iterations. Iterations continue until all features have been examined or until the remaining features can account for less than 1% of the total received information. The final output of SINFA thus consists of a sequence of the features that are most salient at each successive iteration. In addition, the SINFA results indicate the relative contribution of each feature (in the same sequence) to the pattern of judgments made by the subjects.

SINFA results for the Iowa consonant test are presented in Figure 21.7. For each of the three conditions the order of identified features is indicated from left to right (where the leftmost bar in the panel for each condition shows the first-identified or most salient feature for that condition), and the relative contribution of each feature is indicated by the length of its bar. The full width of each panel corresponds to 100%. Thus,

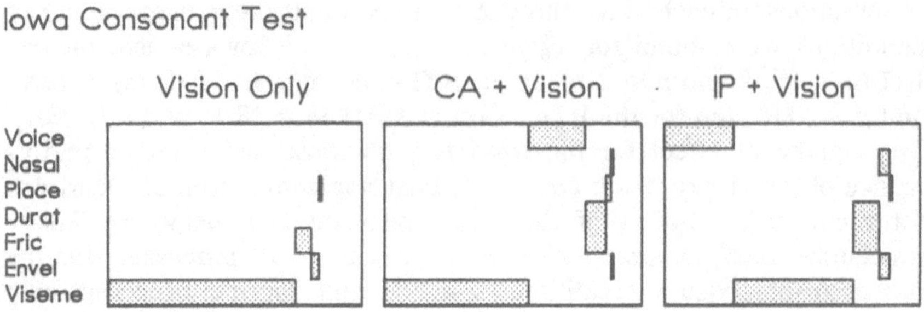

FIGURE 21.7. Sequential information analyses of results from the three conditions of the Iowa consonant test.

the rightmost extent of the bar for the last-identified feature indicates the proportion of the received information that is explained by all identified features. This proportion, in turn, indicates how completely the identified features can account for the subjects' observed judgments. The assignments across phonemes for two or more features (see Appendix 21.2) can become identical in subsequent iterations of SINFA as more and more features are held constant. In cases where multiple features with identical assignment patterns are identified as most salient in a SINFA iteration, bars are shown for all such features for that iteration. For example, the third bar (from left to right) in the panel for the CA-processor-plus-vision condition indicates that (*a*) the features of duration and frication had identical assignment patterns at the third SINFA iteration and (*b*) the combined "duration/frication" feature was most salient for that iteration.

Returning now to the results of Figure 21.7, SINFA demonstrates large contributions of visual inputs to the judgments made for all three conditions. For the vision-only condition the viseme feature accounts for 74% of the received information, and for the CA-processor-plus-vision and IP-processor-plus-vision conditions this feature accounts for 56% and 47% of the received information, respectively. As might be expected, the viseme feature is most salient for the vision-only condition. In addition, the remaining features identified by SINFA for this condition account for only 10% of the received information.

The viseme feature is also most salient for the CA-processor-plus-vision condition. However, other features now make substantial contributions to the judgments. Most salient among these other features are voicing (22%) and frication/duration (8%).

In contrast to the dominance of the viseme feature for the judgments of the vision-only and CA-processor-plus-vision conditions, the first-identified feature for the IP-processor-plus-vision condition is voicing (27%). This finding suggests that an auditory cue is most important for making the judgments of this latter condition, even when speech-reading information is presented. Other auditory cues contributing to the judgments are frication/duration (10%) and nasal/envelope (4%).

As can be appreciated from the rightmost extents of the final bars in each panel of Figure 21.7, the selected features account well for the patterns of judgments. The proportion of received information explained by these features for the vision-only condition is 84%, and the proportions for the two processor-plus-vision conditions are both 89%.

SINFA results for the five conditions of the RTI consonant test are presented in Figure 21.8. Large contributions of visual inputs are again demonstrated for the three conditions with a visual component. The viseme feature is the most salient feature for each of these conditions. The proportions of received information accounted for by this feature are 68%, 57%, and 54% for the vision-only, CA-processor-plus-vision, and IP-processor-plus-vision conditions, respectively. As might be expected, the greatest proportion is found for the vision-only condition.

In addition to the contributions made by visual inputs, results for the two processor-plus-vision conditions show that substantial contributions are made by auditory inputs. In the CA-processor-plus-vision condition these latter contributions include place (13%), frication/duration (10%), and voicing (11%), and in the IP-processor-plus-vision condition these contributions include place (11%), frication/duration (17%), nasality (6%), and voicing/envelope (6%). Note that place and frication/duration are salient features for both processor-plus-vision conditions. Also note that features other than the viseme feature make a greater contribution to the judgments made for the IP-processor-plus-vision condition (40%)

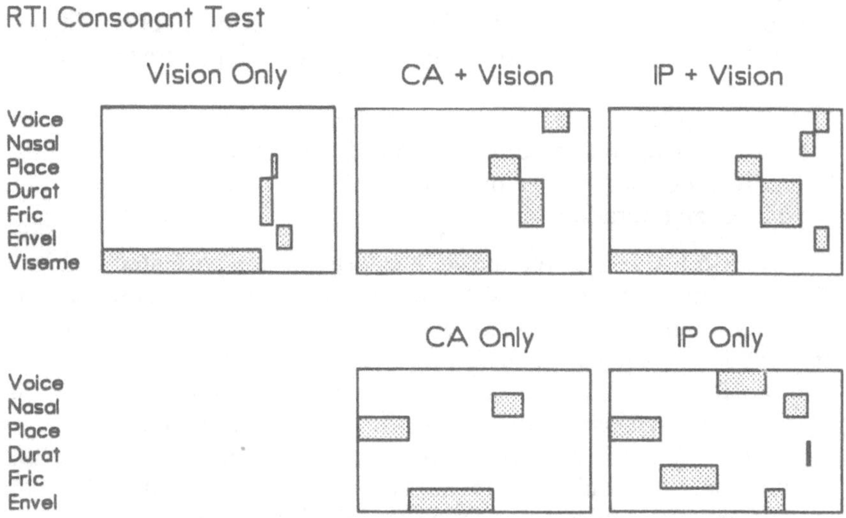

FIGURE 21.8. Sequential information analyses of results from the five conditions of the RTI consonant test.

compared with the contribution for the CA-processor-plus-vision condition (34%). A large part of the difference between the two conditions is the demonstrated access to the nasality feature with the IP processor, which is not found with the CA processor. The IP processor also appears to provide greater access to frication/duration information and to envelope information.

Greater access to nonvisual features of consonants is also demonstrated for the IP processor in the processor-only conditions. Three features are identified by SINFA for the CA processor (place, 22%; envelope, 36%; and nasality, 13%), while all six nonvisual features are identified for the IP processor (place, 22%; frication, 24%; voicing, 21%; envelope, 8%; nasality, 10%; and duration, 1%). In addition, the identified features explain a greater proportion of the received information with the IP processor (86%) than with the CA processor (71%).

To summarize the SINFA results for the consonant tests, we note the following:

1. The viseme feature accounts for a large percentage of the received information for all conditions with a visual component.
2. The viseme feature is the most salient feature for all of these conditions except the IP-processor-plus-vision condition, for which the feature of voicing is most salient.
3. The addition of processor inputs increases access to features other than the viseme feature.
4. Among the most salient of these other features are voicing (both processors, Iowa test), duration/frication (both processors, Iowa and RTI tests), and place (both processors, RTI test).
5. The IP processor further provides access to the features of nasality and envelope for the processor-plus-vision conditions (Iowa and RTI tests).
6. Both processors provide access to place, nasality, and envelope features for the processor-only conditions (RTI test).
7. The IP processor further provides access to the features of frication, voicing, and duration.

Finally, SINFA results for the RTI vowel test are presented in Figure 21.9. As with the consonant tests, the viseme feature is most salient, and accounts for the great majority of received information, for the vision-only condition. Unlike the results from the consonant tests, however, an acoustic feature (F2) is more salient than the viseme feature for the processor-plus-vision conditions. Also, an identical pattern of feature rankings is found for these latter conditions, i.e., F2, viseme, and F1/duration. The only difference between the processors is in the proportions of received information explained by the different features. The proportions of the F2 and viseme features are higher for the IP processor (53% versus 48% for F2, and 28% versus 26% for viseme), and

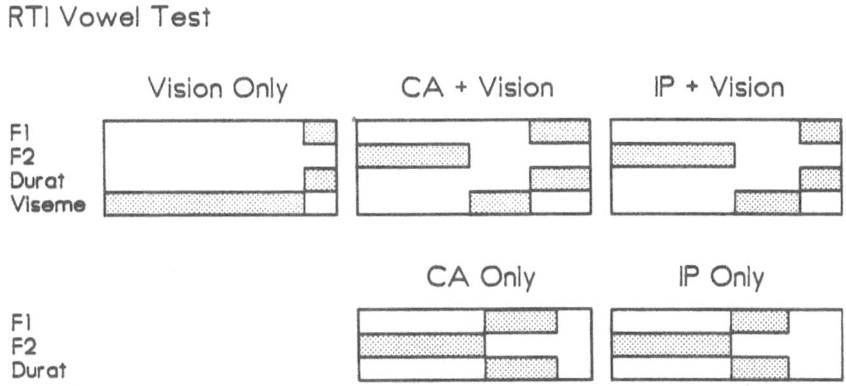

FIGURE 21.9. Sequential information analyses of results from the five conditions of the RTI vowel test.

the proportion of the combined F1/duration feature is substantially higher for the CA processor (26% versus 18%). These differences are consistent with the clearly superior IT scores of the CA processor for F1 and duration (Figure 21.6).

Greater access to F1 and duration cues is also demonstrated for the CA processor in the SINFA results for the processor-only conditions. As shown in the bottom panels of Figure 21.9, the amount of received information accounted for by the combined F1/duration feature is substantially higher for the CA processor (31%) than for the IP processor (25%). Also, the amount of received information explained by the F2 feature is somewhat higher for the CA processor (54% versus 51%).

In summary, the CA processor provides greater access to the combined F1/duration feature in both the processor-plus-vision and processor-only conditions. This processor may also provide greater access to the F2 feature in the processor-only conditions.

Open-Set Recognition Scores

The most difficult tests normally administered to assess the performance of patients with cochlear implants are tests of open-set recognition. Good performance on these tests probably requires a host of linguistic and cognitive skills that are not tapped in tests of consonant and vowel identification. That is, the open-set tests help to evaluate the integration of segmental identification (consonants and vowels), prosodic cues, and contextual information. The open-set tests thus provide complex measures of the representation of speech sounds at the auditory periphery and the interpretation of this representation in the central nervous system. Also, in terms of the "bottom line" for implant patients, the open-set tests mimic many aspects of everyday listening situations.

Results from the open-set tests of the MAC battery for the subjects and processors of this study are presented in Figure 21.10. The tests include those of spondee recognition (Sp), recognition of monosyllabic words from Northwestern University list 6 (NU6), recognition of everyday sentences from lists prepared at the Central Institute for the Deaf (CID), and recognition of single words in the context of sentences (WIC). The results for the CA processor are indicated by the stippled bars, and the results for the IP processor are indicated by the vertically lined bars.

Comparison of the results across subjects for each of the open-set tests demonstrates that there are no significant differences between processors (paired $t < 1.71$ and $p < .10$ for all tests). However, substantial differences are found among subjects both in terms of overall performance and in terms of the scores for the two processors. Subjects MC1, RC, and MC2 have excellent performance with both processors, while the remaining subjects have either moderate (HE and JM) or poor (ET) performance with both processors. Between processors, subject RC has higher scores with the CA processor for all four tests and subject MC2 has higher scores with the IP processor for all four tests. Paired-t comparisons between processors for these tests show that the CA processor is significantly

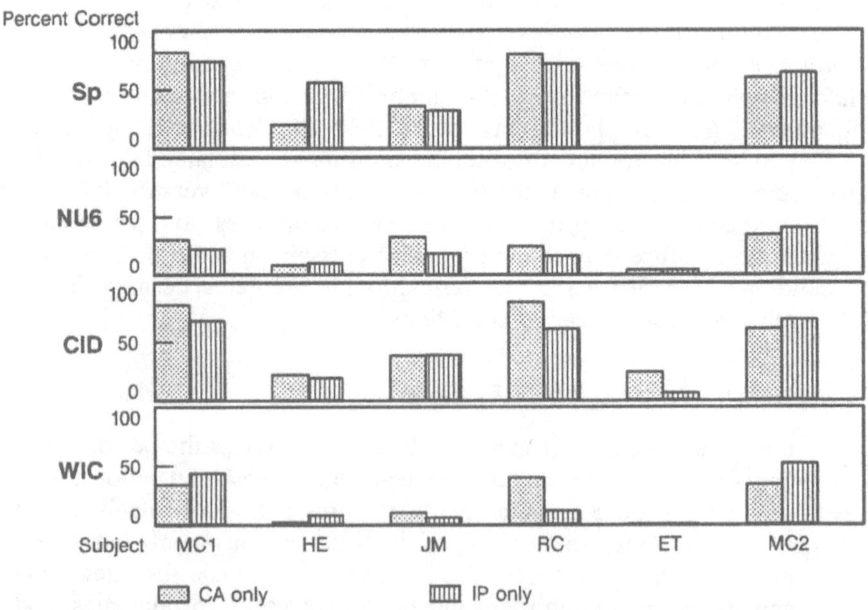

FIGURE 21.10. Results from subtests of the MAC battery designed to measure open-set recognition of speech. Abbreviations for the subtests are Sp for spondee recognition, NU6 for recognition of monosyllabic words from Northwestern University list 6, CID for recognition of everyday sentences from lists prepared at the Central Institute for the Deaf, and WIC for recognition of words in context.

better for subject RC (paired $t = 3.25$; $p < .05$) and that the IP processor is marginally better for subject MC2 (paired $t = 2.90$; $p < .10$). No significant differences are found between processors for the remaining subjects (paired $t < 1.67$; $p > .10$).

Discussion

In this study the CA and IP processors were compared in tests with six subjects implanted with the UCSF/Storz cochlear prosthesis. The tests included those of consonant and vowel identification and of open-set recognition. Each subject had the use of two to four channels of intracochlear stimulation via the UCSF/Storz transcutaneous transmission system (TTS). Also, each subject had had considerable experience with the CA processor when the processors were compared.

Large differences between processors were demonstrated in the results from the consonant and vowel tests. In general, the IP processor produced superior results for consonant identification and the CA processor produced superior results for vowel identification. The principal gains for consonants were in the transmission of information on voicing, nasality, envelope, frication, and duration, and the principal gains for vowels were in the transmission of information on F1 and duration. Results from the tests of open-set recognition indicated an overall equivalence of the two processors across subjects. For particular subjects, however, one processor provided better performance than the other. Subject RC obtained higher scores with the CA processor for all four open-set tests, and subject MC2 obtained higher scores with the IP processor for all four tests.

Representations of Speech Features

The differences in results for the consonant and vowel tests are consistent with differences in the ways in which each processor presents speech stimuli. The CA processor simultaneously presents continuous analog waveforms to all of the stimulation channels in a multielectrode array, while the IP processor presents nonsimultaneous pulses to the same channels. In addition, the type of IP processor used in the present study provides explicit coding of fundamental frequency (F0) and voiced/unvoiced intervals. F0 is coded by initiating stimulation cycles in synchrony with the detected F0 during voiced intervals, and unvoiced intervals are signaled by initiating stimulation cycles at randomly varied times or at rates above the normal range of F0.

A possible advantage of the CA processor is in the preservation of details in the stimulus waveforms. Details that may be perceived by some implant patients include (*a*) frequency changes up through the range of F1

(Eddington, 1983; Hochmair-Desoyer and Burian, 1985; White, 1983), (*b*) rapid temporal variations in the envelopes of speech and speechlike stimuli (Hochmair-Desoyer, Hochmair, and Stiglbrunner, 1985), and (*c*) subtle waveshape changes produced by the addition of frequency components beyond F1 (Hochmair and Hochmair-Desoyer, 1985).

The results from the vowel test are consistent with the observation that at least some patients can discriminate frequency changes through the range of F1 with CA stimuli. This ability would explain the high information transmission (IT) scores obtained with the CA processor for the F1 feature. Because waveform details are discarded in the IP processor, one might also expect lower scores for F1 with that processor. Differences in scores for transmission of F1 information thus may be attributed to the presence (CA processor) or absence (IP processor) of details in analog waveforms.

Improved perception of F1 also could explain the high IT scores found for the duration feature with the CA processor. The roles of the F1 and duration features are highly correlated for the vowels in the RTI test. This leads to assignment redundancies (see Appendix 21.2) that could produce high IT scores for duration even if duration per se were not well transmitted. The present results do not allow discrimination among three possibilities: (*a*) excellent transmission of F1 information only, (*b*) excellent transmission of duration information only, or (*c*) excellent transmission of both. Results from previous studies, on the perception of F1 information with CA waveforms (Eddington, 1983; Hochmair-Desoyer and Burian, 1985; White, 1983), support possibilities (*a*) and (*c*).

The chief advantage of the IP processor may be the reduction of channel interactions through the use of nonsimultaneous stimuli. This reduction may increase the salience of channel-related cues and therefore improve the representation of frequency components across the speech spectrum. An increased salience of channel cues is likely to become progressively more important as the number of stimulation channels is increased. Thus, this advantage of the IP processor may be more evident in subjects with many channels (e.g., six to ten) than in subjects with relatively few channels (e.g., two to four). Indeed, results from previous studies conducted by our group, using a subject fitted with a percutaneous cable, demonstrated large increases in both consonant and vowel identifications when the number of stimulation channels in an IP processor was increased from four to six (Wilson et al., 1988a).

For the subjects of the present study, with only two to four channels of stimulation, the representation of frequency components with channel cues is necessarily coarse. However, even a coarse representation may provide a significant advantage for the perception of overall spectral shape. This advantage might be reflected in the improved IT scores for many of the consonant features, especially nasality and voicing. The nasals are characterized by an intense formant at approximately 250 Hz and a relatively weak set of higher formants above 800 Hz. The spectral region between the first and second formants is almost devoid of energy. Recognition of this spectral shape could allow identification of the nasals as a class in the consonant identification tests.

A superior representation of spectral shape also would provide greater access to voicing information. An important cue to voicing is the ratio of energy at low frequencies (e.g., below 1500 Hz) to energy at high frequencies (e.g., above 1500 Hz). A high ratio is typically found for voiced intervals of speech, and a low ratio is typically found for unvoiced intervals. Faithful transmission of the relative energies in these bands would help to produce correct voiced/unvoiced decisions.

The voiced/voiceless distinction might also be aided by the explicit coding of voiced and unvoiced intervals used in the IP processor. Indeed, percepts produced during unvoiced intervals—with stimulus pulses presented at randomly varied times or at rates above the normal range of F0—should be easily discriminated from the percepts produced during voiced intervals—with stimulus pulses presented at the F0 rate (see, e.g., Dobie and Dillier, 1985; Pfingst, 1985; Shannon, 1983). Such coding of voiced and unvoiced intervals complements the representation of spectral balance between low and high bands. This multiplicity of cues to voicing could increase the subjects' access to voicing information. Improved transmission of voicing information would be expected to produce increases in the IT scores for voicing, envelope, and frication.

A final difference that may favor the IP processor involves the stimuli used for the high-frequency (basal) channels. The presence of speech energy at high frequencies is signaled in the CA processor by the delivery of high-frequency analog stimuli to these channels. In contrast, low-frequency pulse trains are used in the IP processor for all channels, avoiding a potential problem with adaptation. Results from both psychophysical (Shannon, 1983) and single-unit (Moxon, 1971; Parkins, 1986; van den Honert and Stypulkowski, 1987; see also Javel, Chapter 17, this volume) studies have demonstrated strong adaptation to stimuli with frequencies much above 300 Hz. Thus, the use of such stimuli in the CA processor could produce substantial temporal distortions in the representation of sustained high-frequency components in speech, a problem that may be avoided through the use of an IP processor. A faithful representation of sustained high-frequency components would allow discrimination of the long-duration consonants /ʃ, s, z/ from the remaining consonants in the Iowa and RTI tests. This discrimination would improve the IT score for the duration feature. The IT scores for the envelope and frication features may also be enhanced by a representation that maintains perception of sustained high-frequency sounds.

To summarize the observations on the consonant and vowel results, we note that (*a*) waveform cues may be used to perceive the F1 feature of vowels with the CA processor and (*b*) reduced channel interactions and explicit coding of voice/unvoiced information may produce increased scores for the voicing, nasality, frication, and envelope features of consonants with the IP processor. In addition, the use of low-frequency pulse trains for the stimulation of basal channels in the IP processor may reduce or eliminate possible deleterious effects of adaptation. This last advantage of IP processors would be expected to produce increases in the transmission of duration, frication, and envelope information for consonants.

Comparison of Tests

Although the consonant and vowel tests show clear differences between the CA and IP processors, results from the open-set tests do not demonstrate an overall superiority of one processor over the other. This latter finding is a little surprising in that consonant identification is more important than vowel identification for overall speech intelligibility (see, e.g., Denes, 1963; Miller and Nicely, 1955; Minifie, 1953). Thus, in the absence of other factors, one might expect that the IP processor would produce superior scores on the open-set tests. Many other factors, however, may have affected the results of the present open-set tests. These factors include (*a*) the disparity in the subjects' experience with the two processors and (*b*) the fact that good performance on the open-set tests probably involves a host of linguistic and cognitive skills that are not tapped in tests of consonant and vowel identification. In addition, the superior performance obtained with the CA processor for vowel identification may have offset to some degree the superior performance obtained with the IP processor for consonant identification. Finally, the results from the consonant and vowel tests may not be fully representative inasmuch as only a limited number of consonant and vowel tokens were used.

Among these possibilities, we regard the last as least likely because (*a*) the results from all consonant tests were highly consistent with each other and together included most of the consonants with high frequencies of occurrence in English (Denes, 1963) and (*b*) the formant space sampled by the vowels in the vowel test spanned a considerable portion of the range of formant frequencies for all vowels in English (Peterson and Barney, 1952). The remaining factors are all likely contributors to the open-set results.

The one of these factors that may have favored one processor over the other is the disparity in experience. For the subjects of this study typical experience with the CA processor approximated 1 year of daily use, while experience with the IP processor was limited to the tests conducted with that processor (among several) during a 1-week period. Results from many previous studies have demonstrated large learning effects associated with the experience gained from using a particular prosthesis system (see, e.g., Table 21.2 and Schindler and Kessler, 1987; Tyler et al. 1986; Wilson et al. 1988d). To the extent that such learning is not transferred to a new system (in this case, a different speech processor) (Powell et al., 1987; Tyler et al., 1986), one might expect the disparity in experience to influence test scores in favor of the CA processor. In any event, equivalent or superior results on the open-set tests are found with the IP processor for five of the six subjects in the present study. This finding suggests (*a*) that the IP processor could be applied to these five subjects without any initial deficit and (*b*) that, with equivalent experience, the IP processor might emerge as the superior processor for most subjects.

An additional observation from the open-set results is that the performance of the IP processor appears to be highly sensitive to limitations on the optimization of processor parameters. In particular, the subject with the consistently better performance using the IP processor (MC2) had the best fulfillments of the fitting criteria established for that processor (Wilson et al., 1988a; Wilson et al. 1988b; Wilson et al., 1988d). Reference to Table 21.3 shows that she had the use of all four stimulation channels, a relatively low time between sequential pulses (0.5 ms), and a relatively short time for a complete stimulation cycle (5.2 ms).

In contrast, the subject with the consistently better performance using the CA processor (RC) had only two functional channels of intracochlear stimulation. This number is certainly too few for even a gross representation of the speech spectrum with an IP processor. The relatively poor performance of the IP processor therefore could be attributed at least in part to a poor match to its fitting criteria.

Another possible explanation for RC's superior performance with the CA processor is that he made especially good use of the information present in the CA stimulus waveforms. Indeed, the impressive results obtained with RC (two channels), MC1 (three channels), certain patients in the Vienna series (one channel; see Hochmair-Desoyer and Burian, 1985; Hochmair-Desoyer, Hochmair, and Stiglbrunner, 1985), and certain patients in the Symbion series (four monopolar channels with relatively poor isolation; see Eddington, 1983) support the hypothesis that the major bearer of information in CA processors is the waveform itself. Although results from studies conducted at UCSF demonstrate that additional information can be provided with four channels of CA stimulation using the UCSF electrode array (Ochs et al., 1985; Schindler et al., 1987; White et al., 1985). This additional information is not required for excellent performance in some patients. Most likely, the best results are obtained for patients who have the greatest access to information in the CA waveform(s).

If this second interpretation is pertinent to RC's case, then patients with such special abilities might be best served with a CA processor. Optimal implementations of this processor would provide any additional information the patient might be able to utilize in multiple channels of stimulation. The maximum number of useful channels is likely to be limited, however, by the severe interactions that can occur among channels when simultaneous stimuli are used.

In summary, the results from the open-set tests provide additional insights into the processors and patients of this study. They demonstrate an overall equivalence of the two processors despite considerable experience with the CA processor, and they indicate that performance with the IP processor is highly sensitive to the choice of processor parameters. Finally, the open-set results show that either processor can be superior for particular subjects. This last finding further suggests that substantial gains in speech recognition can be made across a population of implant patients by (*a*) selecting the best type of processor for each patient and (*b*) using implanted and external hardware capable of supporting a wide range of processor options.

Hybrid Processor

The results of the consonant and vowel tests show that both the CA and IP processors have strengths. The main strength of the CA processor may be in its presentation of waveform details, and the main strength of the IP processor may lie in its reduction of channel interactions with the use of nonsimultaneous stimuli. It may be possible to combine these strengths in a single "hybrid" processor using both CA and IP stimuli. Recall that the principal advantages of the CA strategy may be realized in a single channel of stimulation. If so, one channel of CA stimulation could be used in a hybrid processor to good effect, while leaving the remaining channels available for IP stimuli. The channel for CA stimulation could be selected on the basis of the tonotopic position corresponding to the range of F1 (i.e., the apical-most channel for present prostheses) or on the basis of some desirable combination of low threshold, wide dynamic range, and measured access to waveform details (such as discrimination of frequency changes in the F1 range). If the channel used for the CA stimulus has a relatively low threshold, the presence of the continuous CA signal might not interfere too much with the IP stimuli. That is, the advantage of having a CA stimulus may outweigh the increased level of channel interactions that it introduces. The IP stimuli could be used to code either the entire spectrum of speech or the spectrum above F1. In the first case, frequency components in the F1 range would be redundantly coded by CA and IP stimuli, and the region above F1 would be coded with a relatively coarse resolution using the IP stimuli. In the second case, the redundancy of coding in the F1 range would be traded for a higher resolution of coding (with IP stimuli) for frequency components above the F1 range. One or more of these possible implementations of hybrid processors may produce results that are superior to those obtained with either parent processor. The hybrid processor might be most useful for patients who (*a*) can discriminate frequency changes throughout a substantial portion of the F1 range and (*b*) have low thresholds of stimulation for at least one channel.

Although the hybrid processor may provide significant benefits for certain patients, we believe the number of such patients is likely to be small. First, the lack of waveform detail in the IP processor will be of little or no consequence to the many patients who cannot discriminate frequency changes above 300 Hz (Pfingst, 1985; Wilson et al., 1988b). Also, patients with high thresholds for all channels, or with high levels of measured interactions among channels, probably will obtain superior results with the IP processor (Wilson et al., 1988a; Wilson et al., 1988b). Finally, when four or more channels are available, the IP processor may be superior for all patients because (*a*) the resolution of frequency representation in the F1 range will approximate or exceed the resolution obtained under optimal conditions with CA stimuli, (*b*) the resolution of frequency representation above the F1 range is likely to be much better than that obtained with single or multichannel CA processors, and (*c*) the additional advantages of IP processors, such as explicit coding of voicing information and the use of low-frequency stimuli for the basal channels, will be retained as the number of channels is increased.

Conclusions

Major conclusions from the studies reviewed in this paper are the following:

1. For the present subjects, each of whom had two to four channels of intracochlear stimulation with the UCSF/Storz cochlear prosthesis, consonant identification is superior with an IP processor and vowel identification is superior with a CA processor.
2. Strengths of the IP processor for consonant identification include better representations of voicing, nasality, envelope, frication, and duration; and strengths of the CA processor for vowel identification include better representations of F1 and duration.
3. These strengths might be combined in a hybrid CA/IP processor that could be superior to either parent processor for some subjects (e.g., subjects with two to four channels of stimulation and with a low threshold for at least one of these channels).
4. Even in the face of considerable experience with the CA processor, five of the six subjects immediately had similar (four subjects) or superior (one subject) performance on tests of open-set recognition using the IP processor. The subject with the superior performance using the IP processor had the best match to the fitting criteria established for that processor, and the subject with the superior

performance using the CA processor had the worst match. The ability to match IP processor parameters to the fitting criteria was limited in the present study by the number of functional channels and by the properties of the UCSF/Storz transcutaneous transmission system.

5. These findings from the open-set tests indicate that different implant patients generally require different processors for optimal performance. This conclusion in turn suggests that improvements across a population of patients can be made by (*a*) selecting the best type of processor for each patient and (*b*) using implanted and external hardware capable of supporting a wide range of processor options.

Acknowledgments. We thank the patients who participated in the described studies for their dedicated effort and pioneering spirit. We are pleased to acknowledge the important scientific contributions of F.T. Hambrecht, D.K. Kessler, G.E. Loeb, M.M. Merzenich, S.D. Soli, and R.D. Wolford. This work was supported by NIH Contract NO1-NS-5-2396, through the Neural Prosthesis Program.

Appendix 21.1

Matrices for the consonant and vowel tests of this study are presented in Tables A1.1–A1.3. The stimuli for each matrix are indicated along the left margin, and the responses for each matrix are indicated along the top margin. Matrix values for the RTI tests (Tables A1.2 and A1.3) are given as the fraction of response for each cell, as described in the Methods section.

Appendix 21.2

Assignments of articulatory and acoustic features for the consonants and vowels of the Iowa and RTI tests are shown in Table A2.1. For the two consonant tests, the assignments for voicing, nasality, duration, and frication are the same as those used by Miller and Nicely (1955) and by Singh and Black (1966). The assignments for place of articulation are identical to those of Singh and Black (1966). Envelope cues are assigned according to the major groupings described by Van Tasell and coworkers (1987). Finally, the visual cues are assigned according to previous findings on viseme groupings for these particular consonants (Owens and Blazek, 1985) and the patterns demonstrated in the vision-only matrices of this study.

TABLE A1.1. Confusion matrices for Iowa consonant test.

(*a*) Vision only

	p	b	m	f	v	ʃ	dʒ	s	z	t	d	n	g	k
p	10	15	5											
b	8	13	8								1			
m	4	13	12								1			
f				18	3		1	2	1	3	1			1
v				18	6					1	3		1	
ʃ			1			7	10	7	3				2	
dʒ				1		9	14	4	1				1	
s		1			1			12	10	2	3			1
z						3	2	7	12	1	4	1		
t					1	2	3	6	2	8	6	1		1
d	1							6	3	4	11	2		3
n				1	1			1	2	5	10	7	2	
g	1						1	3	2	4	10	3	4	2
k								1	1	5	8	7	3	5

(*b*) CA + vision

	p	b	m	f	v	ʃ	dʒ	s	z	t	d	n	g	k
p	28	2												
b	13	16	1											
m	8	11	11											
f				18		1				9		1	1	
v				5	18			3	2	1	1			
ʃ						15		9	1	4				1
dʒ						4	19	1	3	1			2	
s						4		21	2	2				1
z						1	4	3	16	2	2		2	
t								4	2	21	1			2
d							2		3		18	2	4	1
n						1					13	8	8	
g			1			1	1		1	1	19	3	2	1
k								3		6	1		2	18

(*c*) IP + vision

	p	b	m	f	v	ʃ	dʒ	s	z	t	d	n	g	k
p	29	1												
b	1	17	11									1		
m			30											
f		1		8	4	4	1	1		8	3			
v		1		2	19				4	1	3			
ʃ						20	3	5	2					
dʒ						1	22		5		2			
s						7		17	1	1		1	1	2
z						1	2		25		1	1		
t										20				10
d		1							2		18	7	2	
n				1	1				2		7	19		
g									2		20	6	2	
k										4	1		2	23

TABLE A1.2. Confusion matrices for the RTI consonant test.

(*a*) Vision only

	ð	s	z	t	d	n	k	l
ð	1.000							
s		.398	.417	.130	.056			
z		.519	.333	.019	.083	.019	.028	
t		.269	.241	.278	.194	.019		
d	.019	.213	.444	.222	.102			
n	.056	.056		.074	.583	.111		.120
k					.019	.185	.194	.602
l						.056		.944

(*b*) CA + vision

	ð	s	z	t	d	n	k	l
ð	.981		.019					
s	.037	.463	.222	.194	.028		.056	
z	.019	.269	.528	.083	.037	.019	.028	
t	.028		.046	.731	.056		.139	
d		.102	.194	.056	.435	.185		
n	.056		.046	.056	.324	.454		.065
k						.028	.944	.028
l								1.000

(*c*) CA only

	ð	s	z	t	d	n	k	l
ð	.426	.083	.028	.120	.204		.139	
s	.130	.278	.037	.463			.093	
z	.157	.204	.259	.019	.111	.130	.083	.037
t	.074		.056	.500		.019	.352	
d		.111	.213		.250	.278	.148	
n	.074	.056	.111		.222	.463	.056	
k				.019			.981	
l					.019			.981

(*d*) IP + vision

	ð	s	z	t	d	n	k	l
ð	.981	.019						
s		.544	.281	.137	.019		.019	
z		.248	.722	.019	.011			
t		.019		.817	.106	.022	.037	
d		.074	.037	.074	.631	.183		
n	.028		.019		.163	.735		.056
k				.028			.954	.019
l						.011		.989

(*e*) IP only

	ð	s	z	t	d	n	k	l
ð	.417	.218	.102	.069	.120	.037	.009	.028
s	.093	.620	.111	.148	.009		.019	
z	.250	.074	.403	.060	.065	.120		.028
t	.060	.037		.690	.083	.056	.074	
d	.037	.019	.019	.028	.699	.181	.019	
n	.056	.042			.204	.625		.074
k				.171			.829	
l						.019		.981

TABLE A1.3. Confusion matrices for the RTI vowel test.

(*a*) Vision only

	i	I	ɔ	o	u
i	.661	.339			
I	.261	.739			
ɔ			1.000		
o				.967	.033
u				.194	.806

(*b*) CA + vision

	i	I	ɔ	o	u
i	.872	.128			
I	.050	.950			
ɔ			1.000		
o			.028	.933	.039
u				.056	.944

(*c*) CA only

	i	I	ɔ	o	u
i	.900	.083			.017
I	.128	.883			.011
ɔ			.933	.067	
o			.144	.706	.150
u		.011		.089	.878

(*d*) IP + vision

	i	I	ɔ	o	u
i	.828	.172			
I	.217	.783			
ɔ			1.000		
o			.033	.950	.017
u				.194	.806

(*e*) IP only

	i	I	ɔ	o	u
i	.822	.094	.028	.011	.044
I	.189	.744		.033	.033
ɔ			.972	.028	
o			.039	.861	.100
u				.233	.767

The assignments for the vowel features of first and second formant frequencies and of duration reflect the results from direct measurement of these acoustic parameters for the tokens in the RTI vowel test. The viseme groupings are those of Jeffers and Barley (1971).

TABLE A2.1. Classification of phonemes used in the Iowa and RTI tests.

(*a*) Iowa test

	p	b	m	f	v	ʃ	dʒ	s	z	t	d	n	g	k
Voicing	0	1	1	0	1	0	1	0	1	0	1	1	1	0
Nasality	0	0	1	0	0	0	0	0	0	0	0	1	0	0
Place	0	0	0	0	0	1	1	2	2	2	2	2	3	3
Duration	0	0	0	0	0	1	0	1	1	0	0	0	0	0
Frication	0	0	0	1	1	1	1	1	1	0	0	0	0	0
Envelope	0	1	2	3	1	3	1	3	1	0	1	2	1	0
Viseme	0	0	0	1	1	2	2	3	3	3	3	3	3	3

(*b*) RTI tests

	ð	s	z	t	d	n	k	l
Voicing	1	0	1	0	1	1	0	1
Nasality	0	0	0	0	0	1	0	0
Place	0	0	0	0	0	0	1	0
Duration	0	1	1	0	0	0	0	0
Frication	1	1	1	0	0	0	0	0
Envelope	0	1	0	2	0	3	2	3
Viseme	0	1	1	1	1	1	2	2

	i	I	ɔ	o	u
F1	0	1	1	1	0
F2	1	1	0	0	0
Duration	1	0	2	2	1
Viseme	0	0	1	2	2

References

Brimacombe, J.A., Webb, R.L., Dowell, R.C., Mecklenburg, D.J., Beiter, A.L., Barker, M.J., and Clark, G.M. (1988). Speech recognition abilities in profoundly deafened adults using the Nucleus 22 channel cochlear implant system. In *Cochlear Implant: Current Situation,* edited by P. Banfai (Erkelenz, West Germany: Rudolf Bermann GmbH), pp. 487–490.

Clark, G.M., Blamey, P.J., Brown, A.M., Gusby, P.A., Dowell, R.C., Franz, B.K.H., Pyman, B.C., Shepherd, R.K., Tong, Y.C., Webb, R.L., Hirshorn, M.S., Kuzma, J., Mecklenburg, D.J., Money, D.K., Patrick, J.F., and Seligman, P.M. (1987). *The University of Melbourne-Nucleus Multi-electrode Cochlear Implant* (Basel: Karger).

Danley, M.J., and Fretz, R.J. (1982). Design and functioning of the single-electrode cochlear implant. *Ann. Otol. Rhinol. Laryngol.* Suppl. 91, 91:21–26.

De Filippo, C.L., and Scott, B.L. (1978). A method for training and evaluating the reception of ongoing speech. *J. Acoust. Soc. Am.* 63:1186–1192.

Denes, P.B. (1963). On the statistics of spoken English. *J. Acoust. Soc. Am.* 35:892–904.

Dobie, R.A., and Dillier, N. (1985). Some aspects of temporal coding for single-channel electrical stimulation of the cochlea. *Hearing Res.* 18:41–55.

Dowell, R.C., Seligman, P.M., Blamey, P.J., and Clark, G.M. (1987). Evaluation of a two-formant speech-processing strategy for a multichannel cochlear prosthesis. *Ann. Otol. Rhinol. Laryngol.* Suppl. 128, 96:132–134.

Eddington, D.K. (1983). Speech recognition in deaf subjects with multichannel intracochlear electrodes. *Ann. N.Y. Acad. Sci.* 405:241–258.

Finley, C.C., Wilson, B.S., and Lawson, D.T. (1987). Speech processors for auditory prostheses. *Seventh Quarterly Progress Report,* NIH Project NO1-NS-5-2396. Bethesda, Md.: Neural Prosthesis Program, National Institutes of Health.

Gantz, B.J. (1987). Cochlear implants: An overview. *Adv. Otol. Head Neck Surg.* 1:171–200.

Gantz, B.J., Tyler, R.S., Knutson, J.F., Woodworth, G., Abbas, P., McCabe, B.F., Hinrichs, J., Tye-Murray, N., Lansing, C., Kuk, F., and Brown, C. (1988). Evaluation of five different cochlear implant designs: Audiologic assessment and predictors of performance. *Laryngoscope* 98:1100–1106.

Gardi, J.N. (1985). Human brain stem and middle latency responses to electrical stimulation: Preliminary observations. In *Cochlear Implants,* edited by R.A. Schindler and M.M. Merzenich (New York: Raven Press), pp. 351–363.

Grether, C.B. (1970). Psychoacoustic assessment of speech communication systems: The diagnostic discrimination test. Project Themis. Air Force Office of Scientific Research, Contract F44620-69-C-0033.

Hochmair, E.S., and Hochmair-Desoyer, I.J. (1985). Aspects of sound signal processing using the Vienna intra- and extracochlear implants. In *Cochlear Implants,* edited by R.A. Schindler and M.M. Merzenich (New York: Raven Press), pp. 101–110.

Hochmair-Desoyer, I.J., and Burian, K. (1985). Reimplantation of a molded scala tympani electrode: Impact on psychophysical and speech discrimination abilities. *Ann. Otol. Rhinol. Laryngol.* 94:65–70.

Hochmair-Desoyer, I.J., Hochmair, E.S., and Stiglbrunner, H.K. (1985).

Psychoacoustic temporal processing and speech understanding in cochlear implant patients. In *Cochlear Implants,* edited by R.A. Schindler and M.M. Merzenich (New York: Raven Press), pp. 291–304.

Jeffers, J., and Barley, M. (1971). *Speechreading* (Springfield, Ill.: Charles C Thomas).

Loeb, G.E., Byers, C.L., Rebscher, S.J., Casey, D.E., Fong, M.M., Schindler, R.A., Gray, R.F., and Merzenich, M.M. (1983). Design and fabrication of an experimental cochlear prosthesis. *Med. Biol. Eng. Comput.* 21:241–254.

Merzenich, M.M. (1985). UCSF cochlear implant device. In *Cochlear Implants,* edited by R.A. Schindler and M.M. Merzenich (New York: Raven Press), pp. 121–129.

Merzenich, M.M., Leake-Jones, P., Vivion, M., White, M., and Silverman, M. (1978). Development of multichannel electrodes for an auditory prosthesis. *Fourth Quarterly Progress Report,* NIH Project NO1-NS-7-2367. Bethesda, Md.: Neural Prosthesis Program, National Institutes of Health.

Millar, J.B., Tong, Y.C., and Clark, G.M. (1984). Speech processing for cochlear implant prostheses. *J. Speech Hear. Res.* 27:280–296.

Miller, G.A., and Nicely, P.E. (1955). An analysis of perceptual confusions among some English consonants. *J. Acoust. Soc. Am.* 27:338–352.

Minifie, F.D. (1973). Speech acoustics. In *Normal Aspects of Speech, Hearing and Language,* edited by F.D. Minifie, T.J. Hixon, and F. Williams (Englewood Cliffs, N.J.: Prentice-Hall), pp. 235–284.

Moore, B.C.J. (1985). Speech coding for cochlear implants. In *Cochlear Implants,* edited by R.F. Grey (San Diego, Calif.: College-Hill Press), pp. 163–179.

Moxon, E.C. (1971). Neural and mechanical responses to electric stimulation of the cat's inner ear. Doctoral dissertation, MIT, Cambridge, Mass.

Ochs, M.T., White, M.W., Merzenich, M.M., and Schubert, E.D. (1985). Speech recognition in single- and multichannel cochlear implants. *J. Acoust. Soc. Am.* Suppl. 1, 77:S81.

Owens, E., and Blazek, B. (1985). Visemes observed by hearing-impaired and normal-hearing adult viewers. *J. Speech Hear. Res.* 28:381–393.

Owens, E., Kessler, D.K., Raggio, M., and Schubert, E.D. (1985). Analysis and revision of the Minimal Auditory Capabilities (MAC) battery. *Ear Hear.* 6:280–287.

Owens, E., and Raggio, M. (1987). The UCSF tracking procedure for evaluation and training of speech reception by hearing-impaired adults. *J. Speech Hear. Disorders* 52:120–128.

Parkins, C.W. (1986). Cochlear prostheses. In *Neurobiology of Hearing: The Cochlea,* edited by R.A. Altschuler, D.W. Hoffman, and R.P. Bobbin (New York: Raven Press), pp. 455–473.

Peterson, G.E., and Barney, H.L. (1952). Control methods used in a study of vowels. *J. Acoust. Soc. Am.* 24:175–184.

Pfingst, B.E. (1985). Psychophysical data from cochlear implants: Relevance to strategies for rehabilitation. *Sem. Hearing* 6:7–21.

Pfingst, B.E. (1986). Stimulation and encoding strategies for cochlear prostheses. *Otol. Clin. N. Amer.* 19:219–235.

Pfingst, B.E., and Sutton, D. (1983). Relation of cochlear implant function to histopathology in monkeys. *Ann. N.Y. Acad. Sci.* 405:224–239.

Schindler, R.A., and Kessler, D.K. (1987). The UCSF/Storz Cochlear implant: Patient performance. *Am. J. Otol.* 8:247–255.

Schindler, R.A., Kessler, D.K., Rebscher, S.J., Jackler, R.K., and Merzenich, M.M. (1987). Surgical considerations and hearing results with the UCSF/Storz cochlear implant. *Laryngoscope* 97:50–56.

Schindler, R.A., Kessler, D.K., Rebscher, S.J., Yanda, J.L., and Jackler, R.K. (1986). The UCSF/Storz multichannel cochlear implant: Patient results. *Laryngoscope* 96:597–603.

Schubert, E.D. (1985). Some limitations on speech coding for implants. In *Cochlear Implants,* edited by R.A. Schindler and M.M. Merzenich (New York: Raven Press), pp. 269–276.

Shannon, R.V. (1983). Multichannel electrical stimulation of the auditory nerve in man. I. Basic psychophysics. *Hearing Res.* 11:157–189.

Singh, S., and Black, J.W. (1966). Study of twenty-six intervocalic consonants as spoken by four language groups. *J. Acoust. Soc. Am.* 39:372–387.

Tyler, R.S., Preece, J.P., Lansing, C.R., Otto, S.R., and Gantz, B.J. (1986). Previous experience as a confounding factor in comparing cochlear-implant processing schemes. *J. Speech Hearing Res.* 29:282–287.

Tyler, R.S., Preece, J.P., and Lowder, M.W. (1983). The Iowa cochlear-implant test battery. Laboratory Report, University of Iowa at Iowa City, Department of Otolaryngology—Head and Neck Surgery.

van den Honert, C., and Stypulkowski, P.H. (1987). Temporal response patterns of single auditory nerve fibers elicited by periodic electrical stimuli. *Hearing Res.* 29:207–222.

Van Tasell, D.J., Soli, S.D., Kirby, V.M., and Widin, G.P. (1987). Speech waveform envelope cues for consonant recognition. *J. Acoust. Soc. Am.* 82:1152–1161.

Wang, M.D., and Bilger, R.C. (1973). Consonant confusions in noise: A study of perceptual features. *J. Acoust. Soc. Am.* 54:1248–1266.

White, M., Ochs, M., Raggio, M., Morledge, D., and Merzenich, M. (1985). Formant discrimination in a multichannel cochlear prosthesis. *J. Acoust. Soc. Am.* Suppl. 1, 77:S81.

White, M.W. (1983). Formant frequency discrimination and recognition in subjects implanted with intracochlear stimulating electrodes. *Ann. N.Y. Acad. Sci.* 405:348–359.

White, M.W., Merzenich, M.M., and Gardi, J.N. (1984). Multichannel cochlear implants: Channel interactions and processor design. *Arch. Otol.* 110:493–501.

Wilson, B.S., and Finley, C.C. (1985). A computer-based simulator of speech processors for auditory prostheses. *ARO Abstracts, 8th Midwinter Research Conference,* St. Petersburg, Fla., p. 209.

Wilson, B.S., Finley, C.C., Farmer, J.C. Jr., Lawson, D.T., Weber, B.A., Wolford, R.D., Kenan, P.D., White, M.W., Merzenich, M.M., and Schindler, R.A. (1988a). Comparative studies of speech processing strategies for cochlear implants. *Laryngoscope* 98:1069–1077.

Wilson, B.S., Finley, C.C., Lawson, D.T., and Wolford, R.D. (1988b). Speech processors for cochlear prostheses. *Proc. IEEE* 76:1143–1154.

Wilson, B.S., Finley, C.C., Lawson, D.T., and Wolford, R.D. (1988c). Direct comparisons of analog and pulsatile coding strategies with six cochlear implant patients. (In preparation.)

Wilson, B.S., Schindler, R.A., Finley, C.C., Kessler, D.K., Lawson, D.T., and Wolford, R.D. (1988d). Present status and future enhancements of the UCSF cochlear prosthesis. In *Cochlear Implant: Current Situation,* edited by P. Banfai (Erkelenz, West Germany: Rudolf Bermann GmbH), pp. 395–427.

Blake S. Wilson: Discussion

Dr. Josef Miller: I was most bothered by the last slide that you showed. The open-set performance wasn't predicted by the closed-set performance. How about for the patients which have had experience with the compressed analog system? Was their open-set performance predictable on the basis of their closed-set performance on the vowel and consonant discriminations?

Dr. Wilson: The short answer is no. I haven't calculated the correlations among those measures, but I know that there are patients in the series with very good consonant and vowel identification scores and very poor open-set scores. Open-set recognition may involve a whole host of additional features. I believe that you need to conduct both types of studies, where vowel and consonant identification can provide insight into what is being represented at the periphery. Open-set recognition can provide insight into how the patient is utilizing that information. In terms of processor design, perhaps the more direct path is via measurements of vowel and consonant identification; but by itself it is probably insufficient.

Dr. Rabinowitz: First, I want to compliment you on a very nice job summarizing a lot of results. I wanted to follow up on this last point—we've tested a relatively small number of patients thus far, and thus far I have been struck by the consistency between their performance on the segmental level and the open-set tests. Maybe we just haven't tested enough yet. I wonder, though, if the difference has to do with how many stimuli are used in the segmental test. We tend to use larger sets than you, and we also use multiple productions of each stimulus.

Dr. Wilson: I would say that's a possibility. Your finding is consistent with the idea that one possible explanation for our present findings is the large disparity in experience between the two types of processors we use. You're not comparing two processors; you're measuring results with the Symbion processor, right?

Dr. Rabinowitz: One result that you had, I didn't understand. In the vowel data you said the compressed analog processor did somewhat better without vision, and you suggested that was because the patient had better access to F1 and duration. But when you did sequential information analyses, the strongest contributor to their results was F2.

Dr. Wilson: Right. But the proportion of the information contributed by recognition of the F1 feature was substantially larger with the compressed analog strategy, even though identification of F2 was most salient. When you go down the list of features, F1 had a much higher percentage contribution to the overall percept for the compressed analog strategy than for the interleaved pulses strategy. Both did well with F2. The compressed analog strategy did better with F1 and duration.

22
Perceptual Evaluation of a Neurally Based Encoding Strategy for Cochlear Implants

SIGFRID D. SOLI

Introduction

This chapter summarizes research of the Cochlear Implant Research Group, Biosciences Laboratory, 3M, focusing on the development and evaluation of a new cochlear implant electrode and processor system. Most of this research was performed during 1986 and 1987. The implant system is designed to mimic the neural coding of the normal peripheral auditory system in an attempt to restore this coding for individuals with sensorineural deafness. Prototype electrodes and processors have been built, and two local patients have been implanted with a preliminary version of the electrode. Extensive perceptual tests with laboratory and portable versions of the processor have been performed.

The chapter is organized to emphasize the results of these perceptual tests. The chapter begins with a brief description of the physiological background for the neurally based coding strategy. (See van den Honert, Chapter 9, this volume, for a more detailed description.) The implementation of the coding strategy in the processor and the electrode design are also described briefly. Next, the specific objectives of the perceptual tests and the methods of evaluation are discussed. Finally, the results of these tests are presented, followed by concluding comments.

Background

The degeneration of hair cells and the peripheral dendrites that accompanies profound sensorineural deafness eliminates the neural encoding functions normally performed by these processes. When auditory nerve fibers are stimulated electrically with a cochlear implant, these neural encoding functions no longer occur. The success of a variety of present cochlear implant systems for some users suggests that normal neural encoding may not be essential; however, if implant systems are to restore "normal" hearing in a majority of users, it may be necessary for the implant processor and electrode to mimic the normal neural encoding of the peripheral auditory system. The major features of normal peripheral neural encoding and their implications for processor and electrode design are summarized in the following paragraphs.

Spatial Selectivity

The tonotopic organization of the acoustically stimulated cochlea is evident both in its mechanical tuning properties and in the frequency selectivity (i.e., tuning curves) of individual auditory nerve fibers (e.g., Kiang, 1980). Moreover, the spatial selectivity of this tonotopic map is extremely precise. Neural activity in response to low-level sinusoidal acoustic stimulation is limited to only a small population of fibers at the appropriate cochlear place and with the appropriate tuning curve center frequencies. Van den Honert and Stypulkowski (1987a) have shown that with electrical stimulation best spatial selectivity is achieved with a radial bipolar electrode geometry. Longitudinal bipolar and monopolar electrode geometries produce a wider spread of excitation, which may be advantageous in cases where nerve survival is poor or where lower psychophysical thresholds are desired. From a neural coding perspective, however, a radial bipolar geometry is preferred. The electrode should contain many bipolar pairs of contacts positioned on the carrier so that they contact the cochlear region spanning the speech bandwidth from approximately 100 to 6000 Hz. Our design objective was a 10-channel radial bipolar electrode that could be inserted to place all 10 channels within the cochlear region of the speech bandwidth.

Temporal Selectivity

Temporal selectivity in the acoustically stimulated cochlea is seen in the temporal discharge patterns and tuning curves of indiviudal auditory nerve fibers (Geisler, Chapter 2, this volume; Sachs and Blackburn, Chapter 15, this volume). Sachs and Young (1979; Young and Sachs, 1979), for example, have found that the discharge patterns of auditory fibers show phase locking to frequency components near the best frequencies of their tuning curves in response to broadband acoustic speech signals; i.e., these discharge patterns reveal selective temporal periodicities corresponding to the spatial selectivity of these fibers. Auditory nerve fibers also exhibit strong phase locking in response to periodic electrical stimulation (van den Honert and Stylpkowski, 1987b; see also, Javel, Chapter 17, this volume). These observations suggest that each spatially selective, radial bipolar electrode channel should be driven with a signal comprised primarily of components whose temporal periodicities are appropriate to the site of stimulation. A set of narrowly tuned bandpass filters will extract selected periodicities from a broadband waveform, since the output of each filter will consist primarily of sinusoidal components near the center frequency of the filter. We used filter shapes and *Q* factors that match auditory tuning curves to mimic the selectivity of the peripheral auditory system. Our design goal was to implement 10 tuning curve filters, or resonators, in the processor and to map the output of each filter to one bipolar electrode pair, thus mimicking the spatial and temporal selectivity of normal peripheral auditory processes. Figure 22.1 shows a schematic block diagram of the idealized processor design, including 10 filters with half-octave spacing that span the speech bandwidth from approximately 200 Hz to 4 kHz.

Amplitude Compression

The acoustically stimulated cochlea exhibits nonlinear rate-intensity coding, as measured from the discharge rates of auditory fibers (e.g., Kiang, 1968). Moreover, this nonlinearity is compressive–a wide range of input intensities produces a much smaller range of response rates before saturation. The mechanism for this nonlinearity is assumed to play an important role in accounting for the broad acoustic dynamic range of normal auditory systems. The action of this mechanism is clearly absent with electrical stimulation of the cochlea, as seen from the extremely limited electrical dynamic ranges that are common with implant users. Our design goal was to implement highly flexible instantaneous compressive nonlinear input-output functions for each processor channel, which, in conjunction with front-end AGC and syllabic compression, would increase the range of acoustic intensities that could be mapped into the limited electrical dynamic range of the implant user. (See Figure 22.1.)

Electrode and Processor Implementation

The design of the 10-channel radial bipolar electrode was not complete at the time the first patients were ready for implementation. These patients were instead implanted with a four-channel longitudinal bipolar electrode array similar to that used by the Hochmairs (Hochmair-Desoyer and Burian, 1985). The electrode was attached to a percutaneous pedestal and connector, allowing direct access to the implanted contacts. The bipolar contacts were equally spaced on a silastic carrier and separated by 1.75 mm with a monopolar return contact in the base of the pedestal. The electrode could be inserted to an approximate depth of 24 mm to position the bipolar contacts within the cochlear region corresponding to the speech bandwidth.

Both a portable and a lab processor were developed in accordance with the design specifications described above, with several exceptions. Only the details of the portable processor are described, since the lab processor

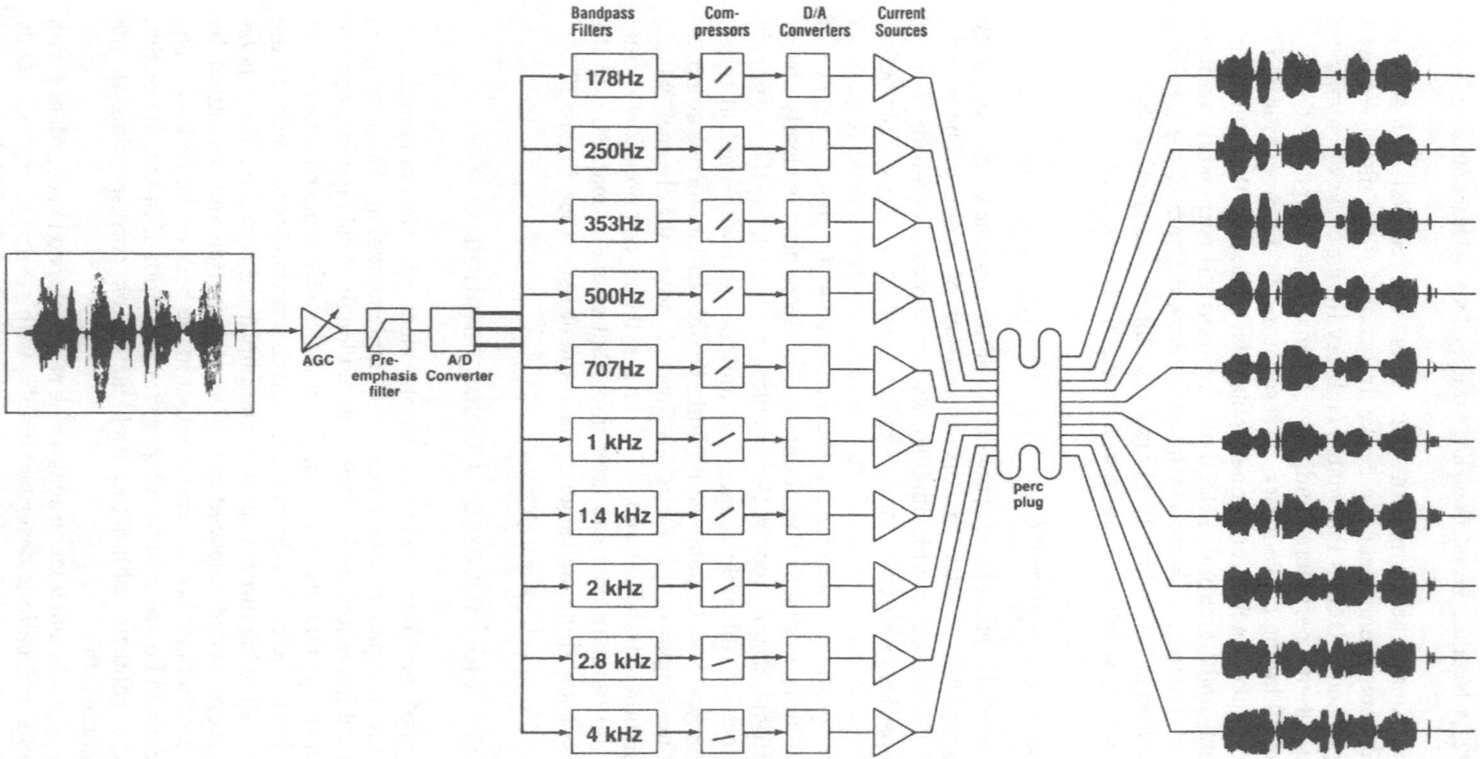

FIGURE 22.1. Schematic block diagram of an idealized processor for a neurally based coding strategy. A broadband input signal is preprocessed by AGC and preemphasis filter, converted to digital form, digitally filtered by 10 tuning curve filters, processed through 10 instantaneous compressive nonlinearities, converted to analog form, and delivered via percutaneous access to 10 radial bipolar electrode pairs.

simulated the portable processor. Nine filter channels, viz., eight resonators and one highpass filter, were implemented digitally using a TMS320C10 signal processing chip running at a 10-kHz sampling rate. The filter outputs were digitally mixed for use with the four-channel electrode, and each mixed filter output was passed through a digital instantaneous compressive nonlinearity which could be programmed to saturate at any specified input level. (See the top panel of Figure 22.6 for additional information on filter and mixing characteristics.) A syllabic compressor was also implemented digitally prior to filtering. Analog preprocessing consisted of a 125-Hz highpass noise rejection filter, AGC with variable sensitivity (patient control), 6-dB/octave preemphasis filter, and 5-kHz anti-aliasing filter. Analog postprocessing consisted of a four-channel demultiplexer, anti-aliasing filter, variable gain (experimenter control), and four current sources.

Objectives of Patient Evaluation

The overall objective of our patient evaluation was to determine the effectiveness of the neurally based encoding strategy described above. Full evaluation of its effectiveness requires patients with good nerve survival in the cochlear region corresponding to the speech bandwidth and with a 10-channel radial bipolar electrode array positioned in this region. Although our research patients were implanted with a four-channel longitudinal electrode array, we believed that it would nonetheless be possible to gain some initial insights into the effectiveness of this strategy by testing these patients.

Four specific issues define the focus of the research reported in this chapter. Separate perceptual tests were performed to address each of these issues. The first three sets of tests relate to key features of normal neural encoding. First, perceptual tests evaluating the effects of the instantaneous compressive nonlinearity on perceptual performance are reported. Second, performance tests addressing spatial selectivity and electrode mapping are described. Third, performance tests related to temporal selectivity and filter characteristics are reported.

The fourth set of perceptual tests compared performance using the neurally based encoding strategy with performance using a pulsatile coding strategy. These tests were performed in collaboration with the Neural Prosthesis Group, Research Triangle Institute, using a modified version of their interleaved pulses processor (Soli and Wilson, 1988; Wilson, Finley, Lawson, and Wolford, 1988; see also Wilson, Finley, and Lawson, Chapter 21, this volume).

Our basic research strategy throughout these tests was to make large changes in the independent variable of interest, e.g., the saturation threshold in tests of the instantaneous nonlinearity or the filter bandwidths in tests of temporal selectivity, and observe their influence on several analytical measures of speech performance in single-subject tests. If performance was significantly better in one configuration, this configuration was implemented in the processor, and the next set of tests was performed. This strategy allowed us to quickly assess the major processing variables with natural speech materials while, at the same time, gaining analytical insights about potential improvements in processing. Details of this strategy are described below.

Method of Evaluation

Subject

All tests were performed with a single implant patient because of the well-known subject variability among implant patients and because of the extensive number of processor configurations tested. A single-subject design was dictated by the time required for fitting each processor configuration, familiarizing the subject with the processor, and performing the tests.

The subject was a 42-year-old female who experienced progressive hearing loss of unknown origin. She was profoundly deaf by the age of 25. She was implanted with the four-channel percutaneous electrode approximately 6 months before the time of testing. Figure 22.2 shows the approximate position of the electrode contacts in her cochlea, based on X-ray photos. Note that the electrode could only be inserted to a depth of approximately 12.25 mm due to an obstruction in the cochlea. Thus, the desired electrode position in the cochlear region corresponding to the speech bandwidth could not be achieved.

Stimulus Materials and Test Method

All tests were sound-only presentations of closed-set consonant or vowel identification administered in randomized order under computer control. For each processor configuration, the subject practiced the consonant or vowel test twice with feedback before being tested without feedback. From 8 to 10 blocks of randomized trials without feedback were obtained in each test condition, with the exception of the pulsatile processor tests where time limitations permitted only half as many blocks to be obtained.

The consonant stimuli consisted of 20 English consonants spoken in an /aCa/ context by a male and a female talker. The vowel stimuli consisted of 10 English vowels spoken in an /hVd/ context by the same male and female talkers. Two tokens of each consonant and vowel utterance were used from each talker. Thus the stimulus sets were comprised of four unique tokens of each utterance (2 talkers × 2 tokens). The consonants

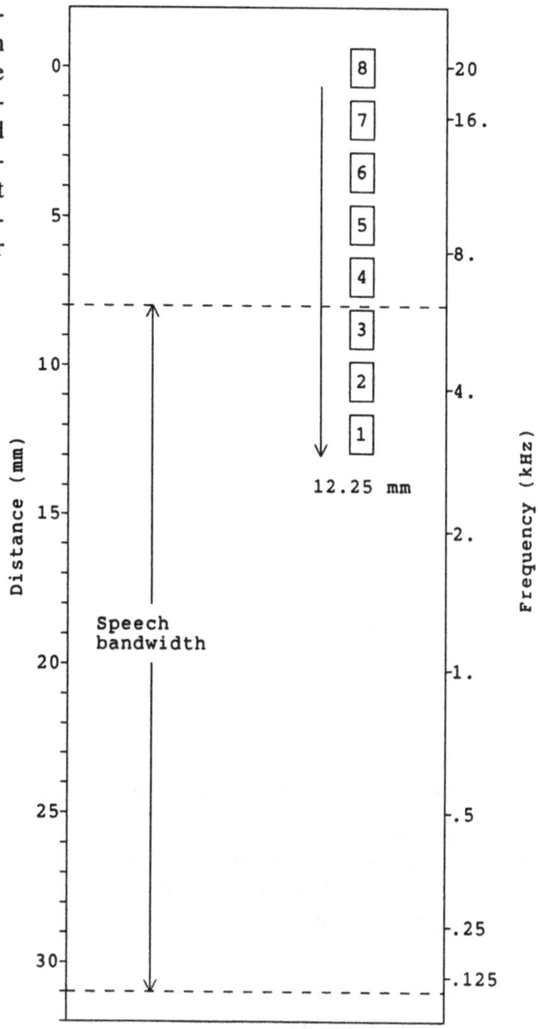

FIGURE 22.2. Estimated position of electrode contacts in patient JS. The left ordinate is the distance in millimeters measured from the round window, and the right ordinate is the approximate best frequency in kilohertz corresponding to the cochlear place.

and vowels and their feature classifications, which will be discussed below, are shown in Tables 22.1 and 22.2, respectively.

Method of Analysis

The raw data from each of the consonant and vowel tests consisted of square confusion matrices. A number of investigators have developed methods of analysis for confusion matrices that can reveal the acoustic cues and features underlying the confusions (e.g., Miller and Nicely, 1955; Soli and Arabie, 1979; Solie, Arabie, and Carroll, 1986; Van Tasell et al., 1987; Wang and Bilger, 1973). A new method based on information

TABLE 22.1. Feature classifications for consonant stimulus set.

	Envelope features			Frequency features			
Stimulus	Voice	Ampli.	Burst	Place	Nasal	Sibil.	Frica.
aba	1	1	1	1	1	1	1
ada	1	1	1	3	1	1	1
apa	2	1	2	1	1	1	1
aka	2	1	2	5	1	1	1
afa	2	1	1	1	1	1	2
asa	2	1	1	3	1	2	2
asha	2	1	1	4	1	2	2
ava	1	1	1	1	1	1	2
azha	1	1	1	4	1	2	2
ama	1	2	1	1	2	1	1
ara	1	2	1	4	1	1	1
aja	1	1	1	4	1	1	1
ata	2	1	2	3	1	1	1
aga	1	1	1	5	1	1	1
ana	1	2	1	3	2	1	1
aza	1	1	1	3	1	2	2
adtha	1	1	1	2	1	1	2
ala	1	2	1	3	1	1	1
atha	2	1	1	2	1	1	2
awa	1	2	1	1	1	1	1
Order of entry into SINFA							
	1	2	3	4	5	6	7

theory, and derived from this previous research, has been used in the present analyses to assess the effectiveness of each processor in conveying specific speech cues and features to the patient.

This method relies on a division of the cues in speech into two broad categories—time-intensity or envelope cues, and spectral or frequency

TABLE 22.2. Feature classifications for vowel stimulus set.

	Envelope feature	Frequency features	
Stimulus	Duration	F1 freq.	F2 freq.
heed	1	1	1
who'd	1	1	2
hod	1	2	2
hood	2	1	2
head	2	2	1
had	1	2	1
hawed	1	2	2
hud	2	2	3
hid	2	1	1
heard	1	2	3
Order of entry into SINFA analysis			
	1	2	3

cues—and on the development of feature classifications based on the two types of cues. Vowel cues fall readily into these categories, with the duration differences between long and short vowels defining an envelope cue and the first and second formant (F1 and F2) frequency differences between vowels defining two frequency cues. The envelope and frequency feature classifications for the 10 vowel stimuli are shown in Table 22.2. Van Tasell et al. (1987; Soli et al., 1985) have also proposed a set of envelope cues for consonants comprised of voicing envelope, amplitude envelope, and burst envelope. Classification of the 20 consonants by the envelope features is shown in Table 22.1 along with their classification by several "traditional" features which presumably are distinguished by both envelope and frequency cues.

The analysis method is a modified version of sequential information transmission analysis (SINFA) developed by Wang and Bilger (1973; Wang, 1976). SINFA performs information transmission analysis using ***conditional*** measures of information rather than ***unconditional*** measures. Most feature classifications are not statistically independent and often can be redundant. For example, the nasal sounds /m,n/ are also voiced consonants and thus are redundantly distinguished from any voiceless consonants by both the nasal and voicing features. SINFA resolves this redundancy by computing conditional information for nasality after partialing out voicing information (or vice versa); however, as with any conditional analyses, the order in which feature information is partialed out has a critical effect on the conditional information scores. SINFA has been modified to overcome this difficulty, allowing the user to specify the order in which features enter the conditional analysis. The modifications to SINFA have two advantages for the present analyses. First, the consonant and vowel envelope features can be forced into the analysis before the other features, so the effects of envelope cues are partialed out of the remaining features to provide a "purer" measure of frequency information. Second, the same order of feature entry can be imposed on each analysis to permit direct comparison of conditional information scores across analyses. (The last row in Tables 22.1 and 22.2 shows the order in which the features were entered into SINFA in all analyses.) These two advantages are important because they produce directly interpretable measures of the effectiveness of frequency coding provided by the neurally based encoding in each configuration.

Evaluation of Instantaneous Compressive Nonlinearity

Design

The nonlinearities follow the resonators and mixers in the processor to compress and limit the filter-mixer outputs so that the resulting signal falls within the patient's electrical dynamic range. [Resonators 1 and 2 were mixed to form channel 1; resonators 3 and 4 were mixed to form channel 2; resonators 5 and 6 were mixed to form channel 3; and resonators 6, 7, 8, and 9 were mixed to form channel 4. (See Figure 22.6 for more details.)] The most critical nonlinearity parameter is the threshold for limiting or saturation which determines the output dynamic range of the signal as well as the proportion of time that the signal is saturated.

Speech samples were processed through the lab simulation of the processor to determine the thresholds for limiting that would produce saturation a predetermined average proportion of the time. Separate limiting thresholds were determined for the four processor channels for each subject. Vowel and consonant tests were performed for several nonlinearity designs. The designs have been divided into two groups in the present analyses: designs with low saturation thresholds producing saturation 50% of the time or more and designs with high thresholds producing saturation 20% of the time or less. A subset of 12 English consonants and 6 vowels was used in these tests to accelerate the testing process.

Results

The results for the consonant tests are shown in Figure 22.3 and for the vowel tests in Figure 22.4. The top panel in each figure displays overall percent correct and overall percent information received for low and high saturation thresholds. Consonant scores improved from 23.8% for low saturation thresholds to 43.8% correct for high thresholds, and vowel scores improved from 44.6% to 71.7%. Large improvements in overall information scores are also evident.

The bottom panel in each figure summarizes the results from the modified SINFA analysis. The columns with solid bases in each figure display information scores for envelope cues, and columns with crosshatched bases display scores for frequency cues which entered the analyses after the envelope cues. The heights of these filled columns indicate ***absolute*** percent information received for each feature or cue, as computed by expressing bits of conditional information received for each feature as a percentage of total information in the stimulus set. The absolute scores allow direct comparisons of processor performance across tests. The heights of the unfilled columns above filled columns indicate ***relative*** percent information received, as computed by expressing bits of conditional information received for each feature as a percentage of total conditional information available for the feature. The relative scores assess the effectiveness of the processor in transmitting whatever conditional information is available for a feature. Both scores should be considered in evaluating a processor. For example, the relative information score for a feature could be high, but if there were only very little total conditional information for the feature, its overall importance—as indicated by its absolute score—would still be small.

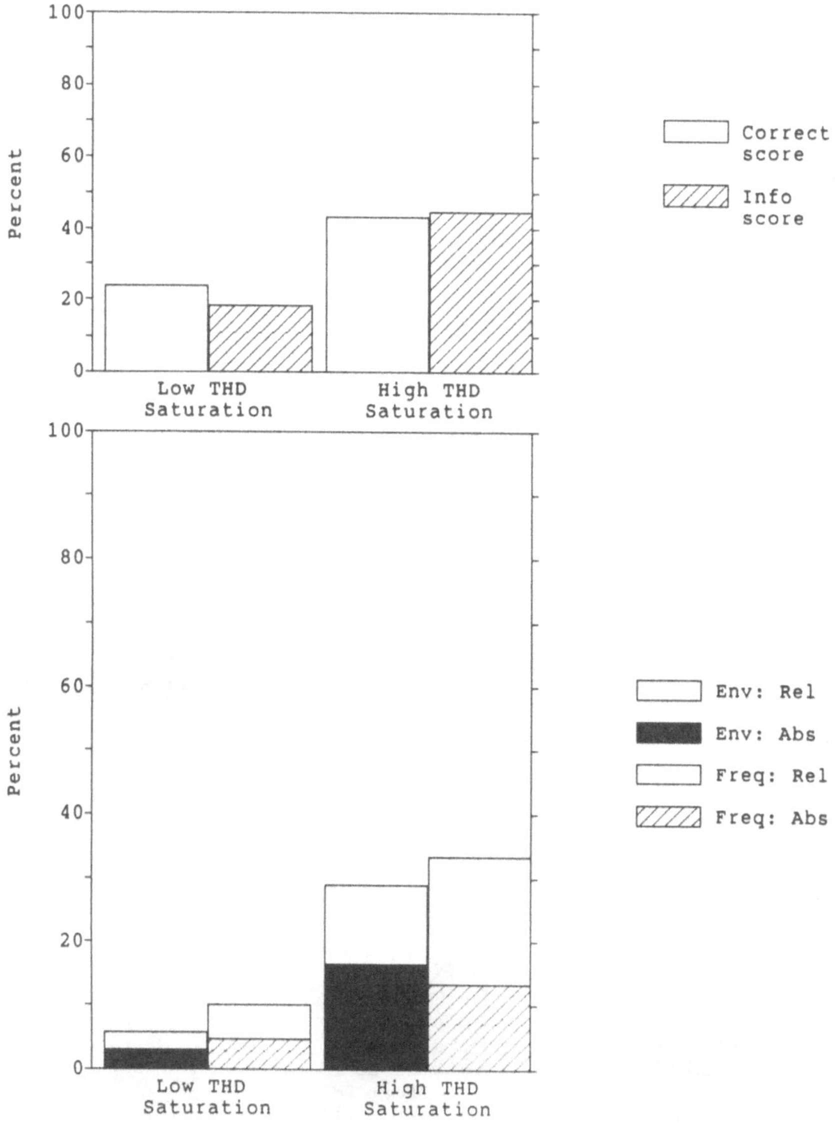

FIGURE 22.3. Percent correct and information scores for consonants as a function of saturation threshold in the instantaneous compressive nonlinearity. The ordinate in the top panel is the percent correct and refers to both the overall correct score and the overall information score. The ordinate in the bottom panel is percent information received and refers to both the relative and absolute information measures.

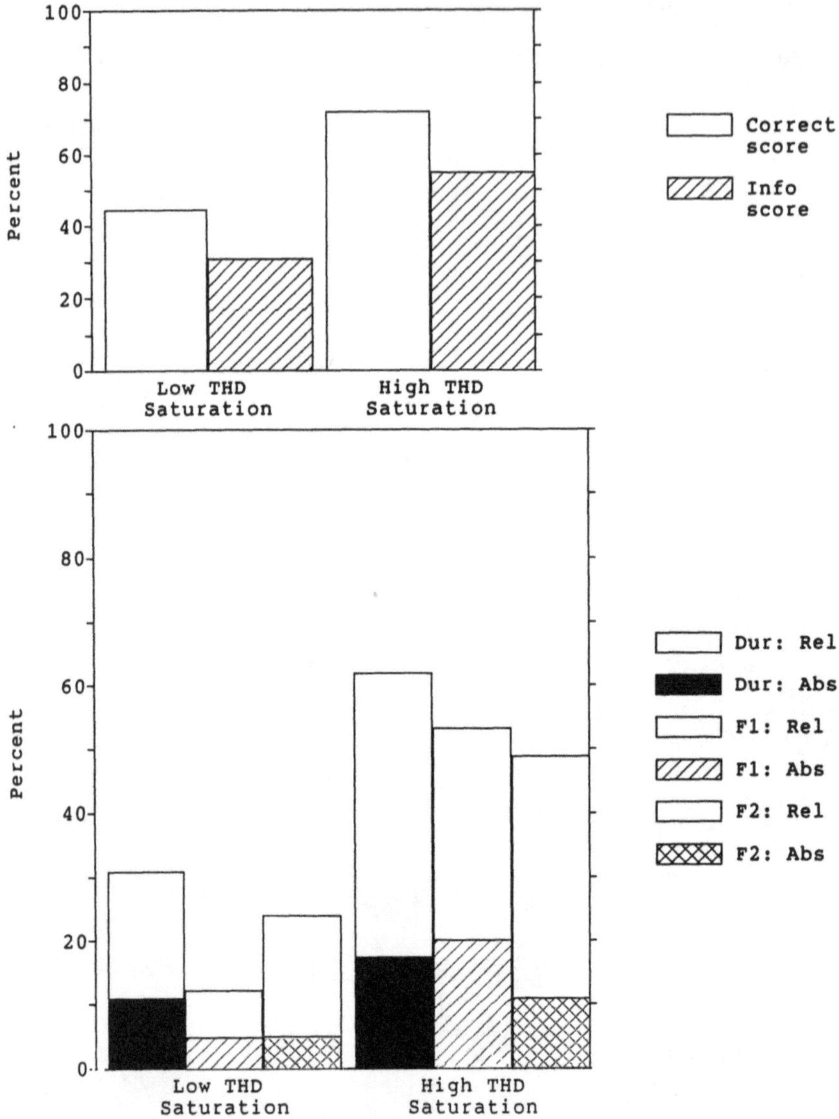

FIGURE 22.4. Percent correct and information scores for vowels as a function of saturation threshold in the instantaneous compressive nonlinearity. (See Figure 22.3 for a description of the ordinates in each panel.)

Figure 22.3 reveals that raising the saturation threshold produced almost a fivefold increase in both absolute and relative envelope information scores for consonants. Raising the threshold also produced approximately a threefold increase in the frequency information scores as well.

Recall that these frequency information scores have had the effects of redundant envelope cues removed. The vowel scores in Figure 22.4 also exhibit large increases, especially in the relative information scores, again for both envelope and frequency cues.

Discussion

Vowel and consonant performance improved substantially as the amount of saturation was decreased, suggesting that relatively high limiting thresholds should be used in programming the nonlinearities. The large improvements in envelope information are perhaps to be expected because low saturation thresholds significantly distort time-intensity cues in the waveform. The similar improvements in frequency information suggest, however, that the harmonic distortion produced with low saturation thresholds may also distort frequency cues.

These results also indicate that the nonlinearities are not an effective means of achieving amplitude compression. Following these tests, the nonlinearities were used primarily as a means of loudness control. Their thresholds were set 12 dB below the average instantaneous peak levels of speech for each channel. These settings produced saturation only 5–7% of the time on the average.

Evaluation of Spatial Selectivity

Design

The mapping of processor channels to electrodes provides a means for evaluation of spatial selectivity. If selectivity is good and the mapping is appropriate, one should observe effective place pitch coding of mid- and high-frequency cues in speech, e.g., F2 cues for vowels and sibilance and burst cues for consonants. Effective spatial selectivity for speech coding requires an appropriate electrode geometry, appropriate electrode placement in the cochlear region spanning the speech bandwidth, and good nerve survival throughout this region. Thus, in our subject neither the electrode geometry nor its placement was ideal for evaluation of spatial selectivity. The current results can only provide a weak test of the importance of spatial selectivity for a neurally based coding strategy.

The subject was asked to rank the pitch sensations associated with each bipolar electrode pair. Although the subject had no difficulty in performing this task, she did not voluntarily described the sensations as pitchlike. Three electrode configurations were generated from the rankings: (1) a "place map" assigning channels to electrodes based on the order of the electrodes on the carrier, (2) a "pitch map" assigning processor channels to electrodes based on the pitch ranking, and (3) a "reverse pitch map" assigning processor channels in the opposite order from the pitch ranking. Vowel performance was tested with each electrode mapping. Of particular interest are the F2 information scores, since they reflect the effects of variations in electrode mappings on frequency cues coded primarily by place information.

Results

Table 22.3 summarizes the results of the pitch-ranking task. The expected pitch ranking based on electrode position is also included for reference. Note that the subject ranked the electrodes in almost exactly the opposite order predicted from the electrode placement: the most basal pair, 7-M, received the lowest pitch rank, while the second most apical pair, 2-3, received the highest pitch rank. The electrode mappings for each test configuration are also shown in the table.

Figure 22.5 shows the vowel test results for the place map, pitch map, and reverse pitch map conditions. Overall percent correct and percent information scores, shown in the top panel of Figure 22.5, are approximately 50% across all conditions. The absolute feature information scores in the bottom panel are generally low, around 10%, and also exhibit very little variation across conditions. The relative information scores are more variable and generally achieve their highest values in the pitch map condition, except for the F2 score, which is slightly higher in the reverse pitch map condition.

Discussion

Comparison of the overall information scores and the absolute feature scores suggests that the subject's spatial selectivity is poor and thus pitch-mapping the electrodes has little effect on vowel performance. The

TABLE 22.3. Pitch ranking of bipolar electrode pairs.

Electrode pair	Place map	Pitch rank	Pitch map	Reverse map
1-2	Ch. 1	5		
2-3		7	Ch. 4	Ch. 1
3-4	Ch. 2	4		
4-5		6	Ch. 3	Ch. 2
5-6	Ch. 3	3	Ch. 2	Ch. 3
6-7		2	Ch. 1	Ch. 4
7-M	Ch. 4	1		

Notes: Electrode contacts are number from apex to base with pair 1-2 the most apical. Pair 7-M pairs contact 7 with the monopolar return. Pitch ranks are numbered from low to high with pair 7-M producing the lowest pitch sensation.

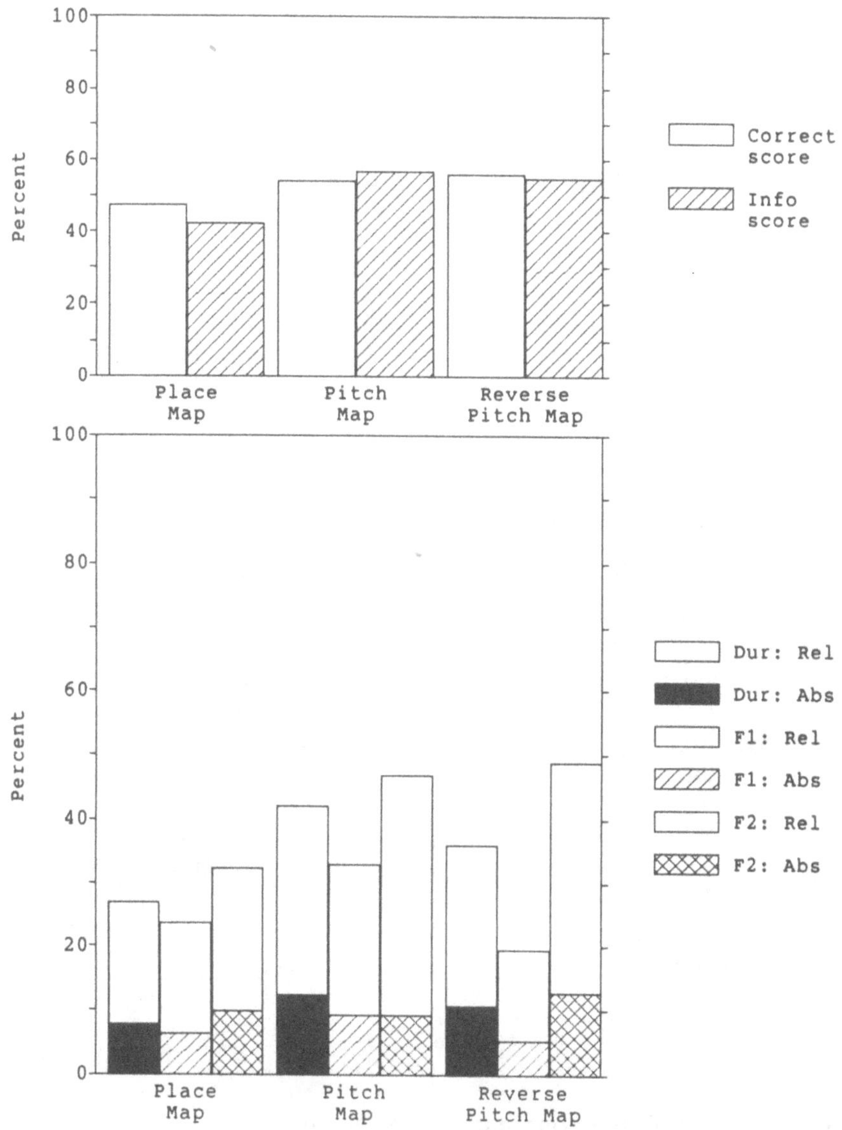

FIGURE 22.5. Percent correct and information scores for vowels as a function of electrode mapping. (See Figure 22.3 for a description of the ordinates in each panel.)

most "appropriate" pitch mapping produced no substantial improvements in F2 information scores. Reversal of the appropriate pitch mapping had little effect on overall performance, even though the pattern of feature scores indicates that the subject received a small amount of frequency information with all of the mappings.

The subject was fitted with the pitch map electrode configuration for subsequent evaluations in hopes that greater long-term improvements might occur with the "best" pitch mapping.

Evaluation of Temporal Selectivity

Design

The filters in the processor were designed as resonators with tuning characteristics very similar to the tuning of auditory nerve fibers in acoustic hearing. A series of tests with different filter designs was undertaken to assess the effects of filter characteristics on speech performance. As with spatial selectivity, the current results provide only a weak test of temporal selectivity because of the electrode design and placement.

The first design, the resonator design, used eight resonators and one high-pass filter with mixed outputs delivered to four bipolar channels. Performance with this design was compared with two other filter designs. The mixes and frequency responses of the resonators in the resonator design are shown in the top panel of Figure 22.6.

The second design, the steep bandpass design, was used to examine the effects on performance of mixing the outputs of the resonators. Filters with approximately the same bandwidth and outer skirts as the mixed resonator outputs were designed for each of the four channels, as seen in the middle panel of Figure 22.6.

The third design, the gradual bandpass design, was based on the filter characteristics from the Symbion processor (Eddington, 1980; 1983). These filters are widely tuned with gradual slopes and substantial overlap, as seen in the bottom panel of Figure 22.6. This design was included because it represents a more-or-less opposite approach from that of the resonator design.

Results

The results from the consonant and vowel tests with each of the filter designs are shown in Figures 22.7 and 22.8. Percent correct scores for consonants remained around 20% for all three filter designs, although overall information scores improved by about 8–12% for the steep and gradual bandpass designs over the resonator design. The absolute and relative information scores for envelope and frequency cues were consistently low for all three filter designs.

Percent correct and overall information scores for the vowels both improved by 13% or more with both bandpass designs, as compared with the resonator design. The vowel feature scores reveal the source of this

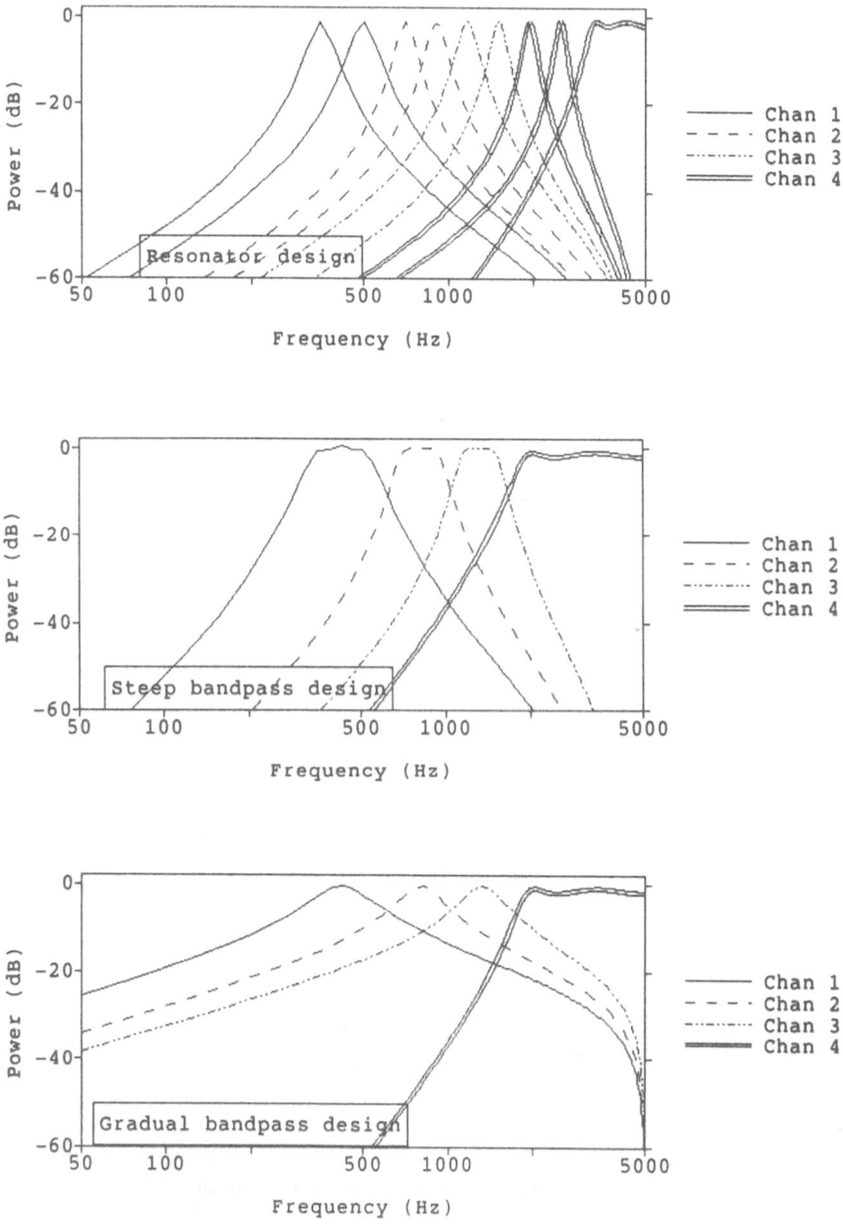

FIGURE 22.6. Frequency responses for filter designs used to evaluate the neurally based coding strategy. The legends for the filter functions in each panel indicate the channel corresponding to each filter. For the resonator design shown in the top panel, the outputs of the resonators displayed with the same legend were mixed to form the channel output. For example, the outputs of resonators 3 and 4 (i.e., the dashed-line filter functions) were mixed to form the channel 2 output.

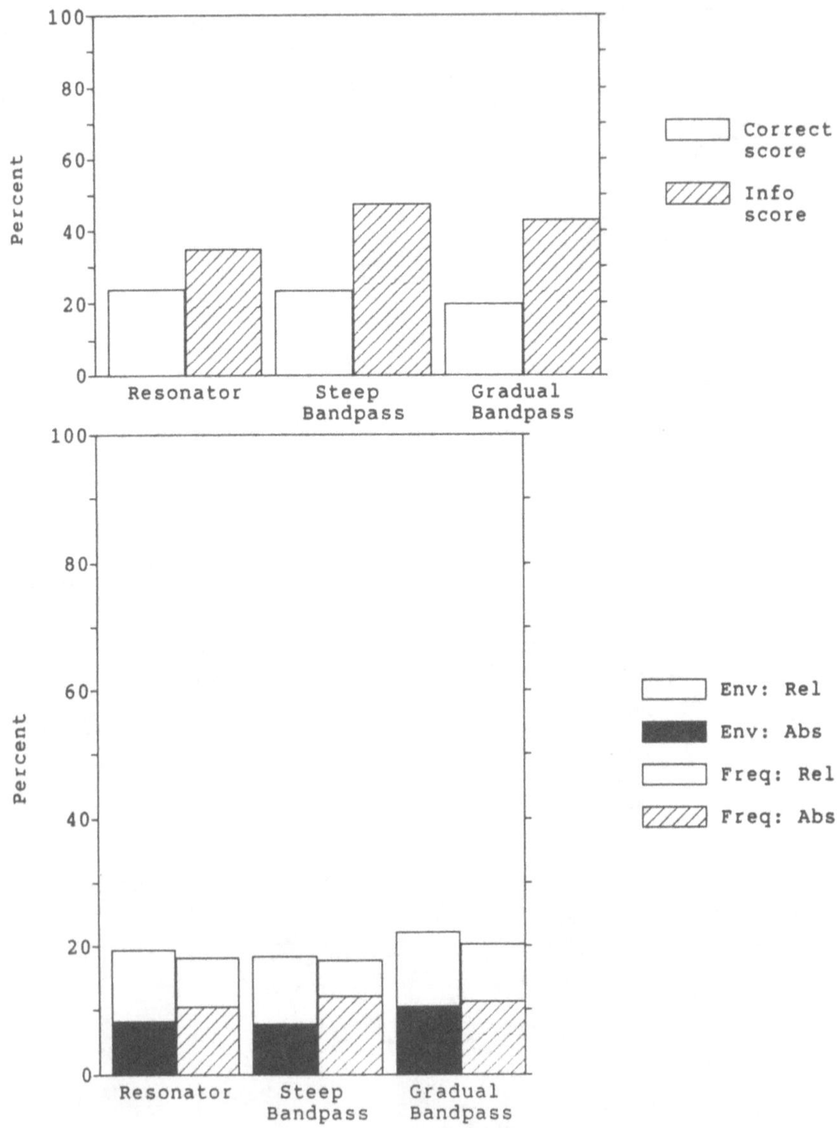

FIGURE 22.7. Percent correct and information scores for consonants as a function of filter bandwidth and mix. (See Figure 22.3 for a description of the ordinates in each panel.).

improvement. The absolute information scores for the duration envelope cue remained about the same across conditions, although relative scores fluctuated more widely, suggesting that the filter designs had little influence on vowel envelope information. Both absolute and relative information scores for F1 frequency cues (with the effects of duration

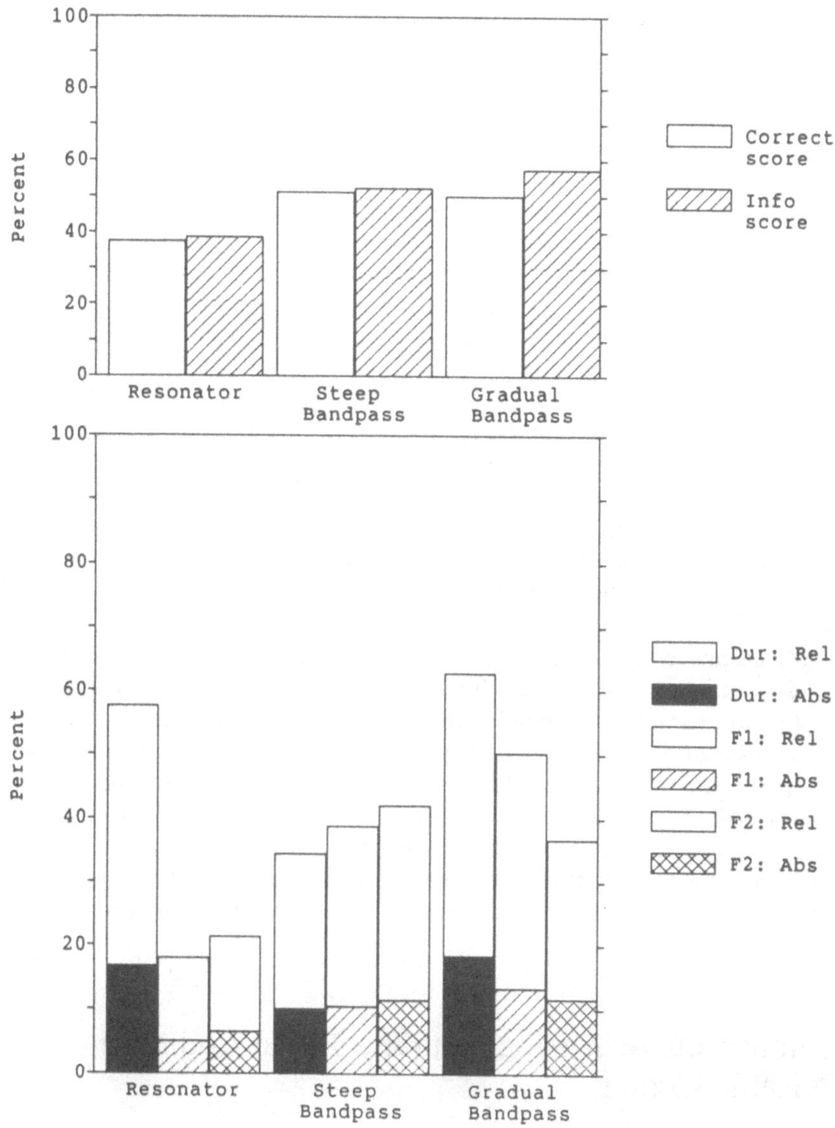

FIGURE 22.8. Percent correct and information scores for vowels as a function of filter bandwidth and mix. (See Figure 22.3 for a description of the ordinates in each panel.)

cues partialed out) improved substantially with increasing bandwidth and overlap. The same is true for F2 frequency cues (with the effects of duration and F1 cues partialed out). Figure 22.8 shows that the resonator design produced absolute information scores for F1 and F2 of about 6% and relative scores of about 20%, while the two bandpass designs produced absolute scores of about 12% and relative scores of about 40%.

Discussion

The results show consistently better vowel performance with the bandpass designs, but no differences in consonant performance. These findings suggest that processors with widely tuned bandpass filter designs may be superior to those with resonator designs in situations where the spatial selectivity of the electrode is limited and where electrode placement is not ideal. These qualifications are important: an appropriate test of the resonator design requires an electrode with radial bipolar geometry placed in the cochlear region spanning the speech bandwidth. Nonetheless, these results point up the importance of matching the processing to the placement and geometry of the electrode.

The observation that most of the improvements with the bandpass designs were seen in the F1 and F2 frequency cues for vowels seems to imply that more broadly tuned filters improve temporal selectivity. In fact, the resonator design processor necessarily exhibits greater temporal selectivity (see van den Honert, Chapter 9, this volume) than the bandpass processors. Since the number of resonators spanning the speech bandwidth is relatively small, however, the resonator design also necessarily undersamples that bandwidth compared with the bandpass designs. This undersampling produces a less uniform representation of the F1 and F2 frequency regions than the bandpass filters designs. In other words, these results suggest that uniform coverage of the F1 and F2 regions, even if this coverage provides "crude" temporal selectivity, may be more useful to the patient than the processing performed by the resonators when electrode geometry, placement, and possibly nerve survival are limiting factors.

Comparison of Analog Neurally Based Coding and Pulsatile Coding

Design

The results of the spatial and temporal selectivity tests, as well as the information about electrode placement (see Figure 22.2), suggest that alternative coding strategies may be more beneficial when spatial selectivity is poor due to either electrode placement or limited nerve survival. The present subject had also participated in other studies at the Hearing Research Laboratory, University of Minnesota, performed in collaboration with members of our laboratory (Kirby et al., 1987). These studies provided further psychophysical evidence of her poor spatial selectivity.

In these studies, a forward-masking task was used to assess channel interactions among signals presented sequentially to different electrode pairs (cf. Shannon, 1983a, 1983b). The results showed strong interactions, i.e., poor spatial selectivity, between all adjacent electrode pairs and most nonadjacent pairs, except for the apical pair 1-2 and the basal pair 6-7. In short, these results suggest that the subject receives only two perceptually distinct channels of information (although four channels of continuous information are presented with the neurally based coding strategy).

Based on these psychophysical test results, a two-channel pulsatile processor design was implemented for this subject in a collaborative effort with the Neural Prosthesis Group, Research Triangle Institute. The basic interleaved pulses processor design, which has been described in detail elsewhere (Wilson et al., 1988); see also Wilson, Finley, and Lawson, Chapter 21, this volume), was simplified to produce only two channels of interleaved pulses. The first channel consisted of interleaved, amplitude-modulated pulses that followed the time-intensity variations of speech below approximately 700 Hz and was presented on electrode pair 1-2. The second channel consisted of similar pulses that followed the time-intensity variations of speech above approximately 3 kHz and was presented on electrode pair 6-7. During voiced intervals of speech, pulses were delivered to both channels at the rate of the voice fundamental frequency. During unvoiced intervals both channels were driven at the maximum possible pulse rate. The first channel was intended to convey low-frequency envelope information, e.g., the voicing and amplitude envelope features for consonants, and the second channel was intended to convey high-frequency envelope information, e.g., the burst envelope and sibilance features for consonants.

The two-channel design is based directly on the work of Breeuwer and Plomp (1984). These investigators developed a similar two-channel coding strategy using amplitude-modulated sinusoids and have found it to be a highly effective method of presenting envelope cues as an aid to lipreading for the hearing impaired. Our use of the two-channel processor, however, was for sound-only stimulation.

The procedure was the same as in previous studies, except that very limited testing time was available, and only four blocks of consonant data could be obtained. Consequently, both tokens from the mail and female talkers were not sampled. The subject's performance with the two-channel pulsatile processor is compared with her performance for only these stimuli, and was obtained with the steep bandpass processor she was wearing at the time.

Results

The results of the consonant tests are summarized in Figure 22.9. Percent correct performance improved by only about 5% with the two-channel

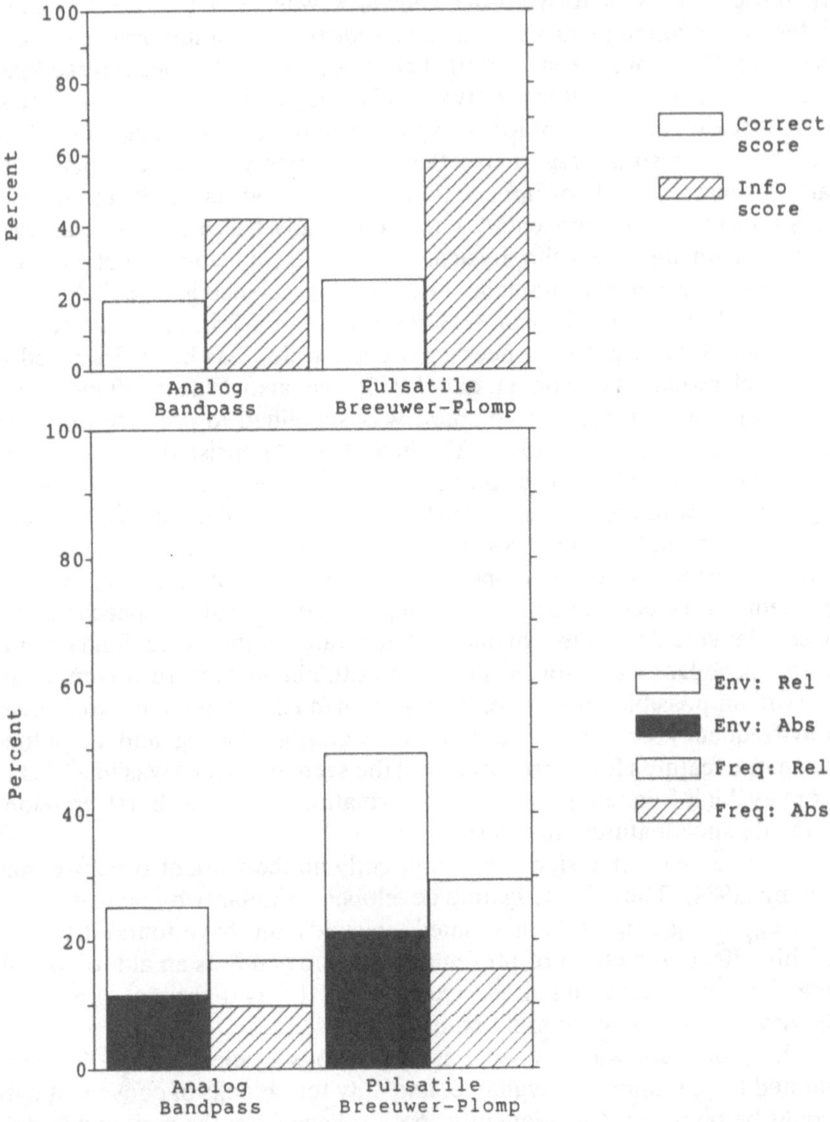

FIGURE 22.9. Percent correct and information scores for consonants with the analog bandpass processor using a neurally based coding strategy and with the pulsatile processor using the Breeuwer-Plomp coding strategy. (See Figure 22.2 for a description of the ordinates in each panel.)

processor over the best performance with the analog bandpass processor, while the overall information score exhibited a substantial improvement of over 16%. The feature information scores also exhibited improvements with the two-channel processor. The largest improvements were seen for the envelope features, where the absolute information score increased by 10% and the relative information increased by 24%. Smaller but consistent improvements were also seen for the frequency feature scores.

Discussion

Although the difference in percent correct performance between the analog and pulsatile processors is fairly small, the consistent and fairly large improvements in both the overall and the feature information scores with the pulsatile processor are noteworthy. These scores clearly indicate that the subject received more consonant information with the pulsatile processor and suggest that with additional experience percent correct performance might also improve. In other words, the subject received consonant information reliably that she had not yet learned to use correctly.

The fact that envelope information scores showed the largest improvements is to be expected, given that the Breeuwer-Plomp coding strategy was designed to provide consonant envelope cues. The small improvements in the frequency information scores suggest either that the subject guessed more accurately given better envelope information or that there are additional envelope cues in consonants beyond those partialed out by SINFA. In either case, two-channel presentation of envelope information was broadly beneficial. One would anticipate, however, that the breadth of this coding strategy may not be as readily extended to vowels because of their important F1 and F2 frequency cues.

To summarize, the reason the two-channel processor was more effective for consonants may be because it provides highly simplified spatial, temporal, and envelope cues for consonants which are best suited to the electrode geometry and placement and to the subject's auditory capabilities.

Conclusions

The results of the studies reported above lead to several general conclusions. First, the neurally based coding strategy remains without a satisfactory experimental test. While the physiological evidence and the theoretical rationale behind this strategy appear sound, the appropriate test awaits a subject with good nerve survival implanted with a radial bipolar electrode array that is positioned in the cochlear region spanning the speech bandwidth. Only then can appropriate spatial and temporal patterns of electrical stimulation be achieved. The neurally based coding strategy is theoretically important, because, if it is correct, it would provide an important link between the physiological, psychophysical, and perceptual research on electrical stimulation. For these reasons, it should be tested further.

Second, the perceptual results in the present four studies, while providing only weak tests of the neurally based coding strategy, were consistent with each other, with the psychophysical tests of channel interaction, and with information on the subject's electrode placement. Even though the results were obtained from a single subject, they provide objective data about the relationships between electrode placement, channel capacity, and the types of speech information that can be effectively coded for an implant user. These relationships have previously been subject to speculation in the implant field. The results also document the effectiveness of the envelope/frequency cue classification and the modified SINFA method as analytical tools for assessing processor designs with speech materials.

Third, the present research suggests a possible alternative approach to the neurally based coding strategy. This approach would be more practically oriented and would incorporate general scientific knowledge of the auditory system as well as specific clinical information about electrode placement, psychophysical abilities, and other characteristics of the individual implant user. The goal of this approach is not necessarily to evaluate a specific coding strategy, but instead to match the nature and complexity of the information provided by the processor to the auditory processing abilities of the subject. The best implant processor for a particular subject should simplify spatial, temporal, and envelope information only enough to match the subject's auditory capabilities—but no more than that. If a processor simplifies and reduces information more than that, it will limit the subject's performance; while if a processor does not simplify the information enough, the most relevant cues may be masked by other parts of the signal. The challenge with this approach is to develop perceptual and psychophysical tests that accurately assess the auditory processing capabilities of the implant user. The theoretical and practical approaches to coding strategies are complementary and can be profitably pursued in parallel.

Acknowledgments. The research reported in this chapter represents the collaborative efforts of members of the Hearing Research Group at 3M, the Hearing Research Laboratory at the University of Minnesota, and the Neural Prosthesis Group at Research Triangle Institute. Chris van den Honert, Virginia Kirby, Paul Stypulkowski, Greg Widin, Heinrich Bantli, Harry Stone, and Linda Johnson at 3M, Dave Nelson at the University of Minnesota, and Blake Wilson, Charlie Finley, and Dewey Lawson at

Research Triangle Institute all made important contributions to this research. The opinions expressed in this chapter, however, are those of the author.

References

Breeuwer, M., and Plomp, R. (1984). Speechreading supplemented with frequency-selective sound-pressure information. *J. Acoust. Soc. Am.* 76:686–691.

Eddington, D.K. (1980). Speech discrimination in deaf subjects with cochlear implants. *J. Acoust. Soc. Am.* 68:885–891.

Eddington, D.K. (1983). Speech recognition in deaf subjects with multichannel intracochlear electrodes, *Ann. N.Y. Acad. Sci.* 405:241–258.

Hochmair-Desoyer, I.J., and Burian, K. (1985). Reimplantation of a molded scala tympani electrode: Impact on psychophysical and speech discrimination abilities. *Ann. Otol. Rhinol. Laryngol.* 94:65–70.

Kiang, N.Y.-S. (1968). A survey of recent developments in the study of auditory physiology. *Ann. Otol. Rhinol. Laryngol.* 77:1–20.

Kiang, N.Y.-S. (1980). Processing of speech by the auditory nervous system. *J. Acoust. Soc. Am.* 68:830–835.

Kirby, V.M., Nelson, D.A., Soli, S.D., and Fortune, T.W. (1987). Channel interactions measured by forward-masking "place" tuning curves with multichannel electrical stimulation. *J. Acoust. Soc. Am.* 82:S72.

Miller, G.A., and Nicely, P.E. (1955). An analysis of perceptual confusions among some English consonants. *J. Acoust. Soc. Am.* 27:338–352.

Sachs, M.B., and Young, E.D. (1979). Encoding of steady-state vowels in the auditory nerve: Representation in terms of discharge rate. *J. Acoust. Soc. Am.* 66:470–479.

Shannon, R.V. (1983a). Multichannel electrical stimulation of the auditory nerve in man. I. Basic psychophysics. *Hearing Res.* 11:157–189.

Shannon, R.V. (1983b). Multichannel electrical stimulation of the auditory nerve in man. II. Channel interactions. *Hearing Res.* 12:1–16.

Soli, S.D., and Arabie, P. (1979). Auditory versus phonetic accounts of observed confusions between consonant phonemes. *J. Acoust. Soc. Am.* 66:46–59.

Soli, S.D., Arabie, P., and Carroll, J.D. (1986). Discrete representation of perceptual structure underlying consonant confusions. *J. Acoust. Soc. Am.* 79:826–837.

Soli, S. D., Kirby, V.M., Van Tasell, D.J., and Widin, G.P. (1985). Time-intensity envelope cues for consonant recognition. *J. Acoust. Soc. Am.* 78:S69.

Soli, S.D., and Wilson, B.S. (1988). Within-subject comparisons of analog and pulsatile speech processors for cochlear implants. *J. Acoust. Soc. Am.* 84:S41.

van den Honert, C., and Stypulkowski, P.H. (1987a). Single fiber mapping of spatial excitation patterns in the electrically stimulated auditory nerve. *Hearing Res.* 82:195–206.

van den Honert, C., and Stypulkowski, P.H. (1987b). Temporal response patterns of single auditory nerve fibers elicited by periodic electrical stimuli. *J. Hearing Res.* 29:207–222.

Van Tasell, D.J., Soli, S.D., Kirby, V.M., and Widin, G.P. (1987). Speech waveform envelope cues for consonant recognition. *J. Acoust. Soc. Am.* 82:1152–1161.

Wang, M.D. (1976). SINFA: Multivariate uncertainty analysis for confusion matrices. *Behav. Res. Methods Instrum.* 8:471–472.

Wang, M.D., and Bilger, R.C. (1973). Consonant confusions in noise: A study of perceptual features. *J. Acoust. Soc. Am.* 54:1248–1266.

Wilson, B.S., Finley, C.C., Lawson, D.T., and Wolford, R.D. (1988). Speech processors for cochlear prostheses. *Proc. IEEE.* 76:1143–1154.

Young, E.D., and Sachs, M.B. (1979). Representation of steady-state vowels in the temporal aspects of the discharge patterns of populations of auditory nerve fibers. *J. Acoust. Soc. Am.* 66:1381–1403.

Sigfrid D. Soli: Discussion

Dr. Pfingst: When Chris presented this type of processor yesterday, we talked about whether it would be better to combine the outputs of adjacent channels or to leave some out. It seems like he was opting for leaving some out, and yet you chose to combine them. Can you comment on why you did that?

Dr. Soli: We have tried both using a monopolar electrode geometry and, thus, seven to eight channels of stimulation. We mapped a single resonator output to each of those channels. Now, granted, it is a monopolar configuration so it is still not ideal. The results we saw were really no better than what I've shown you here. Mapping a single resonator output to a single bipolar electrode is the ideal test, but unless you have enough of those bipolar channels, you are very seriously undersampling the broadband signal by only using four narrowly tuned resonators, and will be missing much of the information falling between the resonators that way. So it is a compromise.

Dr. Dent: Can I go out on a limb and say that many of your results are consistent with the hypothesis that the way the compression was done was interfering with the consonant perception? I didn't see any effect of linear compression on the consonant results. Is that a good summary?

Dr. Soli: Right. The effects as we measured them were negligible.

Dr. Dent: And you were doing the compression after the filtering. Is that correct?

Dr. Soli: But remember that one of the conditions that we tested was a condition where the processor was linear. There was no compression, so the fact that the compression we used did not differ significantly from linear suggests to me that effects of compression were not present in our test.

Dr. Dent: The other point that Mark White has made repeatedly is the importance of cross-coupling among the channels. We finally implemented that strategy and did see an effect. I am referring to Ben Knapp's work. The fact that you get your best results with a linear mapping on the output simply means that you have to preserve the spectral peaks and valleys, if you don't you run into trouble.

Dr. Soli: You are preserving the time-intensity envelope, which I think is important.

Dr. Smoorenburg: Two comments. One with respect to the Breeuwer-Plomp study, I am happy to see that it is being used now. But please bear in mind this study was directed at providing additional auditory information for lip-reading.

Dr. Soli: That's absolutely right. In spite of that, it seems to provide some useful information in a sound-only stimulation condition, at least for consonants. I think Blake Wilson and Charlie Finley have some additional data to support that.

Dr. Finley: I want to comment on one point that you alluded to in your interpretation and results with regard to how accurately you have implemented your overall design in the processors. Chris van den Honert outlined yesterday that the initial design of the processor was to exploit the merits of the radial bipolar electrode configuration, and the configuration that you end up using, for innumerable reasons out of your control no doubt, was a longitudinal bipolar configuration. I have not modeled that configuration, but after seeing the results I reported about the banded longitudinal configuration, I would speculate that the electrode configuration you are using produces an effect, on the population of neurons that are being stimulated, probably like those that you would see with a monopolar electrode like that in the Symbion device, or with the bipolar plus one configuration used with the Nucleus electrode. I find it very interesting that as you work with a patient and optimize the design for overall performance, you gradually evolve back toward a processor structure that is similar to that which Don

Eddington has used with the Symbion device with monopolar electrodes. So I think in regard to testing this hypothesis of a neurally based encoding strategy, the jury is still out.

Dr. Soli: That is one point I would like to leave you with. The other point is that given the practical considerations one has to face in matching processing to patient, it is very wise to explore a range of processing alternatives because of the range of perceptual spaces that we have to work with.

23
Encoding Schemes—Perspectives and Challenges

WILLIAM M. RABINOWITZ

The overall goal is to develop encoding schemes that will provide the greatest speech recognition for subjects using cochlear prostheses. Essentially, the problem is one of matching the important characteristics of speech signals to the limited perceptual space associated with electroauditory stimulation. Because large individual differences occur with electrical stimulation, optimal encodings may need to be chosen on a subject-by-subject basis. Two general approaches are presently being taken to determine optimal encodings.

One approach is focused on beginning with a detailed characterization of the perceptual space obtainable with electrical stimulation. Emphasis is given to performing experiments using elementary nonspeech stimuli and having responses that are nonlinguistic and from limited sets (e.g.,discrimination, identification, scaling, and similarity judgments). Techniques such as multidimensional scaling and metrics derived from communications-theoretical models are then used to reveal underlying perceptual dimensions, their saliency (i.e., resolution and capacity), and the extent of their independence. With this knowledge, stimulus manipulations can then be specified so as to create known perceptual variations. For example, an interdependent manipulation of the physical variables of intensity and frequency may be required for independent variations of the perceptual variables of loudness and pitch. Similarly, detailed manipulations of the dynamic aspects of stimulation may be required to overcome perceptual distortions associated with nonsimultaneous masking and its interaction with limitations on dynamic range. With an adequate understanding of the perceptual space defined from such studies, presumably one can more rationally allocate aspects of the speech signal to be encoded along specific dimensions.

A second approach to encoding comes more directly from the area of speech perception. With or without explicit assumptions and/or knowledge regarding the perceptual space, encoding schemes are studied using speech stimuli. Analyses of errors (i.e., confusion patterns) are then used to develop hypotheses for further encoding refinements. Key issues to address include what are the most important aspects (or "features") of the speech signal to convey and how are they to be encoded. For systems that intentionally represent only specific speech features (e.g., the Nucleus system), further issues include what accuracy is needed in estimating the feature values from the input signal and what incremental benefits result from including additional features (e.g., providing additional formant and better voiced/voiceless representation in a Nucleus-type strategy). To provide information to help interpret as well as bound the performance that might obtain with implant subjects, acoustic simulations tested with normal (or hearing-impaired) listeners can be useful.

In addition to the knowledge we are deriving using these relatively structured approaches to encoding, the experience of patients using existing devices provides information that is valuable and provocative. The recent observation that measurable open-set speech recognition has been obtained by some children (but no adults) using the House/3M single-channel implant raises difficult issues. Clearly, long-term learning and plasticity can dramatically complicate our efforts to determine the efficacy of devices, even devices that are, in some sense, relatively simple and that had been presumed to provide information inadequate to understand speech.

Different approaches to improved encoding need not, of course, be mutually exclusive. In the near term, it seems clear that advances will require the insightful application of ideas across all domains. In addition, we need to better understand the relationships among results along the continuum of different performance measures, ranging from studies of elementary psychophysical percepts to speech reception. For example, the extent to which perception of consonants and vowels from isolated speech segments is predictive of more global measures of open-set reception (i.e., of words, sentences, and continuous discourse) remains controversial.

The problems we face form an exciting set of challenges for the field. Progress as measured by clinical success and research developments, well illustrated by these papers, has been remarkable. However, as the discussions indicate, a great deal more study, integrating basic research strategies with clinical needs, must be performed. We are yet in the infancy of this field; its growth and maturity should provide concepts and tools to assist the profoundly deaf with implantable prostheses as well as the moderately hearing-impaired population with conventional acoustic aids.

24
Session III: General Discussion

Dr. Rabinowitz: I believe Dr. Finley has some comments regarding electrodes and their interface to the neural substrate.

Dr. Finely: I want to avoid a misconception for all of us in thinking about the way that electrodes interface to the system we are trying to stimulate. We have been hearing for the last 2 days, a couple of different messages. One very important message is that one of the things that makes our multichannel devices succeed is that we are achieving a sector-by-sector stimulation of the auditory system. There is no question that in the case of the Symbion system your monopolar elctrodes achieve that. One of the things we heard from the physiologist this morning is our very frustrating inability to mimic the stochastic firing characteristics that we see in acoustically stimulated fibers, but with electrical stimulation we see a very high degree of synchronicity among the fibers we are looking at. It may be thought that the electrode of choice would be something like the monopolar electrode, which would produce a very gradual gradation of stimulus field. But the consequence of that would be that it would access the anatomical variability that exists within the population we are trying to stimulate and may consequently produce a stochastically distributed input into the system, which the physiologists have been unable to achieve with the radial bipolar types of stimulation with pulsatile input. So I think the option of analog for slow varying inputs on a very gradually diffuse field across the population we are trying to stimulate is a very viable option and one that needs to continue to be evaluated.

Dr. Rabinowitz: On another topic, one issue that has come up in several talks is plasticity. Related to this is Greg Wakefield's informational approach, which suggests that we need only ensure that adequate resolution among stimuli exists and the CNS will eventually figure out what to do with it; i.e., we have to have an adequate set of "equivalents classes." A difficulty, however, is how to get insight to determine if learning is occurring in a given case: How long do you wait when you try a radical recoding? You are always up against the problem of knowing whether the information you have chosen to display is inadequate or whether the system can't learn it.

Dr. Smoorenburg: First of all, I think the problem is even more complicated because, from an ethical point of view, you may wonder if you can do something for the patient. If he is accustomed to a certain pattern and you are going to change the pattern, it may be confusing and you don't know whether it's going to work at all and he may be so confused that his original pattern will become less effective. And then how do you know what is going to work? I think you just have to test discrimination. There should be, of course, an increase in performance. I think that you have to do it, not with the real speech stimuli, because they will always interfere with things that have been learned already, but you have to do it with more abstract types of stimuli.

Dr. Soli: We have fielded various processing configurations for as few as a few days or for as long as 6 to 8 weeks. I think, without exception, the performance we measured when the patient first went out the door and then came back weeks later was almost the same. So I have not seen any evidence of this plasticity, at least in that time frame. The other comment I would like to make is that with the two-channel envelope coding scheme we literally saw the results immediately. We saw a fairly large change in at least information scores, which we haven't seen in any of our previous tests.

Dr. Smoorenburg: There are data from Mike, the Nucleus group, and the Viennese group which show learning over a period of more than a year. So I think it's obvious that they are learning.

Dr. Soli: There may be an initial learning period that follows first stimulation.

Question: No, no, not initial. It goes on for a year to a year and a half.

Dr. Josef Miller: Should you wait a year every time you change your processors?

Dr. Smoorenburg: That is indeed the problem.

Dr. Merzenich: Another aspect of it is to think about it in terms of nervous system input, in contrast to acoustic input. One of the fundamental differences is the invariance of input patterns, especially if you use pulsatile stimulation. You have, of course, a distributed pattern that changes as a function of level but in other respects is relatively predictable, relatively invariant. The nervous system is pounded with millions of those inputs from a small number of sites, over time. That's why I think when Blake looks at a patient that's been wearing a compressed analog stimulator for a while and then changes the configuration to an interleaved pulse stimulator, he can still get a good result because the basic distinctions that are being made are distinctions in proportional levels of activity across those channels. And that's got to be pounded into this system to create a relatively robust treatment of it. We have to believe that those millions of repeated and variant stimuli are going to have impact. And they are going to be hard to overcome in time. You are going to have to do a lot to overcome them, and a few days won't work. We did experiments in which we reversed channels in second formant range and the identity went with the location and not with the frequency content.

Dr.Wakefield: Concerning learning, in the frequency discrimination task you see improvements in performance over a 10-week period of time from when you first put your subject in. Now we aren't talking about electrically stimulated patients, just normal acoustic subjects in a psychophysical task. It is not plasticity that speaks to the learning that takes place when you start working with these stimuli. Also in Watson's discrimination of complex sequences experiment, which has been done on normals, long learning time is involved.

Dr. Josef Miller: Do we know from work with pathological ears, either in rehabilitation or in changing schemes for encoding different information, the time it takes to acquire a new sheme, with new rehabilitative devices?

Dr. Smoorenburg: There is a problem of compatability of aided and unaided hearing. You see, I think that situation is quite different from that in which they are stimulated electrically.

Dr. Johnstone: The classic case occurs in stapedectomy, where a patient has had an otosclerotic ear 20 years with a 30-dB loss. Put in a good prothesis and the next day they are hypersensitive: objectively they are very sensitive and their hearing levels are way up. They will fade to normal over a period on the order of 7 to 10 days. That gives you some idea of plasticity in a normal subject.

Dr. Osberger: I think indirect evidence for the role of learning can be found in looking at children's performance with cochlear implants. For example, there are a fair number of children who are outperforming adults with the 3M House device, and performing as well as postlingually deaf adults with a multichannel device. And I think we see that children, after 3 years of using the device, are still showing big improvements with their performance. So it may be that our approach to evaluate different processing schemes in adults may not be the best way to go. It may be that we must try these schemes with children and evaluate them after a period of long learning.

Dr. Rabinowitz: Those are important points. Are there additional experiences with children that address long-term learning effects?

Dr. Osberger: I think we are seeing this both with the Nucleus and with the 3M device. I think the data are most compelling with the 3M device because there are not many adults that do very well with it. So that when you see this very high performance of children, the issue of plasticity and learning is highlighted even more.

Dr. Smoorenburg: Another example of special learning can be seen in Morse code. If you study the people that are very familiar with Morse code, they don't hear dots and dashes. They hear the whole pattern; they hear words.

Dr. Soli: On the other hand, I don't think it's purely plasticity and that people will learn virtually any pattern, which is somewhat what Mary Jo might be suggesting. It is the case in adults that there are processors that they become accustomed to, and once you switch them to another one, which you might think is a theoretically better design, they never get used to the new one. They continually refer to the one they had previously as the one they prefer. Even though they may have much longer experience with the second one, if you give them the first one again they will immediately do better with it and prefer it. It isn't purely adapting to a different processor. There is an influence of the information that's being presented, and we can't assume that because children can learn to use the device better than adults can, that that necessarily makes that processing scheme best.

Dr. Tong: We definitely found that experience is very important. For example, a change in scheme or strategy has a very profound effect on patient performance. Even if you only change the electrode assignments, there is a profound effect. For example, if you normally use six electrodes for F1 and ten electrodes for F2, and then change to eight electrodes for F1 and eight for F2, using the same sixteen electrodes, it will take the patients quite a while to get used to the new electrode assignment.

Dr. Josef Miller: How long?

Dr. Tong: On the order of months, for synthetic vowels. For live speech it could be a little bit faster.

Dr. James Miller: We all have our own experiences with adult patients and evaluating different hearing-aid schemes. In general, there appears to be almost no learning. You come up with a better scheme; they get a better score almost instantly. There is some kind of accommodation to hearing-aid systems that patients report in everyday life. I don't know if this is learning how to set it. As far as this learning goes, Mary Jo Osberger didn't emphasize it, but some of the children wear the implant a long time and nothing happens. So, you have a very severe clinical problem as to when you advise another approach. I think that we all need to identify the indicators that show there might be reorganization or learning, the indicators that show there is progress being made, even though it may not be very obvious. I think we have to learn that.

25
Fundamental Research for Development of Cochlear Prostheses

JOSEF M. MILLER AND FRANCIS A. SPELMAN

The papers presented and discussions that followed stimulated the participants to formulate a set of questions considered to be most important for the development of basic knowledge in the field of electrical stimulation of the ear. It was thought that questions can now be specified at a more rigorous level than they were previously; and these questions permit the formulation of a few clearly defined strategies of investigation which can drive development of our knowledge of prosthesis function and lead to the next generation of improved cochlear prostheses.

Current activities of the field and concerns expressed by these investigators clearly define two general approaches: a behavioral-perceptual approach and a physiological-biophysical approach. The goal of both approaches is to define the fundamental mechanisms that underlie prothesis function. The attainment of that goal will permit basic scientists to develop optimal encoding schemes and clinicians to give subjects optimally structured information, which can, in turn, activate safely multiple clusters of neural elements to provide a robust perception of meaningful acoustic information.

In the category of behavioral-perceptual approaches, three research approaches have been defined. The first approach seeks to characterize the perceptual space generated by electrical stimulation. Investigators attempt to map the basis vectors of this perceptual space onto those of the space defining electrical stimulation. The objective is to determine the similarities between this electrically generated perceptual space and that perceptual space generated with acoustic stimulation. Knowledge of dimensions and characteristics of this electrically generated space may be used to define important features of a speech processor encoding scheme. The second research strategy employs a comprehensive understanding of normal speech reception and discrimination. Implicit in this approach is the assumption that if the electrically generated perceptual space is not similar to the acoustic space, then at least the nervous system is sufficiently adaptable to deal with the differences. Hence, it concludes that the detailed characteristics of the electrically generated perceptual space are not important for a successful encoding scheme. It will be sufficient for the speech processor in a prothesis to provide an analog of the information important for speech understanding that is available in acoustic speech waveforms. The third research strategy is patient-driven. In this strategy it is argued that the encoding scheme must be flexible. Encoding strategies are presumed to be as broad as the variability that exists in the otopathology of profound deafness and the variability that exists in the individual patient's capabilities and needs. This approach assumes that the structure of a speech processing scheme may be derived only over time by the patient. Idealized, this strategy would offer the subject the widest possible menu of signal processing schemes. The designer presumes that with a systematic shaping of this menu, based upon the individual patient's discriminative abilities, an optimal processor will result.

These research strategies are obviously without rigid borders. Behavorial research to determine electrical perceptions frequently represents a marriage of more than one strategy. Two interesting subsets of work are clear in this volume. These include research designed to define the relationship between the perception of complex signals to the sensitivity and dynamic range of performance demonstrated with simple signals, and research designed to relate the psychophysical performance in animal models to structural characteristics of the auditory periphery. These investigations represent a reductionist analysis of speech discrimination performance. They provide an interface between behavioral studies and physiological investigations and basic knowledge of the mechanisms that underlie prosthesis function.

Unlike behavioral strategies which share the immediate goal of enhancing speech discrimination, physiological strategies are best defined by somewhat different goals. Thus, one set of investigations is aimed at specifying the electroanatomy of the tissues of the inner ear. By defining the passive electrical characteristics of all tissues and fluids of the inner ear, it is possible to generate lumped- and finite-element models of the pattern of current flow generated by stimulation at any defined site. This knowledge provides necessary information for the design and development of electrode systems that are capable of exciting specifiable cluster of neural elements at known sites within the inner ear. A second strategy of physiological investigation is based upon the evaluation of the response characteristics of eighth nerve fibers and cells of the cochlear nucleus to electrical stimulation. These studies form two categories, one in which the goal is to define the focus of electrical stimuli on excitable cells, the other in which the goal is to define the range of response characteristics that we can control with electrical stimulation. Studies in these two areas will provide the results to determine and control the spatial distribution of neural excitation, the differential excitation and interactions of excitation patterns of units spatially distributed within the ear, the dynamic range of response of individual units and groups of units, and the responses to sinusoidal complexes and multiple sites of excitation.

These investigations are designed to specify the active biophysical properties of the excitable tissues that determine the responsiveness of elements of the auditory system to electrical stimulation. Coupled with models of current flow in the inner ear, such data should allow us to specify the site of neural excitation and the spread of excitation with change in stimulation site and waveform. With that knowledge, we may be able to specify features of the system that can produce a greater dynamic range of response. Further, we hope to specify stimulus parameters such that we may cause the system to respond to electrical stimulation in a manner similar to that elicited with acoustic stimulation. Coupled with information regarding current flow, knowledge of the physiological control available specifies the features of electrode systems and characteristics of signal processors that may permit us to approximate response features observed with acoustic stimulation. The assumption underlying this work is that more salient perceptions, distributed in a normal acoustic perceptual space, will occur if we can make the system respond as with acoustic stimulation, i.e., mimic the normal system.

An alternative strategy is directed at defining response characteristics with electrical stimulation that appear to be most secure and robust. We then can use these features to encode predetermined acoustic signals considered to be of primary importance for perception. Rather than attempting to shape the response features to meet a model of system responsiveness considered to be optimal (e.g., the "normal" acoustic model), this last approach is but an opportunistic approach. It proposes to take those most obvious and robust electrophysiological characteristics we find and use them to introduce signals considered to be of prime importance for perception. With this strategy we assume that, while we may introduce acoustic signals in a highly unusual manner, the plasticity of the nervous system will permit the patient to extract, meaningfully, the important information. Certainly with the growing application of prostheses to young populations of profoundly deaf and our growing knowledge of the plasticity of the young nervous system, this approach has some face validity.

From this symposium, it seems clear that of these strategies discussed above there is a special interest in (1) those investigations which are aimed at generating systems that will provide for more selective excitation, (2) those which will reduce the redundancy and the deterministic nature of simple electrical signals; and importantly, (3) those which will assess the variety of ways that sensory information may be represented and modified as it is tranferred along the central auditory pathways to higher centers.

Thus, during the last decade, specific strategies of research have evolved for elucidating the basic mechanisms of response of the auditory system to electrical stimulation. The behavioral strategies are aimed at a better understanding of perceptual processes, and the electrical and biophysical studies are aimed at providing selective excitation of units of the auditory periphery to yield the greatest dynamic range of system function. These now work hand-in-hand to provide a base to better understand encoding schemes for the development and optimization of speech processors for cochlear implants. With these well-defined strategies it has been possible to better determine and prioritize the principle research questions facing investigators in the field. This has increased the vitality and excitement of this field. It has provided an enhanced base to determine future research and a means to better specify future developments of prostheses and enhance their benefit for the profoundly deaf.

A Program of Studies of the Cochlear Prosthesis

I. The Electroanatomy of the inner ear.
   A. Define the electroanatomy and geometry of the fluid compartments, soft tissues, and bone of the inner ear.
      1. Measure the three-dimensional geometry of the cochlear compartments and surrounding tissues.
      2. Assess the electrical characteristics of each of these compartments and their boundaries.
      3. Assess the changes in their electroanatomy that occur with pathology.
      4. Assess the changes in cochlear electroanatomy that occur with developments in the normal and pathological ear.
   B. Continue development of lumped- and finite-element models to predict the pattern of current flow through and about excitable tissue of the temporal bone.
      1. Carry on studies to verify current flow patterns predicted from models in biological preparation.
      2. Evaluate alternative schemes for selectively stimulating subpopulations of afferents.
   C. Establish comparative models for animal and human electroanatomy.
II. Electophysiology of electrical excitability.
   A. Identify the site(s) of excitation, with variation in parameters and sites of stimulation, in normal and pathological material.
   B. Identify the limits of channel interaction (i.e., the limits of spatial encoding), with variation in parameters and sites of stimulation, including interactive schemes to provide more restricted or focused excitation patterns (e.g., deconvolution technique).

C. Evaluate redundancy of excitation in the eighth nerve and decoding of redundancy in the cochlear nucleus.
D. Evaluate the importance of stochasticity of response properties in the eighth nerve and brain-stem cells for electrical stimulation.
E. Evaluate the dynamic range for frequency and intensity encoding, including the decoding of the temporal microstructure of the signals and the relationship to the information-carrying capacity of the system for envelope characteristics.
F. Evaluate processing of electrically encoded signals in the CNS with special emphasis on the representation of complex signals, such as speech elements, along the central auditory pathways, and the extraction of these multispectral signals in noise.
G. Examine descending influences on electrically evoked activity.
H. Evaluate these characteristics in normal and pathological preparations.
I. Evaluate the effects of early history of excitation and restricted enviroment during development, including study of changes in representation of signals in central nervous system structures and changes in structural characteristics.
J. Evaluate these characteristics in relationship to the electroanatomy of the inner ear and available models of patterns of current flow through inner ear tissues.
K. Generate models of the electrophysiology of encoding and CNS processing of electrical signals.

III. Behavioral assessment.

A. Identify the dimensionality of the stimulus space for electrical stimulation of the auditory system and determine what partitions can be associated with behavior.
B. Define linear and nonlinear functions of simple percepts of pitch and loudness and their relationship to perception and discrimination of complex signals like speech.
C. Increase information on speech perception with acoustic signals and the identification of essential and important elements, in normal and pathological ears.
D. Assess channel interaction and channel information-carrying capacity with regard to simple and complex signals.
E. Evaluate perceptual abilities in the developing nervous system and effects of limited or restricted early development on perception in mature electroperception in the mature nervous system.
F. Evaluate new encoding and processor technologies to provide robust perception.
G. Evaluate and develop new models for the processing of electrically generated speech information in the central auditory system in different patient populations.

H. Perform systematic comparison of perceptual ability in animal models to identify the role of peripheral excitable elements, and systematically compare with human performance.
I. Evaluate noninvasive physiological measures and new imaging techniques of metabolic activity in the CNS relative to perceptual performance to provide insight into the relation of perception to neural activity.

IV. Technical development.
A. Develop transparent and flexible processors.
B. Continue to develop electrodes for discrete excitation.
C. Develop transcutaneous channels that permit flexible processing and measurement of electrode characteristics during implant use.

V. Otopathology.*
A. Continue and increase efforts to determine the temporal bone pathology associated with various forms of sensorineural hearing loss.

---

*While otopathology was not a specific topic of discussion at this symposium, the importance and relevance of studies in this area for the development of models of the electrically stimulated ear was frequently noted.

B. Increase acquisition of temporal bones, and if possible brain-stem material, from implant patients for systematic morphological assessment.

'Ear's to thousands of 'air cells,
May their cilia always be found,
Waving under tectorial membranes,
To comforting softness of sound.
But if 'air cells get lost in the shuffle,
And NIH sends us fat grants,
We'll zap little dendrites with current,
Through marvelous cochlear implants!

–Burma Shave

Index

SPRINGER NATURE

GPSR Compliance

The European Union's (EU) General Product Safety Regulation (GPSR) is a set of rules that requires consumer products to be safe and our obligations to ensure this.

If you have any concerns about our products, you can contact us on ProductSafety@springernature.com

In case Publisher is established outside the EU, the EU authorized representative is:

Springer Nature Customer Service Center GmbH
Europaplatz 3
69115 Heidelberg, Germany

FSC
www.fsc.org
MIX
Papier | Fördert gute Waldnutzung
FSC® C083411

Kolibri 360 GmbH
Ferdinand-Jühlke-Straße 7
99095 Erfurt, Deutschland
produktsicherheit@kolibri360.de